OSTEOPOROSIS

EDITED BY

Robert Marcus, MD

Professor of Medicine
Division of Endocrinology,
Gerontology, and Metabolism
Stanford University School of Medicine;
Director, Aging Study Unit
Department of Veterans Affairs
Medical Center
Palo Alto, California

Boston
Blackwell Scientific Publications
Oxford   London   Edinburgh
Melbourne   Paris
Berlin   Vienna

Blackwell Scientific Publications

Editorial offices:

238 Main Street, Cambridge, Massachusetts
  02142, USA
Osney Mead, Oxford OX2 0EL, England
25 John Street, London WC1N 2BL,
  England
23 Ainslie Place, Edinburgh EH3 6AJ,
  Scotland
54 University Street, Carlton, Victoria
  3053, Australia
Arnette SA, 1 rue de Lille, 75007 Paris,
  France
Blackwell-Wissenschaft, Düsseldorfer Str.
  38, D-10707 Berlin, Germany
Blackwell MZV, Feldgasse 13, A-1238
  Vienna, Austria

Distributors:

USA

Blackwell Scientific Publications
238 Main Street
Cambridge, Massachusetts 02142
(Telephone orders: 800-215-1000 or
  617-876-7000)

CANADA

Times Mirror Professional Publishing
130 Flaska Drive
Markham, Ontario L6G 1B8
(Telephone orders: 800-268-4178 or
  905-470-6739)

AUSTRALIA

Blackwell Scientific Publications (Australia)
  Pty Ltd
54 University Street
Carlton, Victoria 3053
(Telephone orders: 03-347-5552)

OUTSIDE NORTH AMERICA AND AUSTRALIA

Blackwell Scientific Publications, Ltd.
c/o Marston Book Services, Ltd.
P.O. Box 87
Oxford OX2 0DT
England
(Telephone orders: 44-865-791155)

Typeset by BookMasters, Ashland, Ohio
Printed and bound by Braun-Brumfield,
  Inc., Ann Arbor, Michigan

© 1994 by Blackwell Scientific Publications

Printed in the United States of America
94 95 96 97 5 4 3 2 1

Notice: The indications and dosages of
all drugs in this book have been recommended in the medical literature and
conform to the practices of the general
medical community. The medications described do not necessarily have specific
approval by the Food and Drug Administration for use in the diseases and dosages
for which they are recommended. The
package insert for each drug should be con-
sulted for use and dosage as approved by
the FDA. Because standards of usage
change, it is advisable to keep abreast of
revised recommendations, particularly
those concerning new drugs.

Library of Congress Cataloging-in-
  Publication Data
Osteoporosis / edited by Robert Marcus.
    p. cm.
    Includes bibliographical references and
index.
    ISBN 0-86542-266-4
    1. Osteoporosis. I. Marcus, Robert,
1940–
    [DNLM: 1. Osteoporosis—
physiopathology. 2. Osteoporosis-
-therapy. WE 250 O85112 1994]
RC931.O73O75 1994
616.7'16—dc20
DNLM/DLC
for Library of Congress   94-15572
                                            CIP

Contents

Contents

Contributors

Laura K. Bachrach, MD
Division of Endocrinology
Department of Pediatrics
Stanford University Medical Center
Stanford, California

Lorraine A. Fitzpatrick, MD
Associate Professor of Medicine
Director, Bone Histomorphometry
  Unit
Mayo Clinic and Mayo Foundation
Rochester, Minnesota

Robert L. Jilka, PhD
Research Professor of Internal
  Medicine
Division of Endocrinology and
  Metabolism
University of Arkansas for Medical
  Sciences
Little Rock, Arkansas

Donald B. Kimmel, DDS, PhD
Center for Hard Tissue Research
Creighton University School of
  Medicine
Omaha, Nebraska

Robert F. Klein, MD
Staff Physician
Portland Veterans Affairs Medical
  Center

Assistant Professor of Medicine
Oregon Health Sciences University
Portland, Oregon

Lawrence E. Mallette, MD, PhD
Associate Professor of Medicine
Baylor College of Medicine
Acting Chief, Endocrine Section
Veterans Affairs Medical Center
Houston, Texas

Stavros C. Manolagas, MD
Director, Division of Endocrinology
  and Metabolism
University of Arkansas for Medical
  Sciences
Little Rock, Arkansas

Robert Marcus, MD
Professor of Medicine
Division of Endocrinology, Gerontol-
  ogy, and Metabolism
Stanford University School of
  Medicine;
Director, Aging Study Unit
Geriatric Research, Education and
  Clinical Center
Department of Veterans Affairs Med-
  ical Center
Palo Alto, California

Michael R. McClung, MD
Director, Center for Metabolic Bone
  Disorders
Providence Medical Center
Associate Professor of Medicine
Oregon Health Sciences University
Portland, Oregon

Eric S. Orwoll, MD
Chief, Endocrinology and Metabolism
Portland Veterans Affairs Medical
  Center
Associate Professor of Medicine
Oregon Health Sciences University
Portland, Oregon

Susan Marie Ott, MD
Associate Professor
Department of Medicine
University of Washington
Seattle, Washington

Robert R. Recker, MD
Professor of Medicine

Director, Center for Hard Tissue
  Research
Creighton University School of
  Medicine
Omaha, Nebraska

Charles W. Slemenda, MD
Associate Professor of Medicine
Department of Medicine
Division of Biostatistics
Indiana University School of
  Medicine
Indianapolis, Indiana

Marie Luz Villa, MD
Professor of Medicine
Stanford University School of
  Medicine
Musculoskeletal Research Laboratory
Department of Veterans Affairs Med-
  ical Center
Palo Alto, California

Contributors

Preface

The thirteen chapters of this volume range in approach from epidemiology to therapeutics, addressing a broad variety of topics on the nature and management of osteoporosis. Emphasis has been placed on aspects of this disease that are rarely considered in a systematic fashion, and where substantial progress has been made. Following an introductory overview, the chapter by Manolagas and Jilka relates exciting new information regarding the regulation of bone remodeling by cytokines. Kimmel and Recker next discuss skeletal assessment in both theoretical and practical terms. It recently has been appreciated that acquisition of an adequate bone mass at the time of skeletal maturity may be just as important to subsequent fracture risk as bone loss later. Thus, the contributions from Bachrach on bone acquisition and Slemenda on adult bone loss are particularly timely. With current interest in the relative vulnerability of various ethnic groups to osteoporotic fracture, the chapter by Villa on ethnicity and osteoporosis details the difficulties and ambiguities associated with doing ethnicity-specific research. A chapter by Orwoll and Klein on osteoporosis in men offers many new insights to a problem of steadily increasing dimensions. A chapter by Fitzpatrick discusses the vexing problem of glucocorticoid osteoporosis. Although the goal of "curing" osteoporosis remains elusive, progress has been made over the past decade. This is reviewed in chapters by Ott on calcuim and vitamin D, Marcus on estrogen, and Mallette on bisphosphonates. Given the limitations of current pharmacologic therapy, attention to hygienic and other nonpharmacologic approaches remains of critical importance. The clinical chapters, therefore, include an examination of this topic by McClung. The volume concludes with a chapter by Kimmel on the applicability and drawbacks of several animal models of osteoporosis. With a number of recombinant hormones and biologics on the horizon of future therapy, the development of appropriate models for preclinical testing has become a matter of great interest and this contribution is both important and timely.

x ◄

Robert Marcus, M.D.

1 ▸ Introduction: Organizational and Functional Aspects of Skeletal Health

▶ ▶ ▶ Robert Marcus

Osteoporosis is a condition of generalized skeletal fragility caused by a reduction in the amount of bone as well as by a disruption of skeletal microarchitecture. The chapters of this volume, ranging in approach from epidemiology to molecular biology, address a broad variety of topics concerning the nature of osteoporosis and its treatment. The purpose of this chapter is to introduce some fundamental principles of skeletal organization and function with the hope that they may assist the reader to establish a context for approaching subsequent chapters. The composition of the human skeleton, the process of bone remodeling, the geometric contributions to bone strength are first described. Next, the major factors known to regulate the acquisition and maintenance of bone mass are discussed, and finally, a working definition of osteoporosis will be provided.

Skeletal Organization

The skeleton consists of two types of bone. Most bones of the skeleton arise from secondary transformation of cartilage and are referred to as enchondral bones. The flat bones of the skull and face arise directly from mesenchyme and are called membranous bones. It is useful to consider the enchondral skeleton as composed of two compartments, peripheral and central. The *peripheral* or *appendicular skeleton* constitutes 80% of the skeletal mass and is composed of compact plates of cortical bone, called lamellae, that are organized about central (Haversian) nutrient canals. Bones of the *central* or *axial skeleton* consist of a honeycomb of vertical and horizontal bars, called trabeculae, contained within a cortical shell. Trabecular bone is filled with red marrow and fat. In adult human beings, trabecular bone is the sole repository of red marrow, localized for the most part in the vertebral bodies, the pelvis, and the proximal femur. The metaphyseal ends of adult long bones also contain trabecular bone but no red marrow. Vertebral bodies contain about 35% trabecular bone by weight (1) and about 70% by surface area, which greatly exceeds the trabecular component of peripheral bones. Because alterations in bone mass take place on bone surfaces, the fact that trabecular bone has an increased surface area in close proximity to the cells that participate in bone turnover means that changes in bone mass due to altered turnover occur earlier and to a greater extent in the axial skeleton. In the spine, approximately 50% of bone is cortical, including the transverse and spinous processes. The cortical shells that surround the vertebral bodies may provide as much as 50% of vertebral body compressive strength.

Bone Remodeling

Bone participates in three fundamental activities. *Modeling* refers to the process by which the characteristic shape of a bone is achieved. *Repair* is the regenerative response to fracture. *Remodeling* is a continuous cycle of destruction and renewal that is carried out by individual and independent osteons, otherwise called bone remodeling units. Alterations in remodeling activity constitute the final common pathway through which diverse stimuli, such as dietary or hormonal insufficiency, affect the rate of bone loss (2). The characteristic features of bone remodeling are illustrated in Figure 1-1.

Normally, 90% of bone surfaces are at rest, covered by a thin layer of inactive lining cells. Remodeling is initiated by hormonal or physical signals that cause marrow-derived precursor cells to cluster on the bone surface where they fuse into multinucleated osteoclasts that in turn dig a cavity into the bone. In cortical bone this cavity appears as a resorption tunnel within a Haversian canal. On trabecular surfaces it is a scalloped area called a Howship's lacuna. The resorption front leaves a cavity about 60 μm deep. The extent of deepest resorption appears as a cement line, a region of poorly organized collagen fibrils, as opposed to the osteon itself, which shows lamellar collagen deposition.

Coupled to resorption, bone formation ensues when local release of chemical mediators that are embedded in the bone matrix attracts preosteoblasts into the resorption cavity. The identity of these mediators is not known with certainty, but transforming growth factor β and insulin-like growth factor II may each play a role. The preosteoblasts mature into osteoblasts and replace the missing bone by secreting new collagen and matrix constituents. Matrix pro-

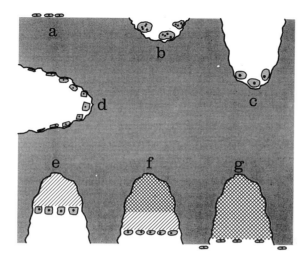

FIGURE 1-1 The remodeling cycle: (a) resting trabecular surface; (b) multinucleated osteoclasts dig a cavity of approximately 20 μm; (c) completion of resorption to 60 μm by mononuclear phagocytes; (d) recruitment of osteoblast precursors to the base of the resorption cavity; (e) secretion of new matrix by osteoblasts; (f) continued secretion of matrix, with initiation of calcification; and (g) completion of mineralization of new matrix. Bone has returned to quiescent state, but a small deficit in bone mass persists. (*Reproduced by permission from Marcus R. Normal and abnormal bone remodeling in man. Ann Rev Med 1987;38:129–141.*)

duction is initially rapid, the new osteoid seam approaching 20 μm in thickness when mineral deposition begins. With time, mineralization catches up to matrix deposition, and the new bone becomes fully mineralized. Resorption and formation are complete within 8 to 12 weeks, several additional weeks being required to complete mineralization.

If the remodeling cycle were completely efficient, bone would be neither lost nor gained. Each remodeling unit would be associated with complete replacement of the packet of bone that was initially lost. However, remodeling, like most biologic processes, is not entirely efficient. The amount of bone replaced by formation is not always equal to the amount previously removed, so that a small bone deficit persists after each cycle. This inefficiency is called *remodeling imbalance* and is minuscule for any single normal bone remodeling event. Unless remodeling dynamics are perturbed, the resulting accumulation of bone deficits may be detected only after many years. The concept of remodeling imbalance is validated by the fact that osteonal thickness decreases with age (3,4). It is not certain whether remodeling imbalance always occurs or whether it develops with aging. Nonetheless, it carries the profound implication that age-related bone loss is a normal, predictable phenomenon, beginning shortly after cessation of linear growth. Any stimulus that increases the overall rate of bone remodeling will increase the rate of bone loss.

For many years, understanding of osteoporosis was predicated on two competing and apparently irreconcilable models, one involving an increase in bone resorption, the other a decrease in formation. In light of the diverse ways in which remodeling can be altered, the naivete of this dichotomy is now evident. Total body remodeling balance encompasses the activation frequency, or birthrate, of new remodeling units, as well as the net activity of each of these units. The latter reflects the balance of individual resorption and formation phases. An acceleration in total bone loss could result from several discrete perturbations of remodeling activity (Figure 1-2). Examples of increased birthrate of remodeling units include thyrotoxicosis, primary hyperparathyroidism, and hypervitaminosis D or A. Immobilization, ethanol abuse, and age all decrease osteoblast efficiency. Dual abnormalities can be seen in some conditions. For example, glucocorticoid inhibition of intestinal calcium absorption is attended by compensatory hypersecretion of parathyroid hormone and an increased birthrate of bone remodeling units. However, the steroid also exerts a toxic effect on osteoblast function that magnifies the degree of remodeling inefficiency

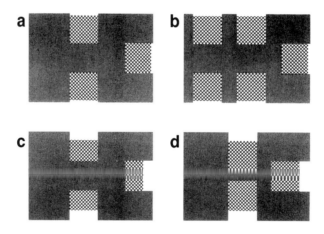

FIGURE 1-2 Schematic model of perturbations in bone remodeling. The upper left, panel a, illustrates a normal trabecular bone surface. Osteoclastic resorption has removed divots of bone from three sites; these have been replaced, but a small deficit persists at each site. In panel b an increased number of active remodeling units is shown. There will be an increase in the overall rate of bone loss, even though there has been no change in the depth to which osteoclasts resorb, or in the efficiency of osteoblast response within any individual remodeling site. The effect of decreased osteoblast efficiency is shown in panel c. Even if osteoclast function and the number of active remodeling units remain stable, bone loss increases. Panel d illustrates the effect of increased osteoclast resorption depth. If osteoblast response does not increase accordingly, accelerated bone loss occurs. (*Reproduced by permission from Marcus R. Normal and abnormal bone remodeling in man. Ann Rev Med 1987;38:129–141.*)

within each remodeling cycle. Estrogen–dependent bone loss is typified by increased osteoclastic activity to the point that resorption cavities perforate trabeculae, leaving no scaffold for an osteoblastic response.

A final point on remodeling concerns the concept of *remodeling space*. This term indicates bone that is temporarily missing because formation has not yet replaced that which was resorbed (5). It is a transient deficit that includes the lacunar space and osteoid tissue awaiting mineralization and was calculated to be about 7.5 g calcium, or 12.5 cm^3 bone when remodeling is normal (6). When bone turnover increases, commensurate expansion of the remodeling space achieves a new stable deficit. When turnover slows, remodeling space contracts. This principle must be remembered when considering the effects of disease on bone mass, since some measurable losses represent simple expansions of the remodeling space that predictably improve upon successful treatment. Conversely, deficits arising from failure of osteoblasts to restore resorbed bone are likely to be permanent.

▶ 5

Since bone remodeling leads ultimately to bone loss, one may ask what useful function it serves. Bone, like any material, accumulates fatigue damage over time. Compared to most building materials, the fatigue properties of bone are not particularly good. It is estimated that running for as little as 100 miles may result in perceptible microdamage to human bone (7). The cumulative nature of fatigue dictates that all human beings should be vulnerable to fatigue fractures over time. Current evidence suggests that remodeling fulfills a scavenger function, by which areas of fatigue microdamage are identified as they develop and are replaced by new lamellar bone. The inefficiency of remodeling may diminish bone mass and strength in the long run, but short-term protection against routine wear is achieved.

Constraints on the Relationship Between Mineral Density and Bone Strength

Most patients with osteoporotic fractures have low bone density compared to age-matched nonfractured control subjects. This is not surprising, in view of the close relationship between the mineral density and strength of bone (8). However, major overlap is seen in the bone densities of fracture patients and non-fractured controls regardless of measurement technique. In prospective studies (9–11) progressive increases in fracture incidence can be demonstrated as levels of bone mass decrease. For example, individuals in the lowest quartile of bone mineral density have a two- to three-fold increase in hip fracture over time (10). Many such individuals may never actually sustain a fracture, so fracture risk must also depend on factors beyond just bone mineral density. Extraskeletal factors such as the susceptibility to falls have been frequently discussed. Less commonly appreciated are skeletal factors other than bone mineral density that influence bone competence. These include bone material and geometric properties. *Material properties* include the brittleness and ultimate breaking strength of bone material. Although mineral content is a primary determinant of material properties, accumulation of cement lines and maturation of bone crystal or collagen over time may all diminish bone strength.

The major *geometric* influence on the competence of long bones is the distribution of bone mass about its bending axis. This can be expressed mathematically as a term called the cross-sectional *moment of inertia*. Briefly summarized, in a given object, the further away the mass is distributed from its central bending axis, the greater its strength. In men, an increase in moment of inertia due to expansion of long bone diameter compensates for the loss of bone mass and maintains bone strength with advancing age. This compensatory mechanism appears to be less robust in women (12,13).

In the axial skeleton, changes in trabecular microstructure are highly relevant to fracture risk. In young people, trabecular bone consists of thick vertical plates that are connected by thinner horizontal trabeculae. The space between adjacent trabeculae increases with age, reflecting the loss of entire trabecular elements (14,15). Parfitt and colleagues (14) suggested that trabecular dropout resulted from perforation during resorption. Perforated trabeculae offer no scaffold for new bone formation to take place. Thus, loss of trabeculae with age leads to deficient trabecular connectivity and, consequently, a substantial decrease in the capacity of trabeculae to withstand bending stress.

The role of trabecular connectivity is central to understanding why measurements of bone mineral density do not adequately predict fracture risk for individuals. Two people may have the same low bone mineral density; in one this reflects diffuse trabecular thinning with maintenance of normal connectivity, whereas the other shows porous bone with trabecular disruption. The first person may have a trivial fracture risk, while the bones of the second person may be in extreme jeopardy. Current noninvasive tools for clinical assessment of bone mass do not distinguish between these two situations. Until methods are developed to make such distinctions, the utility of bone density measurements to predict *individual* fracture risk will be limited.

Peak Bone Mass

Bone density and fracture risk in later years are determined not only by the rate of bone loss during adult life, but also by the maximal bone mineral acquired at skeletal maturity, called the peak bone mass. Only recently has serious attention been given to understanding the acquisition of peak bone mass. It has been frequently stated that "consolidation," or final acquisition of bone continues through the third decade. Recent data suggest that 95% of bone is acquired by late adolescence (16–19) and emphasize the critical importance of the pubertal growth spurt to forming an adequate peak bone mass.

Multiple factors determine peak bone mass. Heredity accounts for much of the variance in bone mass in healthy young populations, with smaller contributions made by such factors as muscle strength, physical activity, circulating reproductive hormone status, and nutritional status. Acquisition of peak bone mass is discussed in this volume by Bachrach (see Chapter 4).

▶ 7

Mechanisms of Bone Mass Regulation

With the exception of heredity, the primary regulators of bone mass in the adult are those that influence peak bone acquisition: physical activity, calcium nutritional state, and endocrine reproductive status. They all exert their effects by altering bone remodeling dynamics.

Physical Activity

Bone adapts to the loads applied to it (Wolff's law), so that an increase in bone density occurs when mechanical loading increases, and loss of bone density follows when customary loads are removed. Loss of bone with immobilization, such as with spinal cord injury, is a frequent and challenging clinical problem. Loss of bone with extended space flight emphasizes the critical role of gravitational stress to the maintenance of bone mass (20). Rubin and Lanyon (21,22) found that application of physiologic loads to isolated turkey ulnae increased bone area after a few weeks. The maximal effect of loading was achieved by a relatively small number of load cycles, and substantial increases beyond that point promoted no additional increase in bone mass. Based on a mathematical model, Whalen and colleagues (23) predicted that load magnitude was a more important determinant of bone density than the number of load cycles. Since muscle contraction is the dominant source of skeletal loading, it is not surprising that significant relationships exist between indices of bone and muscle mass (24) and between bone mineral density and muscle strength (25–28; Figure 1-3).

There is strong support for the notion that bone mass of athletes exceeds that of sedentary individuals (29). Not only is bone density higher in physically active people, but increased activity may slow age-related bone loss. These

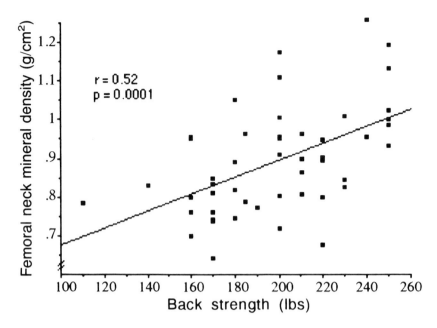

FIGURE 1-3 Relationship between muscle strength and bone density. (*Reproduced by permission from Snow-Harter C, Whalen R, Myburgh K, Arnaud S, Marcus R. Bone mineral density, muscle strength, and recreational exercise in men. J Bone Miner Res 1992;7:1291–1296.*)

cross-sectional studies must be interpreted with caution because genetic and musculoskeletal characteristics may distinguish "athletic" from "sedentary" individuals even before exercise training is initiated. A few intervention trials have examined the effects of exercise on bone density. Once again, interpretation requires caution because most of these have not been randomized trials, and several have applied training routines suited for cardiovascular fitness, but not appropriate for skeletal loading. Nonetheless, results generally confirm that bone density increases with exercise training. However, the increases in bone mass observed during these trials, 1% to 5% on average, have not equalled the 10% to 15% differences that might be predicted from the cross-sectional comparisons.

Contradictory results from two studies offer insight into the type of exercise that is optimal for an osteogenic response. Dalsky and colleagues (30) reported an increase in spinal bone mineral content of elderly women after a 9-month exercise program that included jogging and walking as well as a series of resistance exercises, such as rowing, that specifically loaded the spine. In contrast, Cavanaugh and Cann (31) found that postmenopausal women lost mineral from the spine during a one-year program composed only of brisk walking. The forces produced at the lumbar vertebrae during fast walking and jogging equal 1 and 1.75 times body weight, respectively, whereas resistance activity applies lumbar vertebral stresses as high as 5 to 6 body weights (32). These results suggest resistance exercise to be a more potent stimulus for preserving bone than brisk walking. This notion, if validated, carries important therapeutic implications, because weight-bearing exercises, defined as walking, jogging, running, and dancing, have been the forms of activity traditionally prescribed for skeletal benefit. Although serious weight-loading of frail elders might not safely be carried out, the results of Dalsky lend optimism that lower intensity resistance training could be successfully introduced to this population.

The primary beneficiaries of high weight-loading exercise would be teenage and young adults who are nearing completion of bone acquisition and who could tolerate loading with minimal fracture risk. Nevertheless, recent experience indicates the relatively modest nature of these benefits. Snow-Harter and colleagues (33) randomly assigned a group of young women to a control group or to progressive training programs of jogging or resistance exercise. Exercises were carried out with good compliance and substantial performance gains. After 8 months of training, weight-lifters and joggers each showed a significant increase in lumbar spine mineral of about 1.3%, with no change in the control group and no change at the proximal femur in any group. Perhaps healthy young adults are sufficiently active that the added loads due to exercise training do not provide a major change from habitual levels.

Another observation from the work of Dalsky and coworkers (30) was a return of bone mass toward baseline levels in subjects who stopped the training regimen. Thus, for exercise programs to deliver long-term skeletal benefits, they must be sustained. It is important to remember that exercise is not a way of life for most Americans. Reports from the President's Council on Fitness suggest only one of five adults participates in any regular physical activity. In particular, older men and women often claim regular exercise to be unnecessary at their age, frequently have unrealistic expectations regarding the health benefits of their usual daily activities, and seriously exaggerate the risks of vigorous exercise. Considerable effort is now devoted to understanding the relationship between physical activity and bone health. To gain practical benefits from these insights, we must invest a similar effort into strategies to motivate a sedentary population to adopt exercise as a regular component of daily life.

Calcium Nutritional State

The skeleton contains 99.5% of body calcium and provides a mineral reservoir to support plasma calcium levels at times of need. The preventive and therapeutic aspects of calcium are discussed by Ott (see Chapter 9). However, a few statements summarizing the role of calcium intake during the life cycle are in order.

The daily recommended dietary calcium intake for adolescent boys and girls is 1200 mg, a figure derived primarily from balance studies. Because the 2 or 3 years that define the pubertal growth spurt are accompanied by deposition of 60% of final bone mass, dietary intake should influence bone acquisition more at this time than at other times of life. Johnston and colleagues (34) reported a controlled trial of calcium supplementation in young twins; one twin was assigned placebo and the other calcium. A 3% greater increase in bone mass was observed in the calcium-treated group over 3 years of follow-up. The most striking effect was observed in those children who had not yet entered puberty. In other words, the primary effect of nutritional intervention emerged when sex hormone-dependent bone growth was not simultaneously occurring. It will be interesting to determine whether the skeletal benefit shown in this study will be translated ultimately into an increased peak bone mass.

Consumption figures indicate that the calcium intake of American men corresponds reasonably well to recommended levels at most ages, but that median intakes for girls are well below target levels by age 11 and never recover (35). Thus, calcium undernutrition probably has an important influence on peak bone mass in women.

During the third through fifth decades, growth has stopped, and robust compensatory mechanisms permit rapid adaptation to even severe dietary restriction. Riggs and colleagues (36) found that calcium nutritional state did not affect the rate of bone loss during this period, so that it is unlikely that calcium supplementation will exert important beneficial effects on bone mass at this time. Consensus has not been reached on this point. For example, Baran and coworkers (37) reported that addition of dairy products to the diet of premenopausal women for 3 years attenuated vertebral bone loss.

At menopause, accelerated bone loss reflects loss of endogenous estrogen and has little relationship to dietary calcium. Riis and colleagues (38) and Elders and coworkers (39) showed modest effects on bone loss when early menopausal women were given extra calcium. However, habitual dietary calcium intakes of Danish and Dutch women average 1100 mg, which is considerably higher than in the United States, so what may have been a marginal effect in Northern Europe might be more substantial in North America.

After age 60, the early effects of estrogen deficiency have dissipated, and the compensations to accommodate dietary inadequacy are less efficient. At this time proper attention to calcium intake, be it from diet or supplements, is rational, and has been shown to have beneficial effects on bone turnover and mass (40).

Endocrine Reproductive Status

Formidable evidence supports a critical role for gonadal function in the acquisition and maintenance of bone mass. Hypogonadal boys and girls show important deficits in cortical and trabecular bone mineral, and loss of endogenous androgen or estrogen during adult life accelerates the loss of bone. In women, loss of estrogen has dual effects. Decreased efficiency of intestinal and renal calcium handling increases the calcium requirement (41). In addition, estrogen directly affects bone cell function (42,43), and this interaction may underlie the accelerated bone loss of early deficiency. In terms of bone remodeling, estrogen deficiency enhances the ability of osteoclasts to resorb bone, which increases the risk that any given resorptive event may result in trabecular perforation. In the absence of a suitable scaffold for proliferation of osteoblast precursors, it is not possible to replace the resorbed bone, resulting in the characteristic porous appearance of osteoporosis.

▶ 11

Estrogen replacement at menopause protects bone mass and affords significant protection against osteoporotic fractures. The therapeutic use of estrogen is discussed in Chapter 10. The molecular basis of this protective effect is probably complex, reflecting direct actions of estrogen on bone cells (discussed in Chapter 2 by Jilka and Manolagas), as well as increases in circulating levels of $1,25(OH)_2$ vitamin D (44,45) that improve intestinal calcium absorption efficiency in menopausal women (44).

The skeletal role of androgens is less well understood. Testosterone deficiency is a major cause of osteoporosis in men, in whom hormone replacement restores bone mass. Specific testosterone receptors have been demonstrated in normal human osteoblasts (46). Whether direct actions on bone cells fully account for the effects of androgen on bone mass is unknown. Androgens also increase muscle mass, so effects on bone may be secondary to the increased mechanical loading that would accompany increased muscle bulk. Circulating androgens also make an independent contribution to peak bone mass in women.

THE INTEGRATED NATURE OF BONE MASS REGULATION

Optimal acquisition and maintenance of bone requires sufficiency in physical activity, reproductive status, and nutrition. Deficiency in one is not compensated by excessive attention to another. Women athletes who develop exercise-associated amenorrhea are hypogonadal and lose bone, despite frequent high-intensity exercise (47,48). Therapeutic specificity is a venerable medical tradition. Just as it would be inappropriate to treat iron deficiency with folic acid, it is equally futile to prescribe calcium to an immobilized patient, or to substitute exercise and calcium for estrogen in the hypogonadal patient.

Osteoporosis

Prior to the introduction of noninvasive bone mass measurements, osteoporosis was a clinical and radiologic diagnosis that could be made only after obvious skeletal damage had occurred. Diagnosis based on the presence of fracture proved unworkable because it was too restrictive, excluding individuals whose bones were in jeopardy but had not yet fractured. It is currently fashionable to define osteoporosis more inclusively, as a critical reduction in bone mass to the point that fracture vulnerability increases. In this sense, osteoporosis is analogous to anemia defined as a low red blood cell mass. Although this is a useful definition, it introduces problems of specificity. Bone mineral content does predict fracture risk (9–11), but accounts for only a portion of this risk, so issues beyond simple mineral content must be operative. Some of these have been discussed earlier in this chapter.

To most readers, "osteoporosis" calls to mind specific clinical entities, such as vertebral compression fractures, distal radial (Colle's) fractures, and fractures of the proximal femur, or hip. Although these fractures certainly occur with greater frequency in porotic bone, a diagnosis of osteoporosis implies *generalized* skeletal fragility, with increased risk for all types of fracture. In particular, rib fractures brought about by coughing or sudden torque on the trunk are particularly common, although uncertainty of radiologic diagnosis makes it difficult to assess their prevalence.

Primary osteoporosis is by convention a condition of reduced bone mass and fractures found in menopausal women (postmenopausal osteoporosis) or in older men and women ("senile" osteoporosis). *Secondary osteoporosis* by tradition refers to bone loss resulting from specific clinical disorders, such as thyrotoxicosis or hyperadrenocorticism (Table 1-1; 49). Several clinical states of

TABLE 1-1   Representative Examples of "Secondary" Osteoporosis

Cause	BRU Birthrate*	Resorption	Formation[†]
Glucocorticoids	probably increased	normal to increased	decreased
Hyperthyroidism	increased	increased	increased[‡]
Immobilization	early increase	increased then normal	decreased
Heparin	probably increased	probably increased	uncertain
Hypervitaminosis A	probably increased	increased	uncertain
Anticonvulsants	probably increased	increased	increased[‡]

*Refers to activation, or birthrate, of bone remodeling units
[†]Refers to total bone forming activity
[‡]Despite an increase in overall formation, osteoblastic function for individual bone remodeling units may be impaired
(Reproduced by permission from Marcus R. Secondary forms of osteoporosis. In: Coe FL, Favus MJ, eds. Disorders of bone and mineral metabolism. New York: Raven Press, 1992:889–904.)

estrogen-dependent bone loss, such as the osteopenias resulting from exercise-related amenorrhea and from prolactin-secreting tumors, are conventionally included under primary osteoporosis.

Albright and Reifenstein (50) proposed in 1948 that primary osteoporosis consists of two separate entities, one related to menopausal estrogen loss and the other to aging. Recent support for this concept has been published by Riggs and associates (51) who suggested the terms *type I osteoporosis,* to signify a loss of trabecular bone after menopause, and *type II osteoporosis,* to represent a loss of cortical and trabecular bone in men and women as the end result of age-related bone loss. Whereas the type I disorder is proposed to be directly related to lack of endogenous estrogen, type II osteoporosis would reflect the composite influence of long-term remodeling efficiency, adequacy of dietary calcium and vitamin D, intestinal mineral absorption, renal mineral handling, and parathyroid hormone (PTH) secretion.

► 13

Compelling proof that these are truly distinct entities remains to be offered. Iliac crest biopsies have not shown a characteristic histomorphometric profile of patients whose clinical status suggests the type I disorder (52). The type I-type II model also suffers by its adherence to a bone loss paradigm. For many years, attention of the field has been directed almost exclusively to bone *loss* as a unifying feature of osteoporosis. It has been assumed that postmenopausal women with low bone mass achieved that status because they experienced a drastic menopausal loss of bone. Bone mass at any time in adult life is now understood to reflect the peak investment in bone mineral at skeletal maturity minus that which has been subsequently lost. A woman who experienced interruption of menses, extended bedrest, eating disorder, or systemic illness during her adolescent growth years might enter adult life having failed to achieve the bone mass that would have been predicted from her genetic or constitutional profile. This woman might then undergo a perfectly normal rate of bone loss, but her skeleton would be in jeopardy simply due to the deficit in peak bone mass. It is also possible that differences in fracture patterns from one patient to the next are more indicative of the tendency to fall and the types of falls that are experienced rather than fundamental differences in bone physiology. For the time being, it may be more appropriate to consider osteoporosis the result of multiple physical, hormonal, and nutritional factors acting alone or in concert over a lifetime.

References

1. Nottestad SY, Baumel JJ, Kimmel D, Recker RR, Heany RP. The proportion of trabecular bone in human vertebrae. J Bone Miner Res 1987;2:221–229.

2. Marcus R. Normal and abnormal bone remodeling in man. Ann Rev Med 1987; 38:129–141.

3. Lips P, Courpron P, Meunier PJ. Mean wall thickness of trabecular bone packets in the human iliac crest: changes with age. Calcif Tissue Res 1978;26:13–17.

4. Kragstrup J, Melsen, F, Mosekilde L. Thickness of bone formed at remodeling sites in normal human iliac trabecular bone: variations with age and sex. Metab Bone Dis Rel Res 1983;5:17–21.

5. Jaworski ZFG. Parameters and indices of bone resorption. In: Meunier PJ. Bone Histomorphometry, 2d International Workshop. Paris: Armour Montague, 1976.

6. Parfitt AM. Morphologic basis of bone mineral measurements: transient and steady state effects of treatment in osteoporosis. Miner Electrolyte Metab 1980;4:273–287.

7. Carter DR, Caler WE, Spengler DM, Fankel VH. Fatigue behavior of adult cortical bone: the influence of mean strain and strain range. Acta Ortho Scand 1981;52: 481–490.

8. Carter DR, Hayes WC. The compressive behavior of bone as a two-phase porous structure. J Bone Joint Surg 1977;59-A:954–962.

9. Hui SL, Slemenda CS, Johnston CC Jr. Age and bone mass as predictors of fracture in a prospective study. J Clin Invest 1988;81:1804 1809.

10. Cummings SR, Black DM, Nevitt MC, et al. and the Study of Osetoporotic Fractures Research Group. Appendicular bone density and age predict hip fracture in women. JAMA 1990;263:665–668.

11. Ross PD, Davis JW, Vogel JM, Wasnich RD. A critical review of bone mass and the risk of fractures in osteoporosis. Calcif Tissue Int 1990;46:149–161.

12. Martin RB, Atkinson PJ. Age and sex-related changes in the structure and strength of the human femoral shaft. J Biomech 1977;10:223–231.

13. Ruff CB, Hayes WC. Sex differences in age-related remodeling of the femur and tibia. J Orthop Res 1988;6:886–896.

14. Parfitt AM, Mathews CHE, Villanueva AR, Kleerekoper M, Frame B, Rao DS. Relationships between surface, volume and thickness of iliac trabecular bone in aging and in osteoporosis. Implications for the microanatomic and cellular mechanisms of bone loss. J Clin Invest 1983;72: 1396–1409.

15. Weinstein RS, Hutson MS. Decreased trabecular width and increased trabecular spacing contribute to bone loss with aging. Bone 1987;8:137–142.

16. Gilsanz B, Gibbons DT, Carlson M, Boechat MI, Cann CE, Schulz EE. Peak vertebral density: a comparison of adolescent and adult females. Calcif Tissue Int 1988;43:260–262.

17. Bonjour JP, Theintz G, Buchs B, Slossman D, Rizzoli R. Critical years and stages of puberty for spinal and femoral bone mass accumulation during adolescence. J Clin Endocrinol Metab 1991; 73:555–563.

18. Katzman DK, Bachrach LK, Carter DR, Marcus R. Clinical and anthropometric correlates of bone mineral acquisition in healthy adolescent girls. J Clin Endocrinol Metab 1991;73:1332–1339.

19. Recker RR, Daview KM, Hinders SM, Heaney RP, Stegman MR, Kimmel DB. Bone gain in young adult women. JAMA 1992;268:2403–2408.

20. Mack PB, LaChance PA, Vose GP. Bone demineralization of foot and hand of Gemini-Titan IV, V and VII astronauts during orbital flight. Am J Roentgenol; Rad Ther Nucl Med 1967;100:503–511.

21. Rubin CT, Lanyon CE. Regulation of bone formation by applied dynamic loads. J Bone Joint Surg 1984;66:397–402.

22. Rubin CT, Lanyon LE. Regulation of bone mass by mechanical strain magnitude. Calcif Tissue Int 1985;37:411–417.

23. Whalen RT, Carter DR, Steele CR. The influence of physical activity on the regulation of bone density. J Biomech 1988;21:825–837.

24. Doyle F, Brown J, LaChance C. Relation between bone mass and muscle weight. Lancet 1970;1:391–393.

25. Snow-Harter C, Bouxsein M, Lewis B, Charette S, Weinstein P, Marcus R. Muscle strength as a predictor of bone mineral density in young women. J Bone Miner Res 1990;5:589–595.

26. Snow-Harter C, Whalen R, Myburgh K, Arnaud S, Marcus R. Bone mineral density, muscle strength, and recreational exercise in men. J Bone Miner Res 1992;7:1291–1296.

27. Sinaki M, McPhee MC, Hodgson SF, Merritt JM, Offord KP. Relationship between bone mineral density of spine and strength of back extensors in healthy postmenopausal women. Mayo Clin Proc 1986;61:116–122.

28. Bevier W, Wiswell RA, Pyka G, Kozak K, Newhall K, Marcus R. Relationship of muscle strength and aerobic capacity to bone density in older men and women. J Bone Miner Res 1989;4:421–432.

29. Marcus R, Carter D. The role of physical activity in bone mass regulation. Adv Sports Med Fitness 1988;1:63–82.

30. Dalsky G, Stocke KS, Ehsani AA. Weight-bearing exercise training and lumbar bone mineral content in postmenopausal women. Ann Intern Med 1988;108: 824–828.

31. Cavanaugh DJ, Cann CE. Brisk walking does not stop bone loss in postmenopausal women. Bone 1988;9:201–204.

32. Capozzo A. Force actions in the human trunk during running. J Sports Med 1983;23:14–22.

33. Snow-Harter C, Bouxsein ML, Lewis BT, Carter DR, Marcus R. Effects of resistance and endurance exercise on bone mineral status of young women: a randomized exercise intervention trial. J Bone Miner Res 1992;7:761–769.

34. Johnston CC Jr, Miller JZ, Slemenda CW, et al. Calcium supplementation and increased in bone mineral density in children. N Engl J Med 1992;327:82–87.

35. Carroll MD, Abraham S, Dresser CM. Dietary intake source data, 1976–1980. Washington, DC: Department of Health and Human Services; March 1983. DHHS Publication #PHS 83–1681.

36. Riggs BL, Wahner HW, Melton LJ III, Richelson LS, Judd HL, O'Fallon WM. Dietary calcium intake and rate of bone loss in women. J Clin Invest 1987;80:979–982.

37. Baran D, Sorenson A, Grimes J, et al. Dietary modification with dairy products for preventing vertebral bone loss in premenopausal women: a three-year prospective study. J Clin Endocrinol Metab 1990; 70:264–270.

38. Riis B, Thomsen K, Christianssen C. Does calcium supplementation prevent postmenopausal bone loss? A double-blind, controlled clinical study. N Engl J Med 1987;316:173–177.

39. Elders PJM, Netelenbos JC, Lips P, et al. Calcium supplementation reduces vertebral bone loss in perimenopausal women: a controlled trial in 248 women between 46 and 55 years of age. J Clin Endocrinol Metab 1991;73:533–540.

40. Dawson-Hughes B, Dallal GE, Krall EA, Sadowski L, Sahyoun N, Tannenbaum S. A controlled trial of the effect of calcium supplementation on bone density in postmenopausal women. N Engl J Med 1990; 323:878–883.

41. Heaney RP, Recker RR, Saville PD. Calcium balance and calcium requirements in middle-aged women. Am J Clin Nutr 1977;30:1603–1611.

42. Eriksen EF, Colvard DS, Berg NJ, et al. Evidence of estrogen receptors in normal human osteoblast cells. Science 1988;241:84–86.

43. Komm BS, Terpening CM, Benz DJ, et al. Estrogen binding, receptor mRNA, and biologic response in osteoblast-like osteosarcoma cells. Science 1988;241:81–84.

44. Gallagher JC, Riggs BL, DeLuca HF. Effect of estrogen on calcium absorption and serum vitamin D metabolites in postmenopausal osteoporosis. J Clin Endocrinol Metab 1980;51:1359–1364.

45. Cheema C, Grant BF, Marcus R. Effects of estrogen on circulating "free" and total 1,25-dihydroxyvitamin D and on the parathyroid-vitamin D axis in postmenopausal women. J Clin Invest 1989;83:537–542.

46. Colvard DS, Eriksen EF, Keeting PE, et al. Identification of androgen receptors in normal human osteoblast-like cells. Proc Natl Acad Sci USA 1989;86: 854–857.

47. Drinkwater BL, Nilson K, Chestnut CH III, Bremner WJ, Shainholtz S, Southworth MB. Bone mineral content of amen-

orrheic and eumenorrheic athletes. N Engl J Med 1984;311:277–281.

48. Marcus R, Cann C, Madvig P, et al. Menstrual function and bone mass in elite women distance runners: endocrine metabolic features. Ann Intern Med 1985, 102:158–163.

49. Marcus R. Secondary forms of osteoporosis. In: Coe FL, Favus MJ, eds. Disorders of bone and mineral metabolism. New York: Raven Press, 1992:889–904.

50. Albright F, Reifenstein EC Jr. The parathyroid glands and metabolic bone disease: selected studies. Baltimore: Williams & Wilkins, 1948:162.

51. Riggs BL, Wahner HW, Seeman E, et al. Changes in bone mineral density of the proximal femur and spine with aging. Differences between the postmenopausal and senile osteoporosis syndromes. J Clin Invest 1982;70:716–723.

52. Eriksen EF, Hodgson SF, Eastell R, Cedel SL, O'Fallon WM, Riggs BL. Cancellous bone remodeling in type I (postmenopausal) osteoporosis: quantitative assessment of rates of formation, resorption, and bone loss at tissue and cellular levels. J Bone Miner Res 1990;5:311–320.

2 ▸ The Cellular and Biochemical Basis of Bone Remodeling

▶ ▶ ▶ Robert L. Jilka

Stavros C. Manolagas

Bone is remodeled continuously throughout adult life. This is accomplished by the resorption of old bone by osteoclasts and the subsequent formation of new bone by osteoblasts (1). These two processes are tightly coupled to each other and are responsible for the renewal of the skeleton while maintaining its anatomic and structural integrity. Under normal physiologic circumstances, bone remodeling proceeds in highly regulated cycles in which osteoclasts adhere to bone and subsequently remove it by acidification and proteolytic digestion. After osteoclasts have left the resorption site, osteoblasts invade the area and begin the process of new bone formation by secreting osteoid (a matrix of collagen and other proteins), which is eventually mineralized into new bone. Remodeling is carried out by a group of osteoblasts and osteoclasts termed the *bone remodeling unit*. This group of cells represents the functional cellular unit of the bone tissue, and it is analogous to the nephron in the kidney. After bone formation ceases, the surface of the bone is covered by lining cells, at which time the surface appears to be quiescent.

During the last decade, major advances have been made in our understanding of the ontogeny of osteoclasts and osteoblasts, the interplay between them, and the systemic and local factors that regulate their development and the coupling of their function. This information has provided a much clearer picture of bone metabolism and new insights into the pathophysiology of several disease states.

In this chapter, we address the cellular and biochemical basis of bone remodeling. First, we describe the morphologic and biosynthetic features of osteoclasts and osteoblasts. Then, we discuss the origin of osteoclasts and osteoblasts and their relationship to the hematopoietic tissue, and the role of systemic hormones, as well as local agents such as cytokines and growth factors, in their development. Finally, we highlight some new insights into the pathophysiology of disease states characterized by abnormal bone remodeling, such as postmenopausal osteoporosis.

Morphologic, Biosynthetic, and Functional Features of Osteoclasts

Osteoclasts are cells unique to bone and are always found on endosteal or trabecular bone surfaces tightly associated with the calcified bone matrix (2). They are usually large (50 to 100 μm diameter) multinucleated cells with abundant mitochondria, numerous lysosomes, free ribosomes, and extensive Golgi complexes. The most remarkable morphologic feature of these cells is the ruffled border and its surrounding clear zone, which is formed by a specialization of the plasma membrane. The ruffled border is a complex system of finger-shaped or flat plate-shaped projections of the membrane, the function of which is to mediate the resorption of the calcified bone matrix. This structure is completely surrounded by another specialized area, namely, the clear zone. The cytoplasm in the clear zone area has a uniform appearance and contains bundles of actin-like filaments. The clear zone delineates the area of attachment of the osteoclast to the bone surface and seals off a distinct area of the bone surface that lies immediately underneath the osteoclast and which eventually will be excavated. The ability of the clear zone to seal off this area of bone surface allows the formation of a microenvironment suitable for the operation of the resorptive apparatus of the osteoclast.

The initial phase of osteoclastic bone resorption involves the attachment of osteoclasts to the calcified bone surface. In trabecular and endosteal bone, the surface of bone is covered by an unmineralized layer of collagenous organic material covered by bone lining cells. Osteoclasts cannot degrade this collagenous layer. Therefore, enzymes from other cell types must remove this material before osteoclasts can attach to the mineralized surface (3). Osteoblastic cells secrete collagenases and it is likely that these enzymes are responsible for removal of this collagen layer (4). This scenario is supported by evidence that inhibitors of neutral collagenase suppress bone resorption in organ cultures containing a calcified bone surface covered by collagen. However, inhibitors of neutral collagenase do not affect bone resorption by isolated osteoclasts placed onto calcified bone lacking a collagenous surface (4).

The targeting and attachment of osteoclasts to the bone surface, following removal of the collagenous layer, is mediated by vitronectin receptors expressed on the surface of osteoclasts. Indeed, antibodies to this protein have been shown to inhibit osteoclastic bone resorption and cause detachment of isolated osteoclasts from bone. The vitronectin receptor of osteoclasts likely recognizes osteopontin and thrombospondin present in the bone matrix (5,6).

Once they are attached to the bone surface, osteoclasts secrete protons and enzymes that are capable of resorbing, respectively, the mineral and protein components of the bone matrix (4). Specifically, osteoclasts dissolve bone mineral by secreting acid into the subosteoclastic extracellular compartment (7). This process is catalyzed by a proton pump localized at the ruffled border (8,9). The hydrogen ions required for acidification are derived from the hydration of carbon dioxide carried out by carbonic anhydrase isozyme II in the cytoplasm of the osteoclast (10,11).

The protein components of bone matrix are degraded by the action ▶ 19 of lysosomal cysteine proteases secreted by osteoclasts. These enzymes are transported via primary lysosomes to the ruffled border membrane and are directionally secreted into the bone-resorbing lacuna. The principal protein component of bone, fibrillar collagen, is denatured under acidic conditions. Thus, in the subosteoclastic compartment where bone resorption occurs, collagen becomes susceptible to the action of the lysosomal catheptic enzymes, including cathepsin B, a cysteine proteinase. Because specific inhibitors of cysteine proteinases suppress bone resorption both in vivo and in vitro, it is likely that these lysosomal enzymes play a critical role in the process (4).

A prominent feature of osteoclasts is the presence of high amounts of the phosphohydrolase enzyme, tartrate-resistant acid phosphatase (TRAPase) (12). In fact, this feature is frequently used as an identifier in the detection of osteoclasts in bone specimens (13). In contrast to the role of the lysosomal proteolytic enzymes, little is known about the role of TRAPase in osteoclastic bone resorption. Preliminary evidence indicates that TRAPase could dephosphorylate bone and nonbone phosphoproteins (14). Indeed, antibodies against TRAPase inhibited the bone resorptive activity of isolated osteoclasts, suggesting an important role for acid phosphatases in bone resorption (15).

Osteoclasts bear on their surface several antigens that are also present on hematopoietic cells (16). These include CD54, the cellular ligand for certain integrin proteins; CD45, the common leukocyte antigen; and the CD49b and CD29 antigens that constitute the collagen receptor. In addition, osteoclasts express CD9 (function unknown); CD13, which is the aminopeptidase N that regulates the tissue half-life of small peptides in the case of inflammatory cells; CD71, the transferrin receptor, which may be related to the presence of high levels of the iron-containing TRAPase present in osteoclasts; and CD51 and CD61, which constitute the vitronectin receptor responsible for mediating the attachment of osteoclasts to the bone surface.

Because of a common ancestry with macrophages and some similarity in their functional capabilities, osteoclasts have been thought to be a type of specialized tissue macrophage. As in the case of osteoclasts, macrophages are well endowed with acid hydrolases. Nonetheless, the surface antigens of macrophages and osteoclasts are quite distinct. More important, antigens crucial for the phagocytic and antigen-presenting functions of macrophages are absent from osteoclasts (16). In any event, macrophages might be able to resorb bone (17). However, the mechanism of bone resorption mediated by macrophages is quite distinct from the mechanism of osteoclastic bone resorption. Thus, when osteoclasts are placed onto smooth slices of bone, they excavate the surface of the bone to form pits that are up to 10 μm deep (18,19; Figure 2-1). The bottoms of the pits vary in appearance; some have relatively smooth surfaces with small nodules, whereas others contain fibrillar material that is most likely undegraded collagen. In contrast, macrophages are incapable of excavating the surface of bone slices in vitro (20).

A wide variety of agents can influence osteoclast function. However, the majority of them appear to exert their effects on osteoclasts indirectly, via effects on cells of osteoblastic lineage. The exception to this is calcitonin, a hormone produced by the C cells of the thyroid gland. Osteoclasts express high-affinity (K_d 1-6 × 10^{-10} M) receptors for calcitonin on their surface (21,22); and calcitonin, acting via these receptors, inhibits the motility of the osteoclast and its ability to resorb bone (23,24). The expression of calcitonin receptors occurs

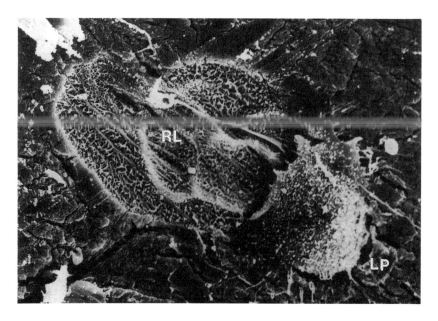

FIGURE 2-1   Scanning electron micrograph of a human osteoclast cultured on a bone slice. The osteoclast exhibits characteristic lamellipodia (LP), and has excavated a resorption lacuna (RC) from the surface of the bone. (*Reproduced by permission from Murrills PJ, Shane E, Lindsay R, Dempster DW. J Bone Miner Res 1989;4:259–268.*)

early in the development of osteoclasts (25) and is another unique feature of osteoclasts among the other cell types present in bone.

Morphologic, Biosynthetic, and Functional Features of Osteoblasts

The term "osteoblast phenotype" is used loosely in the literature to describe cells of the same lineage. However, one needs to appreciate the fact that osteoblasts occur in a continuum of many different stages of functional differentiation, and that at each of these stages, the phenotype, including the morphology as well as the biosynthetic activity, is different (26,27).

▶ 21

Osteoblasts engaged in bone formation are polarized cuboidal mononuclear cells with an average diameter of 20 to 30 µm, whereas quiescent osteoblasts are flat and elongated (2). Bone-forming osteoblasts contain a well developed secretory apparatus of rough endoplasmic reticulum and Golgi complexes oriented toward the bone surface. Some osteoblasts are eventually buried within lacunae of mineralized matrix. These cells are defined as osteocytes and are characterized by extensions of their plasma membrane into the osteoid and mineralized bone matrix through canaliculi. In fact, these extensions represent means of communication between the osteocytes and the bone-forming osteoblasts through gap junctions. Similar gap junctions or cell-to-cell contacts exist between stromal cells of the marrow and osteoblasts. As will be discussed below, stromal cells of the marrow are thought to be of the same lineage as osteoblasts. Hence, bone-forming osteoblasts, osteocytes, and marrow stromal cells are in physical contact with each other. This provides a continuous network of communication between the cells of this lineage, which probably coordinates their function (28).

A major product of the bone-forming osteoblast is type I collagen (29). This polymeric protein is initially secreted in the form of a precursor, which contains peptide extensions at both the N terminal and carboxyl ends of the molecule. The propeptides are proteolytically removed at the time of exocytosis. Further extracellular processing results in mature three-chained type I collagen molecules, which then assemble themselves into a collagen fibril. Individual collagen molecules become interconnected by the formation of pyridinoline cross-links, which are unique to bone (30,31).

Bone-forming osteoblasts synthesize a number of other proteins that are incorporated into the bone matrix. Of these, the most abundant are osteocalcin and osteonectin, which constitute 40% to 50% of the noncollagenous proteins of bone. Osteocalcin (also termed bone gla protein) is a bone-specific protein distinguished by three residues of γ-carboxyglutamic acid (32). Another protein made by osteoblasts also contains γ-carboxyglutamic acid. This so-called matrix gla protein is otherwise unrelated to osteocalcin (33). The γ-carboxyglutamic acid residues provide these proteins with the ability to bind calcium and hydroxyapatite. The expression of osteocalcin coincides with the mineralization process. Osteocalcin, however, may also play a role in bone resorption, as evidenced by its chemotactic and mitogenic influence on cells of osteoclast lineage. Osteocalcin is also chemotactic for osteogenic cells (34,35). Osteonectin is another abundant product of osteoblasts. However, unlike osteocalcin, which is a specific product of osteoblasts, osteonectin is also found in many other developing tissues (36,37).

Osteoblasts also synthesize and secrete several other proteins found in bone. These include glycosaminoglycans, which are attached to one of two small core proteins: PG-I (or biglycan) and decorin (38). Decorin is capable of binding to collagen fibrils and has been implicated in the regulation of collagen fibrillogenesis. In addition, osteoblasts secrete bone acidic glycoprotein, a phosphoprotein found in osteoid undergoing calcification (39).

Osteoblasts produce several more minor proteins, which may serve as attachment factors. These include osteopontin, bone sialoprotein, fibronectin, vitronectin, and thrombospondin (40–45). This group of proteins interacts with integrins present on the cell surface of most differentiated cells. The adhesion proteins contain a specific sequence of amino acids, namely arginine-glycine-aspartate (RGD), which is intimately involved in the interaction with integrins. Interestingly, these attachment proteins play an important role in hematopoietic stem cell differentiation (46,47).

Osteoblasts also produce a variety of growth factors including transforming growth factor-β (TGFβ), basic fibroblast growth factor (bFGF), insulin-like growth factors I and II (IGF-I, IGF-II), as well as several bone morphogenetic proteins (BMP). All these proteins are incorporated into the bone matrix (48–51). Their function in the bone matrix may be related to fracture repair and, possibly, to the coupling of bone resorption and bone formation. Some of these factors are also involved in hematopoiesis, as indicated by evidence that bFGF plays an important role in the proliferation of hematopoietic progenitors (52).

Finally, osteoblasts express relatively high amounts of alkaline phosphatase (53). The particular isoform of alkaline phosphatase present in osteoblasts is the same as that found in the liver and the kidney. Alkaline phosphatase acts as an ectoenzyme, that is, its active site is on the surface of the plasma membrane. This enzyme is anchored to the external surface of the plasma membrane by phosphoethanolamine covalently bound to phosphatidylinositol through an oligosaccharide (54,55). Alkaline phosphatase is released from the surface of the osteoblast and reaches the circulation. Bone-derived alkaline phosphatase constitutes approximately one half of the total alkaline phosphatase activity present in adult serum (56).

Alkaline phosphatase has been long thought to play a role in bone mineralization. However, the precise mechanism of mineralization and the role of alkaline phosphatase in this process remain unclear. In any event, mineralization is due to deposition of hydroxyapatite crystals in the collagenous matrix. This process lags behind matrix production and, in remodeling sites in the adult bone, occurs at a distance of 8–10 μm from the osteoblast (1,2). Osteoblasts are thought to regulate the local concentrations of calcium and phosphate in such a way as to promote the formation of hydroxyapatite. In view of the highly ordered, well-aligned, collagen fibrils complexed with the noncollagenous proteins formed by the osteoblast in lamellar bone, it has been proposed that mineralization proceeds in association with, and perhaps governed by, the heteropolymeric matrix fibrils themselves (57). Matrix vesicles derived from the plasma membrane of osteoblasts might provide a locus of hydroxyapatite crystal formation in lamellar bone as they appear to do in cartilage calcification (58). However, matrix vesicles are rarely seen in sites of lamellar bone formation.

▶ 23

Alkaline phosphatase may promote mineralization by the hydrolysis of phosphate esters, resulting in increased inorganic phosphate at the site of mineralization. Alternatively, alkaline phosphatase may facilitate mineralization by hydrolyzing inorganic pyrophosphate, which acts as an inhibitor of mineralization in the extracellular fluid of bone (59). In the latter scenario, the controlled removal of pyrophosphate would promote the formation of an environment suitable for the precipitation of hydroxyapatite crystals. Consistent with this, lack of alkaline phosphatase due to genetic defects leads to a condition called hypophosphatasia, which is associated with defective bone mineralization. Patients with this condition have increased levels of pyrophosphate, pyridoxal-5′-phosphate, and phosphoethanolamine, suggesting that in normal individuals alkaline phosphatase is responsible for the hydrolysis of these compounds (55).

Besides the proteins and factors discussed above, it is now established that osteoblastic cells produce a variety of cytokines and colony-stimulating factors. This aspect of the biosynthetic activity of osteoblasts will be described in the following section.

Ontogeny of Osteoclasts and Osteoblasts

In the previous sections, we discussed the morphologic, biosynthetic, and functional characteristics of osteoclasts and osteoblasts at their fully differentiated state. Such a description, although useful for didactic purposes, does not convey the dynamism of the system in terms of the continuous formation of new cells from their undifferentiated progenitors. Moreover, it does not convey the importance of this cellular replenishment for bone physiology and pathophysiology.

The Role of the Bone Marrow in Bone Cell Development

Evidence accumulated during the last few years has revealed that both osteoclasts and osteoblasts are derived from precursors occurring in the bone marrow, and that besides their anatomic juxtaposition, the bone marrow and bone interact extensively and are critical for each others' function. Indeed, it is now appreciated that osteoclasts are derived from hematopoietic progenitors of the bone marrow, whereas osteoblasts are of the same lineage as the mesenchymal stromal cells of the bone marrow.

The intersinusoidal spaces of the bone marrow are filled with a variety of cell types, including fibroblastoid, adventitial reticular, adipocytic, macrophagic, and endothelial cells, as well as cells with osteogenic potential; these are collectively referred to as the stromal tissue (28,60). The mesenchymal fibroblastic and reticular cells have extensive cytoplasmic extensions that make intimate contact with hematopoietic progenitors, as well as with cellular processes of reticular cells present in the nearby intersinusoidal spaces. These cells are generally alkaline phosphatase positive and are considered the major stromal cell type that regulates hematopoiesis.

It is now well established that the bone marrow stromal cells are essential for the formation of various types of blood cells such as lymphocytes, granulocytes, platelets, and erythrocytes, as well as monocytes, macrophages, and osteoclasts (61,62). These specialized cell types appear to derive from self-renewing totipotential cells (63). The formation of fully differentiated cells from a single progenitor involves the progression from a state of less differentiated, nonlineage-specific cells to a state of greater differentiation and highly restricted lineage specificity. This process is controlled by cytokines and growth factors that are synthesized and released locally by stromal cells of the bone marrow. Indeed, specialized colonies derived from a single cell can be identified when marrow cells are cultured in the presence of the appropriate cytokines and growth factors. The single progenitor is termed a colony-forming unit (CFU). The designation that follows CFU is determined depending on the phenotype or phenotypes contained in the colony, for example, CFU-M (macrophages) or CFU-GM (granulocytes and macrophages).

Origin of Osteoclasts

It is now widely accepted that osteoclasts are derived from progenitors that originate from hematopoietic cells of the bone marrow (Figure 2-2). Specifi-

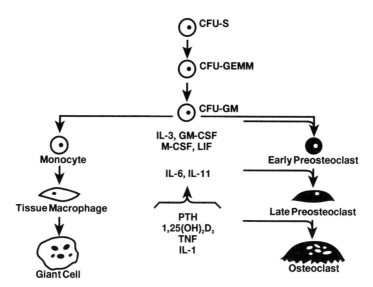

Figure 2-2 Parallels between hematopoiesis and osteoclastogenesis. Mulitpotential hematopoietic progenitor cells (CFU-S, CFU-GEMM, CFU-GM) give rise to a variety of cell types including macrophages and osteoclasts. The differentiation of osteoclasts from progenitor cells is influenced by some of the same cytokines and growth factors that regulate hematopoiesis; these factors include IL-3, GM-CSF, M-CSF, LIF, IL-6 and IL-11. The osteoclastogenic effects of PTH, $1,25(OH)_2D_3$, IL-1 and TNF may be mediated, at least in part, by these factors.

cally, osteoclasts develop from cloned pluripotent stem cells, as well as the mulitpotential hematopoietic cells CFU-granulocyte/erythrocyte/megakaryocyte/macrophage (CFU-GEMM) and CFU-GM; but not the unipotential CFU-M and CFU-granulocyte (64–67). Nonetheless, the point at which the committed osteoclast progenitor in the marrow diverges from the macrophage lineage is not clear. Intriguingly, monocyte/macrophage preparations obtained from tissues such as lung, spleen, and peripheral blood, cultured in the presence of the appropriate supportive stromal cells, can give rise to osteoclasts (68).

The sequence of events (and the precise route) whereby osteoclast progenitors from the bone marrow move to bone where they appear as fully differentiated osteoclasts is unknown. It appears, however, that osteoclasts may reach bone either via the circulation or by chemotaxis; the latter is probably more relevant to areas of bone that are in direct contact with the marrow. That osteoclasts can reach bone via the circulation is evidenced by the results of parabiosis studies in which two experimental animals are joined along their lateral body wall, allowing the exchange of blood cells between them (69). Blood cells from a normal mouse can correct the paucity of functional osteoclasts of an osteopetrotic mouse. Consistent with the evidence that osteoclast progenitors can arise from the blood stream, CFU–GM have been recently identified in peripheral blood (70).

The Cellular and Biochemical Basis of Bone Remodeling

Origin of Osteoblasts

The stromal cells of the bone marrow, as well as osteoblastic cells, also originate from pluripotent stem cells. As opposed to most hematopoietic cells, stromal and osteoblastic cells adhere to plastic surfaces. Stromal cells with osteogenic potential, as well as with the potential to become fibroblasts, chondrocytes, adipocytes, and muscle cells, are formed in marrow cell cultures as adherent colonies. The common progenitor that gives rise to these colonies is termed CFU-fibroblast (CFU-F) (27). Cells present in CFU-F colonies can induce both bone formation and hematopoiesis when transferred under the kidney capsule (71). In addition, bone can be formed in diffusion chambers containing bone marrow cells or CFU-F harvested from cultures of marrow cells (72). Furthermore, stromal cells can form calcified nodules in vitro in the appropriate milieu (73).

Marrow stromal cells and osteoblastic cells exhibit an extensive overlap in their phenotypic properties. Indeed, bone marrow–derived stromal cell lines express phenotypic markers of osteoblasts such as alkaline phosphatase and type I collagen (74,75). Conversely, osteoblastic cells are capable of secreting the same colony-stimulating factors and cytokines secreted by stromal cells such as interleukin-6 and -11 (IL-6, IL-11), granulocyte/macrophage–colony-stimulating factor (GM-CSF), and macrophage–colony-stimulating factor (M-CSF) (76). At this stage, it is not known whether the stromal cells responsible for the control of hematopoiesis and the stromal cells that give rise to osteoblasts represent distinct lineages or different maturation stages along the differentiation pathway of a single cell lineage.

Regulation of Osteoclast Development

A major advance in our understanding of osteoclast development has been the elucidation of the paramount importance of stromal/osteoblastic cells for osteoclast formation. Indeed, it is now established that the development of osteoclasts from hematopoietic precursors cannot be accomplished unless stromal/ osteoblastic cells are present. Moreover, it is established that cells of the stromal/ osteoblastic lineage mediate the effects of both systemic hormones and locally produced factors that stimulate osteoclast development (77,78).

The two major hormones of the calcium homeostatic system, namely, parathyroid hormone (PTH) and 1,25-dihydroxyvitamin D_3 [$1,25(OH)_2D_3$], are potent stimulators of osteoclast formation in vitro as well as in vivo (79–84). The ability of these hormones to stimulate osteoclast development and to reg ulate calcium absorption and excretion from the intestine and kidney, respectively, are the key elements of extracellular calcium homeostasis.

Administration of PTH to animals causes an increase in the number of osteoclasts present on bone surfaces between 0.5 and 4 hours. In addition, PTH administration enhances the appearance of ruffled borders in osteoclasts (81–83). Interestingly, PTH receptors have not been detected on fully differentiated mammalian osteoclasts (85,86); however, such receptors have been demonstrated in avian osteoclasts (87). Whether this represents a real difference in the expression of this receptor among species, as opposed to an apparent difference caused by methodologic reasons, remains unclear. In any event, in vitro addition of PTH to cultures of fully differentiated mammalian osteoclasts does not affect osteoclast motility nor does it stimulate the ability of these cells to resorb bone. However, when mammalian osteoclasts are cultured in the presence of osteoblastic cells, increased osteoclastic bone resorption can be induced by the addition of PTH to these cultures (88). PTH stimulates osteoclast development from hematopoietic progenitors such as those found in bone marrow cultures (79). However, similar to evidence from studies with fully differentiated osteoclasts, this effect requires the presence of stromal/osteoblastic cells (89,90). Consistent with the contention that PTH regulates either osteoclast development or the activity of fully differentiated osteoclasts via its actions on stromal/osteoblastic cells, PTH receptors have been found on both adventitial reticular cells of the marrow stroma as well as mature bone-forming osteoblasts (85,86).

▶ 27

1,25-Dihydroxyvitamin D_3 stimulates the fusion and differentiation of hematopoietic precursors of osteoclasts into mature osteoclasts (79). This cell fusing property of $1,25(OH)_2D_3$ is not specific for cells of the osteoclast lineage. $1,25(OH)_2D_3$ can also cause fusion (as well as promote the differentiation) of peripheral blood monocytes (91). Similar to the case with PTH, $1,25(OH)_2D_3$ stimulates the activity of differentiated mammalian osteoclasts. This effect however, requires the presence of stromal/osteoblastic cells (92). This, and the observation that stromal cells express the receptor for, and respond to, $1,25(OH)_2D_3$, indicate that the prodifferentiating effects of $1,25(OH)_2D_3$ on hematopoietic progenitors alone may not account for the effects of the hormone on osteoclastogenesis (93). Hence, additional actions on the cells of stromal/osteoblastic lineage are involved in the osteoclastogenic effects of this hormone.

Besides the systemic hormones PTH and $1,25(OH)_2D_3$, an array of factors produced locally in the bone microenvironment can stimulate osteoclast development. Since the early stages of hematopoiesis and osteoclastogenesis proceed along identical pathways, it is not surprising that this group of factors includes the same cytokines and colony-stimulating factors that are involved in hematopoiesis. To date, the list of cytokines and colony-stimulating factors implicated in the regulation of osteoclast development includes the interleukins IL-1, IL-3, IL-6, IL-11, and tumor necrosis factor (TNF), GM-CSF, M-CSF, and the leukemia inhibitory factor (LIF) (see Figure 2-2).

Interleukin-1 and TNF represent the original paradigms of cytokines that can influence the bone resorption process. IL-1 refers to two proteins (IL-1α and IL-1β) that display a wide spectrum of properties, including actions on the immunologic and hematopoietic systems (94). TNF also exists in two forms, namely TNFα and TNFβ (95). IL-1, TNF, and IL-6 are interacting cytokines, the induction of which is orchestrated by a variety of stimuli including the cytokines themselves (96). In addition, some IL-1- and TNF-induced responses, such as production of acute phase proteins, cachexia, anemia, and human chorionic gonadotropin production by trophoblasts are mediated by IL-6 (97–99).

Administration of IL-1 or TNF to rodents causes increased bone remodeling (100,101). In addition, IL-1 and TNF stimulate osteoclast development from hematopoietic progenitors in vitro (102). Further, IL-1 and TNF can stimulate the release of calcium from bone explants (103,104). The effects of IL-1 and TNF on osteoclastic cells, however, seem to be mediated indirectly through the actions of these cytokines on stromal/osteoblastic cells (105–107). Indeed, neither of these agents can stimulate isolated osteoclasts to excavate pits from the surface of smooth cortical bone slices. TNF is 100-fold less potent than IL-1 in inducing bone resorption, but TNF strongly synergizes with IL-1 to promote this process (108).

Several studies have suggested that osteoblasts isolated from adult human trabecular bone, neonatal murine calvaria cells, or osteoblastic cell lines, are capable of producing IL-1 and TNF constitutively or in response to stimulation by lipopolysaccharide or other cytokines (109–113). It is important to note, however, that the production of IL-1 and TNF by these cells appears to be very small (in the 1–10 pM range) and it is not regulated by the systemic hormones PTH or 1,25(OH)₂ Nevertheless, it appears that despite the very low level of production of TNF in the bone microenvironment, this particular cytokine may serve as an important amplifier for the effects of other local cytokines and systemic hormones that stimulate osteoclast development (114).

During the last 5 years, IL-6 has gained prominence among the cytokines that are relevant to bone. Indeed, it has been established that IL-6, besides its important role in the early stages of hematopoiesis, can also stimulate osteoclastogenesis. Thus, IL-6 synergizes with IL-3 to stimulate the development of CFU-GM (115,116) and stimulates early osteoclast precursor formation from cells present in CFU-GM colonies (117). IL-6 also enhances osteoclast formation and bone resorption in cultures of fetal mouse bone in vitro (118,119) and stimulates bone resorption cooperatively with IL-1 in vivo (120). However, IL-6 does not appear to affect bone resorption in cultured neonatal calvariae (121), which contain a predominance of postmitotic osteoclast progenitors and relatively few of the primitive myeloid progenitors, which are the principal targets for IL-6.

Unlike IL-1 and TNF, which are produced in picomolar concentrations, IL-6 is produced in nanomolar quantities by both stromal cells and osteoblastic cells in response to stimulation by both locally produced cytokines, such as IL-1 and TNF (113,118,122,123), growth factors, such as TGFβ (124), and systemic hormones, such as PTH (114,119,125,126). Interestingly, among bone marrow-derived stromal cells there is a phenotype-related specificity in the IL-6 response to PTH as a result of a phenotype-specific expression of the PTH receptor. Furthermore, there is evidence that calcitonin gene-related peptide (CGRP), a neuropeptide, regulates IL-6 production by bone marrow stromal cells (127). This raises the possibility that IL-6 might be relevant to an interplay between neuronal stimuli and bone metabolism. Receptors for IL-6 have recently been demonstrated in human osteoclastoma cells, and IL-6 was shown to stimulate the resorptive activity of these cells (128), suggesting that IL-6 may affect not only the early stages of osteoclast development but also mature osteoclasts. However, it is unclear whether normal osteoclasts, as opposed to osteoclastoma cells, also respond to IL-6.

▶ 29

At this stage, the physiologic role of IL-6 in osteoclast development is unclear. In fact, existing evidence suggests that IL-6 may not be involved in osteoclast development under physiologic circumstances either because this cytokine is redundant in terms of osteoclast development, or its levels in the bone marrow are kept below a critical threshold relative to the sensitivity of the osteoclastogenesis process for IL-6 (129). On the other hand, IL-6 seems to attain major importance for osteoclastogenesis in pathologic states characterized by the dysregulated production of this cytokine. Indeed, as will be discussed in the following section, IL-6 seems to play a causative role in the pathologic bone resorption associated with multiple myeloma (130), Paget's disease (131), and postmenopausal osteoporosis (129).

Interleukin-11 is a newly discovered cytokine that was cloned from stromal cells (132). Recent evidence from our laboratory indicates that IL-11 is also produced by osteoblastic cells (133). IL-11 acts synergistically with IL-3 to stimulate CFU-GM formation and increases the number of progeny of CFU-GEMM both in vitro and in vivo (134–136). IL-11 induces the formation of osteoclasts in cultures of murine bone marrow and calvarial cells, and it stimulates bone resorption (137). Unlike IL-6, which attains its importance for osteoclastogenesis in pathologic conditions, IL-11 appears to be essential for osteoclastogenesis at large, as evidenced by the demonstration that an IL-11 neutralizing antibody suppresses osteoclastogenesis induced by 1,25(OH)$_2$D$_3$, PTH, IL-1, or TNF in both estrogen-replete and estrogen-deplete animals (138).

Macrophage-CSF is critical for osteoclastogenesis. This has been well illustrated by evidence that in osteopetrotic op/op mice, there is a paucity of osteoclasts due to a deficiency in M-CSF bioactivity (139). Lack of M-CSF in this condition is caused by an insertion mutation in the M-CSF gene, resulting in the formation of an incomplete coding region (140). Administration of M-CSF to op/op mice increases osteoclast numbers, restores bone resorption, and cures the skeletal sclerosis (141). M-CSF is also essential for both the proliferation and differentiation of osteoclast progenitors induced by $1,25(OH)_2D_3$ (142); and incubation of fetal bone with M-CSF causes increased osteoclast formation and bone resorption (143). Osteoblastic cell lines, as well as cultures of osteoblastic cells from neonatal calvaria, secrete M-CSF (144,145).

Granulocyte/macrophage-CSF is another factor capable of inducing the proliferation and maturation of hematopoietic progenitors, such as CFU-GEMM, CFU-GM, and their progeny; and this factor stimulates osteoclast formation (146–148). Nevertheless, GM-CSF can also inhibit osteoclast formation (147,149,150). This latter effect is probably due to a GM-CSF-mediated downregulation of receptors for M-CSF (151). GM-CSF is secreted by osteoblastic cells on stimulation with PTH or lipopolysaccharide (152,153).

Leukemia inhibitory factor is another multifunctional cytokine that influences certain aspects of hematopoietic cell differentiation (154) and stimulates bone resorption (155,156). However, unlike IL-6, evidence indicates that LIF can also stimulate bone formation. Mice injected with tumor cells expressing LIF exhibit increased bone turnover and increased osteoblast formation (157). LIF also potentiates retinoic acid-induced expression of alkaline phosphatase in preosteoblasts (158). Osteoblasts produce LIF following stimulation by IL-1 and TNF; but neither PTH nor $1,25(OH)_2D_3$ affects LIF production by osteoblasts (155,159). LIF is produced constitutively by human bone marrow cells and can be further stimulated by IL-1 and TGFβ (160).

Transforming growth factor-β stimulates bone resorption as well as bone formation. Administration of TGFβ to mice causes an increase in the number of CFU-M and CFU-GM in the marrow (161). Further, injection of TGFβ into the subcutaneous tissue that overlies the calvaria of adult mice causes increased bone resorption accompanied by the development of unusually large osteoclasts, as well as increased bone formation (162). At low concentrations (less than 10 pM), TGFβ also enhances $1,25(OH)_2D_3$-induced osteoclast development in murine bone marrow cultures (163). Interestingly, neutralizing antibodies against TGFβ completely suppress $1,25(OH)_2D_3$-stimulated osteoclast development in marrow cell cultures. The effects of TGFβ might be mediated by other cytokines involved in osteoclastogenesis because TGFβ has recently been shown to stimulate both IL-6 and IL-11 (124,133). Intriguingly, results of in vitro studies suggest that TGFβ has inhibitory effects on the response of hematopoietic progenitors to colony-stimulating factors and cytokines (164) and that at high concentrations, TGFβ suppresses osteoclast formation (163).

It is apparent from the preceding discussion that cytokines and growth factors that influence osteoclast formation have synergistic, overlapping, and sometimes opposing effects. More important, however, it appears that the stringent control of cytokine and growth factor production may be essential for the appropriate operation of the bone remodeling unit and that deficiency or inappropriate production of these factors has dramatic effects on bone remodeling.

Regulation of Osteoblast Formation

As was discussed above, osteoblasts are derived from primitive mesenchymal cells, which are also capable of giving rise to chondrocytes, adipocytes, and the stromal cells and fibroblastic cells of the hematopoietic marrow (27,165,166). As in the case of osteoclast development, a variety of growth regulatory factors and systemic hormones stimulate the proliferation and differentiation of osteoblast progenitors. These include TGFβ, bone morphogenetic proteins, IGF-I and IGF-II, bFGF, epidermal growth factor (EGF), and transforming growth factor-α (TGFα). Most of these factors are present in the bone matrix (48–51).

▶ 31

Transforming growth factor-β can be produced by osteoblastic cells in response to stimulation by PTH and 1,25(OH)$_2$D$_3$ (167,168). The form of TGFβ that is produced by osteoblasts is latent, but can be activated under acidic conditions or by proteolysis (169). TGFβ is not only produced by osteoblasts but, as a classical autocrine factor, acts directly on osteoblasts. Indeed, injection of TGFβ into the subcutaneous tissue over the calvaria of normal rats or mice causes the accumulation of large osteoblasts, which subsequently form new woven bone (162). In addition, TGFβ has mitogenic effects on some osteoblastic cells in vitro (167,170), whereas it can inhibit the proliferation of others (171,172). Further, TGFβ increases the synthesis of matrix proteins including fibronectin, collagen, osteopontin, and osteonectin by osteoblastic cells (40,167,170,172–174).

Besides TGFβ, several more members of the superfamily of growth factors that includes TGFβ are made by osteoblasts and can stimulate bone formation (49,175). These proteins include BMP-2, also isolated as osteogenic protein-2; BMP-3, which was originally described as osteogenin; BMP-4; BMP-6, which is identical to another developmentally regulated protein (VG-1) found in frog oocytes; and BMP-7, also isolated as osteogenic protein-1. Although BMP-1 has osteogenic activity, its structure appears unrelated to TGFβ.

Osteoblasts are capable of synthesizing IGFs (50,51). IGFs are growth hormone-dependent peptides with a molecular eight of 7600. Two IGFs have so far been characterized: IGF-I, or somatomedin C, and IGF-II. Besides IGFs, osteoblastic cells produce several IGF-binding proteins, which regulate IGF activity (176–178). IGF-I modulates the differentiated function of the osteoblast via its effects on bone cell receptors for IGF-I, which, along with the IGF-binding proteins, are regulated by hormonal and local factors (177,179–181). As in the case of TGFβ, IGF-I enhances the bone collagen and matrix synthesis and stimulates the replication of cells of the osteoblastic lineage (50,51). Interestingly, IGF-I stimulates IL-6 production and bone resorption (182).

Both bFGF and acidic fibroblast growth factor (aFGF) stimulate the proliferation of osteoblastic cells (183–186). However, these factors do not seem to influence the differentiated function of the osteoblast. FGFs are present in the bone matrix; but only bFGF has been shown to be synthesized by osteoblasts. Acidic FGF is also capable of stimulating bone resorption (186).

Platelet-derived growth factor (PDGF) is composed of two polypeptide chains (A and B), but homodimeric (AA or BB) chains may also form. Human osteoblastic cells produce PDGF-AA, but not PDGF-BB, despite the fact that PDGF-BB is present in the bone matrix (187). The principal effect of PDGF on bone is the stimulation of preosteoblast proliferation (188). Interestingly, PDGF also stimulates bone resorption (189).

Two more growth factors, EGF and TGFα, exhibit mitogenic effects on osteoblastic cells; in addition, these two factors can stimulate bone resorption (190). At this stage, there is no evidence that EGF or TGFα is produced by osteoblastic cells. However, because macrophages are capable of producing TGFα (191), it is possible that TGFα is present in the bone microenvironment following its release by macrophages that reside in bone and, therefore, may indeed play a role in osteoblast proliferation.

Although the bone anabolic properties of factors and systemic hormones discussed here have been deduced from the demonstration of their stimulatory effects on the proliferation of osteoblastic cells, it is possible that some of these agents might indeed act at very early stages of osteoblast development, namely, on the proliferation and differentiation of stromal cells of the bone marrow. Indeed, receptors for both PTH and $1,25(OH)_2D_3$ are present in stromal cells, and preliminary evidence raises the possibility that $1,25(OH)_2D_3$ may promote the differentiation of these cells toward the osteoblastic phenotype (93).

The Coupling of Osteoclastic and Osteoblastic Activity

As discussed at the beginning of this chapter, the resorption of old bone by osteoclasts and the subsequent formation of new bone by osteoblasts are closely linked processes. The term "coupling" is used to define this tight linkage.

Because of the evidence for the dependency of osteoclast formation on cells of the osteoblastic lineage, it is possible that besides "coupling," bone formation and bone resorption may also be coordinated at the early stages of osteoblast and osteoclast differentiation within the bone marrow. The contention that part of the coordination of bone resorption and bone formation may occur at the early stages of progenitor cell development in the bone marrow is supported by the fact that dysregulation of the early stages of osteoclast formation resulting, for example, from estrogen deficiency, is associated with a disruption of the coupling between resorption and formation.

Given the sequence of the bone remodeling cycle, that is, resorption followed by formation, coupling is thought to be mediated by factors generated during the resorption phase. For coupling to occur, such factors should, in turn, provide the signals that cause the recruitment or the functional activation of the bone-forming cells.

Several factors released from the bone matrix during the resorption phase exhibit the above-mentioned properties. Indeed, TGFβ is produced during bone resorption and can be activated by isolated osteoclasts (192,193). Furthermore, TGFβ might serve as a chemoattractant for osteoblastic cells at the resorption site (194) and, as discussed above, might stimulate the proliferation or differentiation of osteoblastic cells. Besides TGFβ, IGF-I and IGF-II have also been implicated in coupling because these factors are produced in response to stimulation of bone organ cultures or osteoblastic cells by PTH, and these IGFs can also stimulate osteoblastic activity (50,51).

Systemic hormones such as PTH and $1,25(OH)_2D_3$ might also play a role in the coupling of bone resorption and bone formation. Indeed, PTH and $1,25(OH)_2D_3$ are potent bone-resorbing agents. However, both have anabolic effects on bone. Intermittent administration of low amounts of PTH causes increased osteoblast activity and enhances bone formation in experimental animals and human beings, without stimulating osteoclastic bone resorption (195). On the other hand, continuous administration of PTH causes excessive bone resorption and hypercalcemia. In view of the fact that PTH stimulates the production of several growth factors by osteoblastic cells, the effects of PTH in the coupling process may be mediated by local factors.

$1,25(OH)_2D_3$ is essential for normal bone growth and mineralization, as evidenced by the fact that vitamin D deficiency is associated with a dramatic impairment in bone formation and mineralization. Receptors for $1,25(OH)_2D_3$ have been identified on both stromal and osteoblastic cells (93,196), and the hormone can exert stimulatory effects on their activity, including the production of alkaline phosphatase, osteocalcin, and several more specialized osteoblast products (197–199). On the other hand, $1,25(OH)_2D_3$ is also a potent bone resorbing agent and, as discussed in the previous section, plays an important role in osteoclast development.

The frequency with which bone undergoes remodeling differs with the site and the macroscopic organization of the bone tissue involved. Indeed, bone is remodeled with higher frequency in trabecular bone as compared to cortical bone. This is due to the higher rate of osteoclast activation (1,200) in the former.

▶ 33

In fact, it has been calculated that approximately 26% of the trabecular bone is resorbed and replaced every year, compared to only 3% of the cortical bone. The precise reason for this striking difference is not established. However, these differences favor the contention that remodeling is primarily controlled by local factors. In view of the fact that osteoclasts originate from the bone marrow, it is also possible the difference in remodeling rates between trabecular and cortical bone reflects the intimate juxtaposition between trabecular bone and bone marrow. Indeed, trabecular bone has a high surface-to-volume ratio compared to cortical bone, and 70% to 85% of the bone surface in trabecular bone interfaces with the bone marrow (1). Another reason might be the high susceptibility of the more delicate (fine structured) trabecular bone to microdamage and, therefore, the need for more frequent repair.

New Insights on the Pathophysiology of Abnormal Resorption

Most disease states of the adult skeleton are characterized by a disturbance of the normally balanced remodeling. In fact, some of the most common states of abnormal bone metabolism are characterized by excessive bone resorption or insufficient bone formation or both. Appreciation of the relationship between the cells of the bone marrow and the cells of bone, and of the role of local factors in the development of osteoclasts and osteoblasts, has provided a clearer understanding of the pathophysiology of such states.

Multiple Myeloma

Focal osteolysis is a cardinal feature of multiple myeloma. In fact, the osteolytic lesions of multiple myeloma represent one of the most dramatic illustrations of bone resorption. Histomorphometric studies demonstrate that the early stages of multiple myeloma are associated with an increase in the frequency of bone remodeling (201). However, in the late stages of the disease, there is a dramatic increase in osteoclastic bone resorption, while bone formation is decreased, thus leading to a major bone deficit. Osteolysis associated with multiple myeloma is due to enhanced osteoclast formation at the sites of the tumor. This is most likely caused by the production of the cytokines TNF, IL-1, and IL-6 by myeloma cells (202–204). In fact, IL-6 produced by the myeloma cells is an important autocrine factor responsible for the proliferation of the tumor cells. In line with this evidence, it has been recently demonstrated that administration of an IL-6 neutralizing antibody to a hypercalcemic patient with multiple myeloma caused a precipitous decrease of the serum calcium concentration (130). When antibody treatment was interrupted, there was a rapid rebound of serum calcium, followed by a decrease on resumption of antibody administration. Administration of the antibody was also associated with an inhibition of myeloma cell proliferation, reduction of C-reactive protein, and decreased blood platelet and neutrophil counts. These observations strongly suggest that IL-6 is an important factor in the increased osteoclastic bone resorption that characterizes this condition.

Paget's Disease

Paget's disease of bone is another common condition characterized by intense focal bone resorption consisting of increased Howship's lacunar spaces filled with giant osteoclasts (205). It is thought that pagetic lesions are the result of delayed activation or an infection by an altered or, as yet, uncharacterized virus, which may initially lodge in osteoclast progenitors. The initial stages of the disease are associated with an increase in the number, size, and activity of osteoclasts. Osteoblasts appear morphologically normal but must work at an increased level to keep up with the excessive osteoclastic activity. The deposition of new bone matrix and its mineralization by the osteoblast, however, is abnormal, resulting in a disorganized mixture of lamellar bone and woven bone.

Recent studies demonstrated that osteoclast formation in long-term cultures of bone marrow obtained from affected sites in patients with Paget's disease is significantly greater than osteoclast formation in cultures from normal individuals. Moreover, conditioned medium from the pagetic cultures could stimulate osteoclast development in bone marrow cultures from normal individuals (131). More important, both the marrow from the affected site and the serum from individuals with Paget's disease contained dramatically higher levels of IL-6, compared to the marrow from normal sites and serum from normal individuals. Consistent with a critical role for IL-6 in the osteoclast-stimulating activity of the marrow of the pagetic bone, a neutralizing antibody against IL-6 blocked the osteoclast-stimulating capability of conditioned medium from marrow cultures obtained from Paget's patients. This evidence strongly supports the possibility that the osteoclast-stimulating activity in Paget's marrow may be IL-6. In line with this contention and the viral etiology of Paget's disease are the recent observations that the IL-6 promoter contains response elements that can be induced by products of viral genes (206–209).

Postmenopausal Osteoporosis

The hallmark of the syndrome of fractures in postmenopausal osteoporosis is a reduction of skeletal mass caused by an imbalance of bone resorption over bone formation. The deficit in bone tissue causing the osteoporosis exists primarily where bone is in contact with the bone marrow. In fact, the rapid loss of trabecular bone precipitated by the postmenopausal state is associated with perforation of individual trabecular plates caused by increased frequency of remodeling activity and an increase in osteoclastic resorption depth (210). Thus, loss of estrogens appears to cause an imbalance in the normally coupled bone resorption and bone formation processes, due to the combination of increased bone resorption and inadequate compensation by bone formation (211). Consistent with this, evidence from experimentally induced loss of ovarian function (ovariectomy) in rodents indicates that the loss of bone that follows ovariectomy is associated with an increase in the number of osteoclasts present in trabecular bone (212,213).

36 ◄

It has been recently demonstrated that 17β-estradiol inhibits the production of IL-6 by cultured bone marrow stromal and osteoblastic cell lines, as well as primary bone cell cultures from rodents and human beings (122). Estradiol inhibits IL-6 production by inhibiting the stimulated expression of the IL-6 gene through an estrogen receptor-mediated indirect effect on the transcriptional activity of the proximal 225 bp sequence of the promoter, perhaps through an interference with events along the signaling pathways initiated by the IL-6 stimulating agents (214).

Based on the in vitro findings for the inhibition of IL-6 production by estrogen, the hypothesis that estrogen loss upregulates osteoclastogenesis through an increase in the production of IL-6 in the microenvironment of the marrow has been tested in vivo using the ovariectomized mouse model (129,215). It has been shown that the number of CFU-GM colonies and the number of osteoclasts is greater in short-term cultures of marrow cells from ovariectomized mice compared to cultures from sham-operated animals. The increased osteoclast formation in the marrow cultures is mirrored by an increase in the number of osteoclasts present in sections of trabecular bone. More important, administration of 17β-estradiol or injections of an IL-6 neutralizing antibody (but not administration of an IgG isotype control antibody) to the ovariectomized animals prevents all these cellular changes. Consistent with these findings, estrogen loss causes an upregulation of IL-6 production by ex vivo bone marrow cell cultures in response to either $1,25(OH)_2D_3$ or PTH (216).

These experimental findings constitute compelling evidence that the production of IL-6 by stromal and osteoblastic cells is inhibited by estrogens. With estrogen loss, this inhibitory effect is removed, resulting in an upregulation of IL-6 which, in turn, upregulates the formation of osteoclasts. The demonstrated ability of an anti-IL-6 antibody to inhibit osteoclast activity in human beings (130), taken together with the inhibitory effect of 17β-estradiol on IL-6 at the protein level and the level of the human IL-6 gene promoter in human cells (122,214), establish the relevance of the experimental evidence to human beings. Based on this, we believe that the interrelationship between estrogen loss, upregulation of IL-6, and increased osteoclastogenesis provides a convincing mechanistic explanation for the pathophysiology of the accelerated bone loss that begins at menopause. Additional evidence for a role of IL-6 in the bone loss caused by estrogen deficiency is provided by the report of Balena and colleagues (217), that mice with IL-6 gene knockout do not lose trabecular bone following ovariectomy.

At present, it remains debatable whether IL-6 is the sole pathogenetic factor responsible for the increased osteoclastogenesis that ensues on estrogen loss, or whether other cytokines, such as IL-1 and TNF, are also upregulated and, therefore, contribute to this pathologic process. The evidence supporting the latter possibility is based on studies conducted primarily in peripheral blood mononuclear cells from human beings (218–220). However, in our opinion this evidence is circumstantial, especially because a mechanistic link between cytokine release by circulating blood mononuclear cells and the bone remodeling process is not apparent. In any event, it is reasonable to expect that the stimulatory signals for increased IL-6 production in the estrogen-deficient state are provided by several agents including PTH, $1,25(OH)_2D_3$, TGFβ, as well as IL-1 and TNF, since all of these are capable of stimulating IL-6 by stromal/osteoblastic cells. Considering this, removal of the inhibitory effect of estrogen on IL-6 is sufficient to account for the increased production of this cytokine and, therefore, the increased osteoclastogenesis irrespective of whether other cytokines are also upregulated. Therefore, one need not invoke estrogenic regulation of other cytokines to explain the upregulation of osteoclastogenesis in the estrogen-deficient state. The substantial quantitative difference in the production levels of IL-6 (nanomolar) versus IL-1 and TNF (picomolar) by stromal/osteoblastic cells, and the evidence that the IL-1 and TNF signals for osteoclastogenesis are mediated via IL-6 and IL-11 (at least in part), renders a putative regulatory effect of estrogens on IL-1 and TNF even less critical. This, of course, does not exclude the possibility that IL-1 and TNF are produced in the marrow in biologically significant quantities by the resident monocytes/macrophages, nor is it inconsistent with an important role of IL-1 and TNF in osteoclastogenesis, especially in inflammatory states such as the arthritides. However, it decreases the likelihood that IL-1 and TNF play a pathogenetic role in triggering the upregulation of osteoclastogenesis following loss of ovarian function.

References

1. Parfitt AM. The physiological and clinical significance of bone histomorpho- metric data. In: Recker RR, ed. Bone histomorphometry: techniques and inter-

pretation. Boca Raton, Fla: CRC Press, 1983:143–223.

2. Jee WSS. The skeletal tissues. In: Weiss L, ed. Cell and tissue biology. Baltimore: Urban and Schwarzenberg, 1988: 213–254.

3. Chambers TJ, Darby JA, Fuller K. Mammalian collagenase predisposes bone surfaces to osteoclastic resorption. Cell Tissue Res 1985;241:671–675.

4. Delaisse JM, Vaes G. Mechanism of mineral solublization and matrix degradation in osteoclastic bone resorption. In: Rifkin BR, Gay CV, eds. Biology and physiology of the osteoclast. Boca Raton, Fla: CRC Press, 1992:289–314.

5. Horton MA, Taylor ML, Arnett TR, Helfrich MH. Arg-Gly-Asp (RGD) peptides and the anti-vitronectin receptor antibody 23C6 inhibit dentine resorption and cell spreading by osteoclasts. Exp Cell Res 1991;195:368–375.

6. Reinholt FP, Hultenby K, Oldberg Å, Heinegård D. Osteopontin—a possible anchor of osteoclasts to bone. Proc Natl Acad Sci USA 1990;87:4473–4475.

7. Baron R, Neff L, Louvard D, Courtoy PJ. Cell-mediated extracellular acidification and bone resorption: evidence for a low pH in resorbing lacunae and localization of a 100-kD lysosomal membrane protein at the osteoclast ruffled border. J Cell Biol 1985;101:2210–2222.

8. Väänänen HK, Karhukorpi EK, Sundquist K, et al. Evidence for the presence of a proton pump of the vacuolar H(+)-ATPase type in the ruffled borders of osteoclasts. J Cell Biol 1990;111:1305–1311.

9. Blair HC, Teitelbaum SL, Ghiselli R, Gluck S. Osteoclastic bone resorption by a polarized vacuolar proton pump. Science 1989;245:855–857.

10. Gay CV, Mueller WJ. Carbonic anhydrase and osteoclasts: localization by labeled inhibitor autoradiography. Science 1974;183:432–434.

11. Sundquist KT, Leppilampi M, Järvelin K, Kumpulainen T, Väänänen HK. Carbonic anhydrase isoenzymes in isolated rat peripheral monocytes, tissue macrophages, and osteoclasts. Bone 1987;8:33–38.

12. Minkin C. Bone acid phosphatase: tartrate resistant acid phosphatase as a marker of osteoclast function. Calcif Tissue Int 1982;34:285–290.

13. van de Wijngaert FP, Burger EH. Demonstration of tartrate-resistant acid phosphatase in un-decalcified, glycomethacrylate-embedded mouse bone: a possible marker for (pre)osteoclast identification. J Histochem Cytochem 1986;34: 1317–1323.

14. Ek-Rylander B, Wendel M, Heinegård D, Andersson G. Osteoclastic tartrate-resistant acid phosphatase/ATPase can act as a bone matrix phosphoprotein phosphatase. J Bone Miner Res 1991;6(S1):S276. Abstract.

15. Zaidi M, Moonga B, Moss DW, MacIntyre I. Inhibition of osteoclastic acid phosphatase abolishes bone resorption. Biochem Biophys Res Commun 1989; 159:68–71.

16. Horton MA, Helfrich MH. Antigenic markers of osteoclasts. In: Rifkin BR, Gay CV, eds. Biology and physiology of the osteoclast. Boca Raton, Fla: CRC Press, 1992:33–54.

17. Bar-Shavit Z, Teitelbaum SL, Reitsma P, et al. Induction of monocytic differentiation and bone resorption by 1,25-dihydroxyvitamin D_3. Proc Natl Acad Sci USA 1983;80:5907–5911.

18. Jones SJ, Boyde A, Ali NN, Maconnachie E. Variation in the sizes of resorption lacunae made in vitro. Scanning Microsc 1986;4:1571–1580.

19. Chambers TJ, Revell PA, Fuller K, Athanasou NA. Resorption of bone by isolated rabbit osteoclasts. J Cell Sci 1984;66:383–399.

20. Chambers TJ, Horton MA. Failure of cells of the mononuclear phagocyte series to resorb bone. Calcif Tissue Int 1984; 36:556–558.

21. Warshawsky H, Goltzman D, Rouleau MF, Bergeron JJ. Direct in vivo demonstration by radioautography of specific binding sites for calcitonin in skeletal and renal tissues of the rat. J Cell Biol 1980;85:682–694.

22. Nicholson GC, Moseley JM, Sexton PM, Mendelsohn FAO, Martin TJ. Abundant calcitonin receptors in isolated rat osteoclasts. J Clin Invest 1986;78:355–360.

23. Chambers TJ, Magnus CJ. Calcitonin alters behavior of isolated osteoclasts. J Pathol 1982;136:27–39.

24. Chambers TJ, McSheehy PM, Thomson BM, Fuller K. The effect of calcium-regulating hormones and prostaglandins on bone resorption by osteoclasts disaggregated from neonatal rabbit bones. Endocrinology 1985;116:234–239.

25. Taylor LM, Tertinegg I, Okuda A, Heersche JN. Expression of calcitonin receptors during osteoclast differentiation in mouse metatarsals. J Bone Miner Res 1989;4:751–758.

26. Owen TA, Aronow M, Shalhoub V, et al. Progressive development of the rat osteoblast phenotype in vitro: reciprocal relationships in expression of genes associated with osteoblast proliferation and differentiation during formation of the bone extracellular matrix. J Cell Physiol 1990; 143:420–430.

27. Owen M. Lineage of osteogenic cells and their relationship to the stromal system. In: Peck WA, ed. Bone and mineral research. Vol 3. Amsterdam: Elsevier, 1985:1–25.

28. Deldar A, Lewis H, Weiss L. Bone lining cells and hematopoiesis: an electron microscopic study of canine bone marrow. Anat Rec 1985;213:187–201.

29. Olsen BR. Collagen biosynthesis. In: Hay ED, ed. Cell biology of extracellular matrix. New York: Plenum Press, 1981: 139–177.

30. Pinnel RS, Fox R, Krane S. Human collagens: difference in glycosylated hydroxylysines in skin and bone. Biochim Biophys Acta 1971;229:119–122.

31. Robins SP, Duncan A. Pyridinium crosslinks of bone collagen and their location in peptides isolated from rat femur. Biochim Biophys Acta 1987;914:233–239.

32. Price PA. Osteocalcin. In: Peck WA, ed. Bone and mineral research. Vol 1. Princeton, NJ: Excerpta Medica, 1983:157–190.

33. Price PA, Williamson MK. Primary structure of bovine matrix Gla protein, a new vitamin K-dependent bone protein. J Biol Chem 1985;260:14971–14975.

34. Malone JD, Teitelbaum SL, Griffin GL, Senior RM, Kahn AJ. Recruitment of osteoblast precursors by purified bone matrix constituents. J Cell Biol 1982;92: 227–230.

35. DeFranco DJ, Glowacki J, Cox KA, Lian JB. Normal bone particles are preferentially resorbed in the presence of osteocalcin-deficient bone particles in vivo. Calcif Tissue Int 1991;49:43–50.

36. Termine JD, Kleinman HK, Whitson SW, Conn KM, McGarvey ML, Martin GR. Osteonectin, a bone-specific protein linking mineral to collagen. Cell 1981;26: 99–105.

37. Holland PWH, Harmper SJ, McVey JH, Hogan BLM. In vivo expression of mRNA for the Ca^{++}-binding protein SPARC (osteonectin) revealed by in situ hybridization. J Cell Biol 1987;105:473–482.

38. Ruoslahti E. Structure and biology of proteoglycans. Annu Rev Cell Biol 1988;4:229–255.

39. Gorski JP, Griffin D, Dudley G, et al. Bone acidic glycoprotein-75 is a major synthetic product of osteoblastic cells and localized as 75- and/or 50-kDa forms in mineralized phases of bone and growth plate and in serum. J Biol Chem 1990; 265:14956–14963.

40. Wrana JL, Kubota T, Zhang Q, et al. Regulation of transformation-sensitive secreted phosphoprotein (SPPI/osteopontin) expression by transforming growth factor-beta. Comparisons with expression of SPARC (secreted acidic cysteine-rich protein). Biochem J 1991;273:523–531.

41. Bianco P, Riminucci M, Bonucci E, Termine JD, Robey PG. Bone sialoprotein (BSP) secretion and osteoblast differentiation: relationship to bromodeoxyuridine incorporation, alkaline phosphatase, and matrix deposition. J Histochem Cytochem 1993;41:183–191.

42. Bianco P, Riminucci M, Silvestrini G, et al. Localization of bone sialoprotein (BSP) to Golgi and post-Golgi secretory structures in osteoblasts and to discrete sites in early bone matrix. J Histochem Cytochem 1993;41:193–203.

43. Weiss RE, Reddi AH. Synthesis and localization of fibronectin during collagenous matrix-mesenchymal cell interaction and differentiation of cartilage and bone

in vivo. Proc Natl Acad Sci USA 1980; 77:2074–2078.

44. Grzesik WJ, Gehron Robey P. Bone matrix RGD glycoproteins: immunoprecipitation and their interaction with human primary osteoblastic bone cells in vitro. J Bone Miner Res 1994.

45. Robey PG, Young MF, Fisher LW, McClain TD. Thrombospondin is an osteoblast-derived component of mineralized extracellular matrix. J Cell Biol 1989;108:719–727.

46. Long MW, Briddell R, Walter AW, Bruno E, Hoffman R. Human hematopoietic stem cell adherence to cytokines and matrix molecules. J Clin Invest 1992; 90:251–255.

47. Teixidó J, Hemler ME, Greenberger JS, Anklesaria P. Role of β_1 and β_2 integrins in the adhesion of human CD34^{hi} stem cells to bone marrow stroma. J Clin Invest 1992;90:358–367.

48. Hauschka PV, Chen TL, Mavrakos AE. Polypeptide growth factors in bone matrix. In: Evered D, Harnett S, eds. Cell and molecular biology of vertebrate hard tissues. Chichester: Wiley, 1988;207–225.

49. Wozney JM, Rosen V, Celeste AJ, et al. Novel regulators of bone formation: molecular clones and activities. Science 1988;242:1528–1534.

50. Canalis E, McCarthy TL, Centrella M. Growth factors and cytokines in bone cell metabolism. Annu Rev Med 1991;42:17–24.

51. Mohan S, Baylink DJ. Bone growth factors. Clin Orthop 1991;263:30–48.

52. Gabbianelli M, Sargiacomo M, Pelosi E, Testa U, Isacchi G, Peschle C. "Pure" human hematopoietic progenitors: permissive action of basic fibroblast growth factor. Science 1990;249:1561–1564.

53. Bourne GH. Phosphatase and calcification. In: Bourne GH, ed. The biochemistry and physiology of bone. Vol II. New York: Academic Press, 1972:79–120.

54. Low MG, Zilversmit DB. Role of phosphatidylinositol in attachment of alkaline phosphatase to membranes. Biochemistry 1980;19:3913–3918.

55. Whyte MP. Alkaline phosphatase: physiological role explored in hypophos-phatasia. In: Peck WA, ed. Bone and mineral research. Vol 6. Amsterdam: Elsevier, 1989:175–218.

56. Millan JL, Whyte MP, Avioli LV, Fishman WH. Hypophosphatasia (adult form): quantitation of serum alkaline phosphatase isoenzyme activity in a large kindred. Clin Chem 1980;26:840–845.

57. Glimcher MJ. Mechanisms of calcification: role of collagen fibrils and collagen-phosphoprotein complexes in vitro and in vivo. Anat Rec 1989;224:139–153.

58. Anderson HC. Matrix vesicle calcification: review and update. In: Peck WA, ed. Bone and mineral research. Vol 3. Amsterdam: Elsevier, 1985:109–149.

59. Fleisch H, Russell RGG, Straumann F. Effect of pyrophosphate on hydroxyapatite and its implications in calcium homeostasis. Nature 1966;212:901–903.

60. Westen H, Bainton DF. Association of alkaline-phosphatase-positive reticulum cell in bone marrow with granulocyte precursors. J Exp Med 1979;50:919–937.

61. Metcalf D. The molecular control of cell division, differentiation commitment and maturation in haemopoietic cells. Nature 1989;339:27–30.

62. Shadduck RK, Waheed A, Greenberger JS, Dexter TM. Production of colony stimulating factor in long-term bone marrow cultures. J Cell Physiol 1983;114:88–92.

63. Emerson SG. The stem cell model of hematopoiesis. In: Hoffman R, Benz EJ, Shattil SJ, Furie B, Cohen HJ, eds. Hematology. Basic principles and practice. New York: Churchill Livingstone, 1991:72–81.

64. Hagenaars CE, van der Kraan AA, Kawilarang-de Haas EW, Visser JW, Nijweide PJ. Osteoclast formation from cloned pluripotent hemopoietic stem cells. Bone Miner 1989;6:179–189.

65. Hattersley G, Kerby JA, Chambers TJ. Identification of osteoclast precursors in multilineage hemopoietic colonies. Endocrinology 1991;128:259–262.

66. Kerby JA, Hattersley G, Collins DA, Chambers TJ. Derivation of osteoclasts from hematopoietic colony-forming cells in culture. J Bone Miner Res 1992;7:353–361.

67. Kurihara N, Chenu C, Miller M, Civin C, Roodman GD. Identification of committed mononuclear precursors for osteoclast-like cells formed in long term human marrow cultures. Endocrinology 1990;126:2733–2741.

68. Udagawa N, Takahashi N, Akatsu T, et al. Origin of osteoclasts: mature monocytes and macrophages are capable of differentiating into osteoclasts under a suitable microenvironment prepared by bone marrow-derived stromal cells. Proc Natl Acad Sci USA 1990;87:7260–7264.

69. Marks SC Jr, Walker DG. Mammalian osteopetrosis—a model for studying cellular and humoral factors in bone resorption. In: Bourne GH, ed. The biochemistry and physiology of bone. Vol IV. New York: Academic Press, 1976:227–301.

70. Serke S, Säuberlich S, Abe Y, Huhn D. Analysis of CD34-positive hemopoietic progenitor cells from normal human adult peripheral blood: flow-cytometrical studies and in-vitro colony (CFU-GM, BFU-E) assays. Ann Hematol 1991;62:45–53.

71. Friedenstein AJ, Chailakhjan RK, Latzinih NV, Panasyuk AF, Keiliss-Borok IV. Stromal cells responsible for transferring the microenvironment of the hemopoietic tissues. Transplantation 1974;17:331–339.

72. Ashton BA, Allen TD, Howlett CR, Eaglesom CC, Hattori A, Owen M. Formation of bone and cartilage by marrow stromal cells in diffusion chambers in vivo. Clin Orthop 1980;151:294–307.

73. McCulloch CA, Strugurescu M, Hughes F, Melcher AH, Aubin JE. Osteogenic progenitor cells in rat bone marrow stromal populations exhibit self-renewal in culture. Blood 1991;77:1906–1911.

74. Benayahu D, Kletter Y, Zipori D, Weintroub S. Bone marrow-derived stromal cell line expressing osteoblastic phenotype in vitro and osteogenic capacity in vivo. J Cell Physiol 1989;140:1–7.

75. Benayahu D, Horowitz M, Zipori D, Wientroub S. Hemopoietic functions of marrow-derived osteogenic cells. Calcif Tissue Int 1992;51:195–201.

76. Horowitz MC, Jilka RL. Colony stimulating factors and bone remodeling. In: Gowen M, ed. Cytokines and bone metabolism. Boca Raton, Fla: CRC Press, 1992:185–227.

77. Burger EH, Van der Meer JWM, Nijweide PJ. Osteoclast formation from mononuclear phagocytes: role of bone-forming cells. J Cell Biol 1984;99:1901–1906.

78. Suda T, Takahashi N, Martin TJ. Modulation of osteoclast differentiation. Endocr Rev 1992;13:66–80.

79. Takahashi N, Yamana H, Yoshiki S, et al. Osteoclast-like cell formation and its regulation by osteotropic hormones in mouse bone marrow cultures. Endocrinology 1988;122:1373–1382.

80. Graves L III, Jilka RL. Comparison of bone and parathyroid hormone as stimulators of osteoclast development and activity in calvarial cell cultures from normal and osteopetrotic (mi/mi) mice. J Cell Physiol 1990;145:102–109.

81. Baron R, Vignery A. Behavior of osteoclasts during a rapid change in their number induced by high doses of parathyroid hormone or calcitonin in intact rats. Bone 1981;2:339–346.

82. Miller SC, Bowman BM, Myers RL. Morphological and ultrastructural aspects of the activation of avian medullary bone osteoclasts by parathyroid hormone. Anat Rec 1984;208:223–231.

83. King GJ, Holtrop ME, Raisz LG. The relation of ultrastructural changes in osteoclasts to resorption in bone cultures stimulated with parathyroid hormone. Metab Bone Dis Rel Res 1978;1:67–74.

84. Holtrop ME, Cox KA, Clark MR, Holick MF, Anast CS. 1,25-Dihydroxycholecalciferol stimulates osteoclasts in rat bones in the absence of parathyroid hormone. Endocrinology 1981;108:2293–2301.

85. Rouleau MF, Warshawsky H, Goltzman D. Parathyroid hormone binding in vivo to renal, hepatic, and skeletal tissues of the rat using a radioautographic approach. Endocrinology 1986;118:919–931.

86. Rouleau MF, Mitchell J, Goltzman D. In vivo distribution of parathyroid hormone receptors in bone: evidence that a predominant osseous target cell is not

the mature osteoblast. Endocrinology 1988; 123:187–192.

87. Agarwala N, Gay CV. Specific binding of parathyroid hormone to living osteoclasts. J Bone Miner Res 1992;7:531–539.

88. McSheehy PM, Chambers TJ. Osteoblastic cells mediate osteoclastic responsiveness to parathyroid hormone. Endocrinology 1986;118:824–828.

89. Akatsu T, Takahashi N, Udagawa N, et al. Parathyroid hormone (PTH)-related protein is a potent stimulator of osteoclast-like multinucleated cell formation to the same extent as PTH in mouse marrow cultures. Endocrinology 1989;125:20–27.

90. Yamashita T, Asano K, Takahashi N, et al. Cloning of an osteoblastic cell line involved in the formation of osteoclast-like cells. J Cell Physiol 1990;145:587–595.

91. Suda T, Miyaura C, Abe E, Kuroki T. Modulation of cell differentiation, immune responses and tumor promotion by vitamin D compounds. In: Peck WA, ed. Bone and mineral research. Vol. 4. Amsterdam: Elsevier, 1986:1–48.

92. McSheehy PM, Chambers TJ. 1,25-Dihydroxyvitamin D_3 stimulates rat osteoblastic cells to release a soluble factor that increases osteoclastic bone resorption. J Clin Invest 1987;80:425–429.

93. Bellido T, Girasole G, Passeri G, et al. Demonstration of estrogen and vitamin D receptors in bone marrow derived stromal cells: upregulation of the estrogen receptor by $1,25(OH)_2D_3$. Endocrinology 1993;133:553–562.

94. Dinarello CA. Interleukin-1 and interleukin-1 antagonism. Blood 1991;77: 1627–1652.

95. Vassalli P. The pathophysiology of tumor necrosis factors. Annu Rev Immunol 1992;10:411–452.

96. Akira S, Hirano T, Taga T, Kishimoto T. Biology of multifunctional cytokines: IL 6 and related molecules (IL 1 and TNF). FASEB J 1990;4:2860–2867.

97. Starnes HF Jr, Pearce MK, Tewari A, Yim JH, Zou J-C, Abrams JS. Anti-IL-6 monoclonal antibodies protect against lethal Escherichia coli infection and lethal tumor necrosis factor-α challenge in mice. J Immunol 1990;145:4185–4191.

98. Neta R, Perlstein R, Vogel SN, Ledney GD, Abrams J. Role of interleukin 6 (IL-6) in protection from lethal irradiation and in endocrine responses to IL-1 and tumor necrosis factor. J Exp Med 1992;175: 689–694.

99. Li Y, Matsuzaki N, Masuhiro K, et al. Trophoblast-derived tumor necrosis factor-alpha induces release of human chorionic gonadotropin using interleukin-6 (IL-6) and IL-6-receptor-dependent system in the normal human trophoblasts. J Clin Endocrinol Metab 1992;74:184–191.

100. Boyce BF, Aufdemorte TB, Garrett IR, Yates AJ, Mundy GR. Effects of interleukin-1 on bone turnover in normal mice. Endocrinology 1989;125:1142–1150.

101. Johnson RA, Boyce BF, Mundy GR, Roodman GD. Tumors producing human tumor necrosis factor induced hypercalcemia and osteoclastic bone resorption in nude mice. Endocrinology 1989; 124:1424–1427.

102. Pfeilschifter J, Chenu C, Bird A, Mundy GR, Roodman GD. Interleukin-1 and tumor necrosis factor stimulate the formation of human osteoclast-like cells in vitro. J Bone Miner Res 1989;4:113–118.

103. Gowen M, Mundy GR. Actions of recombinant interleukin 1, interleukin 2, and interferon-gamma on bone resorption in vitro. J Immunol 1986;136:2478–2482.

104. Bertolini DR, Nedwin GE, Bringman TS, Smith DD, Mundy GR. Stimulation of bone resorption and inhibition of bone formation in vitro by human tumour necrosis factors. Nature 1986;319:516–518.

105. Thomson BM, Saklatvala J, Chambers TJ. Osteoblasts mediate interleukin 1 stimulation of bone resorption by rat osteoclasts. J Exp Med 1986;164:104–112.

106. Thomson BM, Mundy GR, Chambers TJ. Tumor necrosis factors alpha and beta induce osteoblastic cells to stimulate osteoclastic bone resorption. J Immunol 1987;138:775–779.

107. Rodan SB, Wesolowski G, Chin J, Limjuco GA, Schmidt JA, Rodan GA. IL-1 binds to high affinity receptors on human osteosarcoma cells and potentiates prostaglandin E_2 stimulation of cAMP production. J Immunol 1990;145:1231–1237.

108. Stashenko P, Dewhirst FE, Peros WJ, Kent RL, Ago JM. Synergistic interactions between interleukin 1, tumor necrosis factor, and lymphotoxin in bone resorption. J Immunol 1987;138:1464–1468.

109. Keeting PE, Rifas L, Harris SA, et al. Evidence for interleukin-1β production by cultured normal human osteoblast-like cells. J Bone Miner Res 1991;6:827–833.

110. Keeting PE, Scott RE, Colvard DS, et al. Development and characterization of a rapidly proliferating, well-differentiated cell line derived from normal adult human osteoblast-like cells transfected with SV40 large T antigen. J Bone Miner Res 1992; 7:127–136.

111. Gowen M, Chapman K, Littlewood A, Hughes D, Evans D, Russell G. Production of tumor necrosis factor by human osteoblasts is modulated by other cytokines, but not by osteotropic hormones. Endocrinology 1990;126:1250–1255.

112. Rickard D, Russell G, Gowen M. Oestradiol inhibits the release of tumor necrosis factor but not interleukin 6 from adult human osteoblasts in vitro. Osteoporosis Int 1992;2:94–102.

113. Chaudhary LR, Spelsberg TC, Riggs BL. Production of various cytokines by normal human osteoblast-like cells in response to interleukin-1β and tumor necrosis factor-α: Lack of regulation by 17β-estradiol. Endocrinology 1992;130:2528–2534.

114. Jilka RL, Passeri G, Girasole G, Marcus T, Manolagas SC. Antibodies against tumor necrosis factor inhibit IL-1-induced IL-6 production in calvaria cells. J Bone Miner Res 1991;6(S1):S145. Abstract.

115. Ikebuchi K, Wong GG, Clark SC, Ihle JN, Hirai Y, Ogawa M. Interleukin 6 enhancement of interleukin-3 dependent proliferation of multipotential hemopoietic progenitors. Proc Nat Acad Sci USA 1987; 84:9035–9039.

116. Wong GG, Witek JAS, Temple PA, et al. Stimulation of murine hematopoietic colony formation by human interleukin-6. J Immunol 1988;140:3040–3044.

117. Kurihara N, Civin C, Roodman GD. Osteotropic factor responsiveness of highly purified populations of early and late precursors for human multinucleated cells expressing the osteoclast phenotype. J Bone Miner Res 1991;6:257–261.

118. Ishimi Y, Miyaura C, Jin CH, et al. IL-6 is produced by osteoblasts and induces bone resorption. J Immunol 1990;145: 3297–3303.

119. Lowik CWGM, van der Pluijm G, Bloys H, et al. Parathyroid hormone (PTH) and PTH-like protein (PLP) stimulate interleukin-6 production by osteogenic cells: a possible role of interleukin-6 in osteoclastogenesis. Biochem Biophys Res Commun 1989;162:1546–1552.

120. Black K, Garrett IR, Mundy GR. Chinese hamster ovarian cells transfected with the murine interleukin-6 gene cause hypercalcemia as well as cachexia, leukocytosis and thrombocytosis in tumor-bearing nude mice. Endocrinology 1991;128:2657–2659.

121. Al-Humidan A, Ralston SH, Hughes DE, et al. Interleukin-6 does not stimulate bone resorption in neonatal mouse calvariae. J Bone Miner Res 1991;6:3–8.

122. Girasole G, Jilka RL, Passeri G, et al. 17β-estradiol inhibits interleukin-6 production by bone marrow-derived stromal cells and osteoblasts in-vitro: a potential mechanism for the antiosteoporotic effect of estrogens. J Clin Invest 1992;89:883–891.

123. Linkhart TA, Linkhart SG, Mac Charles DC, Long DL, Strong DD. Interleukin-6 messenger RNA expression and interleukin-6 protein secretion in cells isolated from normal human bone: regulation by interleukin-1. J Bone Miner Res 1991;6:1285–1294.

124. Horowitz M, Phillips J, Centrella M. TGF-β regulates interleukin-6 secretion by osteoblasts. In: Cohn DV, Gennari C, Tashjian AH Jr, eds. Calcium regulating hormones and bone metabolism. Vol 11. Amsterdam: Excerpta Medica, 1992:275–280.

125. Feyen JHM, Elford P, Dipadova RE, Trechsel U. Interleukin-6 is produced by bone and modulated by parathyroid hormone. J Bone Miner Res 1989;4:633–638.

126. Littlewood AJ, Russell J, Harvey GR, Hughes DE, Russell RGG, Gowen M.

The modulation of the expression of IL-6 and its receptor in human osteoblasts in vitro. Endocrinology 1991;129:1513–1520.

127. Sakagami Y, Girasole G, Yu X-P, Boswell HS, Manolagas SC. Stimulation of interleukin-6 production by either calcitonin gene-related peptide or parathyroid hormone in two phenotypically distinct bone marrow-derived murine stromal cell lines. J Bone Miner Res 1993;8:811–816.

128. Ohsaki Y, Takahashi S, Scarcez T, et al. Evidence for an autocrine/paracrine role for interleukin-6 in bone resorption by giant cells from giant cell tumors of bone. Endocrinology 1992;131:2229–2234.

129. Jilka RL, Hangoc G, Girasole G, et al. Increased osteoclast development after estrogen loss: mediation by interleukin-6. Science 1992;257:88–91.

130. Klein B, Wijdenes J, Zhang X-G, et al. Murine anti-interleukin-6 monoclonal antibody therapy for a patient with plasma cell leukemia. Blood 1991;78:1198–1204.

131. Roodman GD, Kurihara N, Ohsaki Y, et al. Interleukin 6. A potential autocrine/paracrine factor in Paget's disease of bone. J Clin Invest 1992;89:46–52.

132. Paul SR, Bennett F, Calvetti JA, et al. Molecular cloning of a cDNA encoding interleukin 11, a stromal cell-derived lymphopoietic and hematopoietic cytokine. Proc Natl Acad Sci USA 1990;87:1311.

133. Passeri G, Bellido T, Girasole G, Tkaczyk A, Manolagas SC, Jilka RL. Transforming growth factor-β (TGFβ) and interleukin-1 (IL-1) induce the interleukin-11 (IL-11) mRNA in both bone marrow-derived stromal cells and osteoblasts from humans. J Bone Miner Res 1993;8(S1): S162. Abstract.

134. Tsuji K, Lyman SD, Sudo T, Clark SC, Ogawa M. Enhancement of murine hematopoiesis by synergistic interactions between steel factor (ligand for c-kit), interleukin-11, and other early acting factors in culture. Blood 1992;79:2855–2860.

135. Schibler KR, Yang Y-C, Christensen RD. Effect of interleukin-11 on cycling status and clonogenic maturation of fetal and adult hematopoietic progenitors. Blood 1992;80:900–903.

136. Hangoc G, Yin T, Cooper S, Schendel P, Yang Y-C, Broxmeyer HE. In vivo effects of recombinant interleukin-11 on myelopoiesis in mice. Blood 1993;81:965–972.

137. Passeri G, Girasole G, Knutson S, Yang YC, Manolagas SC, Jilka RL. Interleukin-11 (IL-11): a new cytokine with osteoclastogenic and bone resorptive properties and a critical role in PTH- and 1,25(OH)$_2$D$_3$-induced osteoclast development. J Bone Miner Res 1992;7(S1):S110. Abstract.

138. Girasole G, Passeri G, Knutson S, Jilka RL, Manolagas SC. A distinct and hierarchically central role of interleukin-11 among other cytokines in osteoclast development. J Bone Miner Res 1993;8(S1): S117. Abstract.

139. Wiktor-Jedrzejczak W, Bartocci A, Ferrante AW Jr, et al. Total absence of colony-stimulating factor 1 in the macrophage-deficient osteopetrotic (op/op) mouse. Proc Natl Acad Sci USA 1990; 87:4828–4832.

140. Yoshida H, Hayashi S-I, Kunisada T, et al. The murine mutation osteopetrosis is in the coding region of the macrophage colony stimulating factor gene. Nature 1990;345:442–444.

141. Felix R, Cecchini MG, Fleisch H. Macrophage colony stimulating factor restores in vivo bone resorption in the op/op osteopetrotic mouse. Endocrinology 1990;127:2592–2594.

142. Tanaka S, Takahashi N, Udagawa N, et al. Macrophage colony-stimulating factor is indispensable for both proliferation and differentiation of osteoclast progenitors. J Clin Invest 1993;91:257–263.

143. Corboz VA, Cecchini MG, Felix R, Fleisch H, van der Pluijm G, Löwik CWGM. Effect of macrophage colony-stimulating factor on in vitro osteoclast generation and bone resorption. Endocrinology 1992;130:437–442.

144. Elford PR, Felix R, Cecchini M, Trechsel U, Fleisch H. Murine osteoblastlike cells and the osteogenic cell MC3T3-E1 release a macrophage colony-stimulating activity in culture. Calcif Tissue Int 1987;41:151–156.

145. Horowitz MC, Einhorn TA, Philbrick W, Jilka RL. Functional and molecular changes in colony stimulating factor secretion by osteoblasts. Connect Tissue Res 1989;20:159–168.

146. Sieff CA, Emerson SG, Donahue RE, et al. Human recombinant granulocyte-macrophage colony-stimulating factor: a multilineage hematopoietin. Science 1985; 230:1171–1173.

147. Takahashi N, Udagawa N, Akatsu T, Tanaka H, Shionome M, Suda T. Role of colony-stimulating factors in osteoclast development. J Bone Miner Res 1991;6:977–985.

148. MacDonald BR, Mundy GR, Clark S, et al. Effects of human recombinant CSF-GM and highly purified CSF-1 on the formation of multinucleated cells with osteoclast characteristics in long-term bone marrow cultures. J Bone Miner Res 1986; 1:227–233.

149. Hattersley G, Chambers TJ. Effects of interleukin 3 and of granulocyte-macrophage and macrophage colony stimulating factors on osteoclast differentiation from mouse hemopoietic tissue. J Cell Physiol 1990;142:201–209.

150. Shinar DM, Sato M, Rodan GA. The effect of hemopoietic growth factors on the generation of osteoclast-like cells in mouse bone marrow cultures. Endocrinology 1990;126:1728–1735.

151. Walker F, Nicola NA, Metcalf D, Burgess AW. Hierarchical down regulation of hemopoietic growth factor receptors. Cell 1985;43:269–276.

152. Horowitz MC, Coleman DL, Flood PM, Kupper TS, Jilka RL. Parathyroid hormone and lipopolysaccharide induce murine osteoblast-like cells to secrete a cytokine indistinguishable from granulocyte-macrophage colony-stimulating factor. J Clin Invest 1989;83:149–157.

153. Horowitz MC, Coleman DL, Ryaby JT, Einhorn TA. Differential secretion of granulocyte-macrophage colony stimulating factor by a murine osteoblast cell line MC3T3. J Bone Miner Res 1989;4:911–921.

154. Burstein SA, Mei R-L, Henthorn J, Friese P, Turner K. Leukemia inhibitory factor and interleukin-11 promote maturation of murine and human megakaryocytes in vitro. J Cell Physiol 1992;153:305–312.

155. Ishimi Y, Abe E, Jin CH, et al. Leukemia inhibitory factor/differentiation-stimulating factor (LIF/D-factor): regulation of its production and possible roles in bone metabolism. J Cell Physiol 1992;152:71–78.

156. Reid LR, Lowe C, Cornish J, et al. Leukemia inhibitory factor: a novel bone-active cytokine. Endocrinology 1990;126:1416–1420.

157. Metcalf D, Gearing DP. Fatal syndrome in mice engrafted with cells producing high levels of the leukemia inhibitory factor. Proc Natl Acad Sci USA 1989; 86:5948–5952.

158. Rodan SB, Wesolowski G, Hilton DJ, Nicola NA, Rodan GA. Leukemia inhibitory factor binds with high affinity to pre-osteoblastic RCT-1 cells and potentiates the retinoic acid induction of alkaline phosphatase. Endocrinology 1990;127:1602–1608.

159. Ishimi Y, Abe E, Jin CH, et al. Leukemia inhibitory factor/differentiation-stimulating factor (LIF/D-factor): regulation of its production and possible roles in bone metabolism. J Cell Physiol 1992; 152:71–78.

160. Wetzler M, Talpaz M, Lowe DG, Daiocchi C, Gutterman JU, Kurzrock R. Constitutive expression of leukemia inhibitory factor RNA by human bone marrow stromal cells and modulation by IL-1, TNF-α, and TGF-β. Exp Hematol 1991; 19:347–351.

161. Bursuker I, Neddermann KM, Petty BA, et al. In vivo regulation of hemopoiesis by transforming growth factor beta 1: stimulation of GM-CSF- and M-CSF-dependent murine bone marrow precursors. Exp Hematol 1992;20:431–435.

162. Marcelli C, Yates AJ, Mundy GR. In vivo effects of human recombinant transforming growth factor β on bone turnover in normal mice. J Bone Miner Res 1990;5:1087–1096.

163. Shinar DM, Rodan GA. Biphasic effects of transforming growth factor-β on the production of osteoclast-like cells in mouse bone marrow cultures: the role of

prostaglandins in the generation of these cells. Endocrinology 1990;126:3153–3158.

164. Ruscetti FW, Dubois CM, Jacobsen SEW, Keller JR. Transforming growth factor β and interleukin-1: a paradigm for opposing regulation of haemopoiesis. Bailliere's Clin Haematol 1992;5:703–721.

165. Grigoriadis AE, Heersche JNM, Aubin JE. Differentiation of muscle, fat, cartilage, and bone from progenitor cells present in a bone-derived clonal cell population: effect of dexamethasone. J Cell Biol 1988;106:2139–2151.

166. Leboy PS, Beresford JN, Devlin C, Owen ME. Dexamethasone induction of osteoblast mRNAs in rat marrow stromal cell cultures. J Cell Physiol 1991;146:370–378.

167. Gehron Robey P, Young MF, Flanders KC, et al. Osteoblasts synthesize and respond to transforming growth factor-type β (TGF-β) in vitro. J Cell Biol 1987;105:457–463.

168. Oursler MJ, Cortese C, Keeting P, et al. Modulation of transforming growth factor-β production in normal human osteoblast-like cells by 17β-estradiol and parathyroid hormone. Endocrinology 1991;129:3313–3320.

169. Bonewald LF, Wakefield L, Oreffo ROC, Escobedo A, Twardzik DR, Mundy GR. Latent forms of transforming growth factor-β (TGFβ) derived from bone cultures: identification of a naturally occurring 100-kDa complex with similarity to recombinant latent TGFβ. Mol Endocrinol 1991;5:741–751.

170. Centrella M, McCarthy TL, Canalis E. Transforming growth factor beta is a bifunctional regulator of replication and collagen synthesis in osteoblast-enriched cell cultures from fetal rat bone. J Biol Chem 1987;262:2869–2874.

171. Pfeilschifter J, D'Souza SM, Mundy GR. Effects of transforming growth factor-β on osteoblastic osteosarcoma cells. Endocrinology 1987;121:212–218.

172. Noda M, Rodan GA. Type-β transforming growth factor inhibits proliferation and expression of alkaline phosphatase in murine osteoblast-like cells. Biochem Biophys Res Commun 1986;140:56–65.

173. Rosen DM, Stempien SA, Thompson AY, Seyedin SM. Transforming growth factor-beta modulates the expression of osteoblast and chondroblast phenotypes in vitro. J Cell Physiol 1988;134:337–346.

174. Wrana JL, Maeno M, Hawrylyshyn B, Yao KL, Domenicucci C, Sodek J. Differential effects of transforming growth factor-beta on the synthesis of extracellular matrix proteins by normal fetal rat calvarial bone cell populations. J Cell Biol 1988;106:915–924.

175. Seyedin SM, Rosen DM. Unique bone-derived cytokines. In: Gowen M, ed. Cytokines and bone metabolism. Boca Raton, Fla: CRC Press, 1992:109–113.

176. Mohan S, Strong DD, Lempert UG, Tremollieres F, Wergedal JE, Baylink DJ. Studies on regulation of insulin-like growth factor binding protein (IGFBP)-3 and IGFBP-4 production in human bone cells. Acta Endocrinol (Copenh) 1992;127:555–564.

177. Scharla SH, Strong DD, Mohan S, Baylink DJ, Linkhart TA. 1,25-Dihydroxyvitamin D_3 differentially regulates the production of insulin-like growth factor I (IGF-I) and IGF-binding protein-4 in mouse osteoblasts. Endocrinology 1991;129:3139–3146.

178. Bautista CM, Baylink DJ, Mohan S. Isolation of a novel insulin-like growth factor (IGF) binding protein from human bone: a potential candidate for fixing IGF-II in human bone. Biochem Biophys Res Commun 1991;176:756–763.

179. Centrella M, McCarthy TL, Canalis E. Receptors for insulin-like growth factors-I and -II in osteoblast-enriched cultures from fetal rat bone. Endocrinology 1990;126:39–44.

180. Kurose H, Yamaoka K, Okada S, Nakajima S, Seino Y. 1,25-Dihydroxyvitamin D_3 [$1,25(OH)_2D_3$] increases insulin-like growth factor I (IGF-I) receptors in clonal osteoblastic cells. Study on interaction of IGF-I and $1,25(OH)_2D_3$. Endocrinology 1990;126:2088–2094.

181. Chen TL, Chang LY, Bates RL, Perlman AJ. Dexamethasone and 1,25-dihydroxyvitamin D_3 modulation of insulin-like growth factor-binding proteins in rat

osteoblast-like cell cultures. Endocrinology 1991;128:73–80.

182. Slootweg MC, Most WW, Van Beek E, Schot LPC, Papapoulos SE, Löwik CWGM. Osteoclast formation together with interleukin-6 production in mouse long bones is increased by insulin-like growth factor-I. J Endocrinol 1992;132:433–438.

183. Rodan S, Wesolowski G, Thomas K, Rodan GA. Growth stimulation of rat calvaria osteoblastic cells by acidic fibroblast growth factor. Endocrinology 1987;121:1917–1923.

184. Globus RK, Plouet J, Gospodarowicz D. Cultured bovine bone cells synthesize basic fibroblast growth factor and store it in their extracellular matrix. Endocrinology 1989;124:1539–1547.

185. Canalis E, Centrella M, McCarthy T. Effects of basic fibroblast growth factor on bone formation in vitro. J Clin Invest 1988;81:1572–1577.

186. Shen V, Kohler G, Huang J, Huang SS, Peck WA. An acidic fibroblast growth factor stimulates DNA synthesis, inhibits collagen and alkaline phosphatase synthesis and induces resorption in bone. Bone Miner 1989;7:205–219.

187. Zhang L, Leeman E, Carnes DC, Graves DT. Human osteoblasts synthesize and respond to platelet-derived growth factor. Am J Physiol (Cell Physiol) 1991;261:C348–C354.

188. Centrella M, McCarthy TL, Kusmik WF, Canalis E. Relative binding and biochemical effects of heterodimeric and homodimeric isoforms of platelet-derived growth factor in osteoblast-enriched cultures from fetal rat bone. J Cell Physiol 1991;147:420–426.

189. Tashjian AH Jr, Hohmann EL, Antoniades HN, Levine L. Platelet-derived growth factor stimulates bone resorption via a prostaglandin-mediated mechanism. Endocrinology 1982;111:118–124.

190. D'Souza SM, Ibbotson KJ. Epidermal growth factor and transforming growth factor-α and bone. In: Gowen M, ed. Cytokines and bone metabolism. Boca Raton, Fla: CRC Press, 1992:147–184.

191. Rappolee DA, Werb Z. Macrophage-derived growth factors. Curr Top Microbiol Immunol 1992;181:87–140.

192. Pfeilschifter J, Mundy GR. Modulation of type β transforming growth factor activity in bone cultures by osteotropic hormones. Proc Natl Acad Sci USA 1987;84:2024–2028.

193. Oreffo ROC, Mundy GR, Seyedin SM, Bonewald LF. Activation of the bone-derived latent TGF beta complex by isolated osteoclasts. Biochem Biophys Res Commun 1989;158:817–823.

194. Pfeilschifter J, Wolf O, Naumann A, Minne HW, Mundy GR, Ziegler R. Chemotactic response of osteoblastlike cells to transforming growth factor beta. J Bone Miner Res 1990;5:825–830.

195. Hock JM, Gera I. Effects of continuous and intermittent administration and inhibition of resorption on the anabolic response of bone to parathyroid hormone. J Bone Miner Res 1992;7:65–72.

196. Manolagas SC, Haussler MR, Deftos LJ. 1,25-dihydroxyvitamin D_3 receptor-like macromolecule in rat osteogenic sarcoma cell lines. J Biol Chem 1980;255:4414–4417.

197. Price PA, Baukol SA. 1,25-Dihydroxyvitamin D_3 increases synthesis of the vitamin K-dependent bone protein by osteosarcoma cells. J Biol Chem 1980;255:11660–11663.

198. Mulkins MA, Manolagas SC, Deftos LJ, Sussman HH. 1,25-Dihydroxyvitamin D_3 increases bone alkaline phosphatase isoenzyme levels in human osteogenic sarcoma cells. J Biol Chem 1983;258:6219–6225.

199. Owen TA, Aronow MS, Barone LM, Bettencourt B, Stein GS, Lian JB. Pleiotropic effects of vitamin D on osteoblast gene expression are related to the proliferative and differentiated state of the bone cell phenotype: dependency upon basal levels of gene expression, duration of exposure, and bone matrix competency in normal rat osteoblast cultures. Endocrinology 1991;128:1496–1504.

200. Eriksen EF. Normal and pathological remodeling of human trabecular bone: three dimensional reconstruction of the remodeling sequence in normals and in

metabolic bone disease. Endocr Rev 1986;7:379–408.

201. Bataille R, Chappard D, Marcelli C, et al. Recruitment of new osteoblasts and osteoclasts is the earliest critical event in the pathogenesis of human multiple myeloma. J Clin Invest 1991;88:62–66.

202. Garrett IR, Durie BGM, Nedwin GE, et al. Production of lymphotoxin, a bone resorbing cytokine, by cultured human myeloma cells. N Engl J Med 1987;317:526–532.

203. Gozzolino F, Torcia M, Aldinucci D, et al. Production of interleukin 1 by bone marrow myeloma cells. Blood 1989;74:380–387.

204. Kawano M, Hirano T, Matsuda T, et al. Autocrine generation and essential requirement of BSF-2/IL-6 for human multiple myeloma. Nature 1988;322:83–86.

205. Rubin JE, Catherwood BD. Paget's disease of bone. In: Manolagas SC, Olefsky JM, eds. Metabolic bone and mineral disorders. New York: Churchill Livingstone, 1988:131–150.

206. Yasukawa K, Hirano T, Watanabe Y, et al. Structure and expression of human B cell stimulatory factor-2 (BSF/IL-6) gene. EMBO J 1987;6:2939–2945.

207. Seghal PB, Helfgott DC, Santhanam U, et al. Regulation of the acute phase and immune responses in viral diseases. Enhanced expression of the β2-interferon/hepatocyte stimulating factor/interleukin-6 gene in virus-infected human fibroblasts. J Exp Med 1988;167:1951–1956.

208. Ray A, Tatter SB, May LT, Seghal PB. Activation of the human β2-interferon/hepatocyte stimulating factor/interleukin-6 promoter by cytokines, viruses and second messengers. Proc Natl Acad Sci USA 1988;85:6701–6705.

209. Kaplan FS. Paget's disease of bone: exploring the questions. Calcif Tissue Int 1992;51:1–3.

210. Parfitt AM, Mathews CHE, Villanueva AR, Kleerekoper M, Frame B, Rao DS. Relationship between surface, volume and thickness of iliac trabecular bone in aging and in osteoporosis: implications for the microanatomic and cellular mechanism of bone loss. J Clin Invest 1983;72:1396–1409.

211. Eriksen EF, Hodgson SF, Eastell R, Cedel SL, O'Fallon WM, Riggs BL. Cancellous bone remodeling in type I (postmenopausal) osteoporosis: quantitative assessment of rates of formation, resorption, and bone loss at tissue and cellular levels. J Bone Miner Res 1990;5:311–319.

212. Turner RT, Wakley GK, Hannon KS, Bell NH. Tamoxifen inhibits osteoclast-mediated resorption of trabecular bone in ovarian hormone-deficient rats. Endocrinology 1988;122:1146–1150.

213. Liu C-C, Howard GA. Bone-cell changes in estrogen-induced bone-mass increase in mice: dissociation of osteoclasts from bone surfaces. Anat Rec 1991; 229:240–250.

214. Pottratz ST, Bellido T, Mocharla H, Crabb D, Manolagas SC. 17β-estradiol inhibits expression of human interleukin-6 promoter-reporter constructs by a receptor-dependent mechanism. J Clin Invest 1994;93:944–950.

215. Manolagas SC, Jilka RL. Cytokines, hematopoiesis, osteoclastogenesis, and estrogens. Calcif Tissue Int 1992; 50:199–202.

216. Passeri G, Girasole G, Jilka RL, Manolagas SC. Increased IL-6 production by murine bone marrow and bone cells following estrogen withdrawal. Endocrinology 1993;133:822–828.

217. Balena R, Constantini F, Yamomoto M, et al. Mice with IL-6 gene knockout do not lose cancellous bone after ovariectomy. J Bone Miner Res 1993;8(S1): S130. Abstract.

218. Pacifici R, Rifas L, Teitelbaum S, et al. Spontaneous release of interleukin 1 from human blood monocytes reflects bone formation in idiopathic osteoporosis. Proc Natl Acad Sci USA 1987;84:4616–4620.

219. Pacifici R, Brown C, Puscheck E, et al. Effect of surgical menopause and estrogen replacement on cytokine release from human blood mononuclear cells. Proc Natl Acad Sci USA 1991;88:5134–5138.

220. Pacifici R, Rifas L, McCracken R, et al. Ovarian steroid treatment blocks a postmenopausal increase in blood monocyte interleukin 1 release. Proc Natl Acad Sci USA 1989;86:2398–2402.

3▸ Clinical Assessment of Bone Strength

▶ ▶ ▶ Donald B. Kimmel

Robert R. Recker

Clinical procedures for assessing bone strength are discussed for their utility in diagnosis, risk prediction, and treatment follow-up of osteoporosis. Established techniques measuring bone mass are emphasized, but the need for new methods that provide supplementary information about skeletal strength is set forth.

Skeletal Composition

The adult human skeleton is composed of 80% cortical bone, a surprisingly high proportion (1,2). All cancellous regions are surrounded by a shell of cortical bone whose thickness varies from 0.5 to 10 mm. The radius and ulna are less than 20% cancellous, except for their distal 2 cm. Even in their distal regions, often taken to represent cancellous bone, cancellous content is only 55% to 65% (3). *Whole* vertebrae, often cited as "predominantly" cancellous bone, are actually 20% (4,5), 25% (6), or 40% (7) cancellous in direct measurements. Even vertebral *bodies* are about 40% to 50% cancellous, and the posterior elements, which contribute half the total mineral in vertebrae (6,8), are 5% cancellous (6). Exact proportions for the proximal femur and femoral neck have not been measured, but reasonable estimates are about 15% cancellous. Although it is claimed that the calcaneus is only 90% cancellous, few supportive data exist (9).

The fat content of bone marrow and soft tissues surrounding bone varies widely. In most peripheral bone sites, it is 75% or more. In axial sites, like the vertebrae, it is 40% to 50% (10). This percentage can be changed by medications and age (11,12). Fat content is important because bone mass measuring equipment is often influenced by fat content of surrounding tissues (13).

It should not be surprising that cortical bone, the dominant type of bone in the skeleton, plays a major role in determining bone strength (14). Much is often made of differences in cortical and metabolically more active cancellous bone and their roles in osteoporosis. The utility for fracture risk evaluation of in vivo bone mass measurement devices that do not separate cortical and cancellous bone is the best indirect sign of the prominent role of cortical bone. Today's data suggest that the relentless drive to separate cortical and cancellous bone during mass measurement should slow, and more effort be devoted toward in vivo methods that evaluate structure and materials quality.

Osteoporosis: A Disease of Fractures Signaling Inappropriately Low Bone Strength

Osteoporosis is a disorder of generalized skeletal fragility (15,16). Some argue that osteoporosis is a disease marked not by low trauma fractures, but by measurable osteopenia, and thus amenable to certain detection by mass measurement devices; the American College of Physicians finds those arguments unconvincing (17). Most osteopenic individuals have no fragility fractures (18,19); many more people have measurable osteopenia than develop osteoporotic fractures. Labeling otherwise healthy people with a nonfatal disease that is likely to remain symptomless not only is an unwarranted threat to their well-being, but also is likely to cause overuse of scarce health care resources. When the ability exists to make measurements that identify people with current or certain future skeletal fragility with very high specificity and sensitivity, then it will be appropriate to rely solely on such techniques for diagnoses.

Osteoporotic fractures signal inappropriately low bone strength. The three determinants of structural strength for any structure are its mass, geometric properties, and materials quality, otherwise called the burden of fatigue damage (20,21). Any one or more of the three may be causal when strength is low. With this sound theoretical basis, the clinical utility of in vivo bone mass measurement tools for determining bone strength is not even slightly surprising. Today's bone mass measurement instruments are excellent laboratory devices. At the same time, without an ability to assess geometric properties or materials quality, such tools cannot make a complete assessment of bone strength. The apparent emphasis here on mass measurement reflects the status of currently applied, widely available measurement technologies, and not the relative importance of assessing all three aspects of bone strength.

Diagnosing Osteoporosis

Diagnosing osteoporosis involves demonstrating the coexistence of fractures and a clinical history of minimal trauma without evidence of metastatic disease.

The diagnostic tools for osteoporosis are a medical history, a physical examination, and a lateral spine radiograph. Serial measurement of height is a good clinical aid for tracking crush fracture osteoporosis (22,23). However, today's best tool for identifying vertebral deformity is the lateral spine radiograph. In fact, the *only* tool for identifying progressive spinal osteoporosis is a lateral spine film. Deformities are most common in the lower thoracic spine, but are well known in both the mid-thoracic and lumbar regions (24–28). Bone mass measurement devices, on the other hand, do poorly at detecting lumbar vertebral deformities; their proper operation is generally impeded (29). Our focus on osteoporosis should not hide the fact that metastatic disease is also a common cause of vertebral deformity.

In vivo bone mass measurement cannot diagnose osteoporosis (30,31), but it is an excellent estimator of future fracture risk (32–36). Thirty-nine percent of sixth decade postmenopausal women with normal spinal or wrist bone density develop an osteoporotic fracture during their lifetime (32–36). For every .01 g/cm^2 (10% of population standard deviation) change in bone mineral density (BMD) this percentage changes 5% (32,36). A woman with BMD .05 g/cm^2 above the population mean has only a 1 in 7 chance (14%) of developing an osteoporotic fracture during her lifetime. However, a woman with a BMD 0.1 g/cm^2 below the population mean has a 9 in 10 chance (89%) of developing an osteoporotic fracture. Despite its lack of diagnostic ability, densitometry used with proper care and explanation to patients thus provides the clinician with useful information. The divergence of risk assessment and diagnostic capabilities occurs because osteoporosis is characterized by low bone *strength*, a problem in the osteoporotic skeleton caused in practice not only by low bone mass but also by poor bone geometry and quality (37). Both geometry and quality are untested by current applications of bone mass measurement.

The main uses for clinical bone mass measurements today are to assess risk of future fracture and to follow treatment outcomes in groups of patients (38–41). An opportunity also exists to assist the speedy and accurate diagnosis of the otherwise healthy individual with a single vertebral compression. The following discussion gives the current perspective on these techniques and offers future directions.

Clinical Bone Mass Measurement Techniques

Radiographs

The simplest widely available tool for evaluating bone mass is a radiograph. However, a relatively large decline in bone mineral (~30% to 40%) must occur before changes in density are apparent. A radiograph's most useful feature is the morphology it reveals, not the bone density. Microradioscopy of fine screen hand radiographs offers enhanced diagnostic ability (42). Radiogrammetry hand and femur films can detect both cortical thinning and changes in geometry that offer an evaluation of future fracture risk (43–45). Greater femoral neck length and angulation are positively related to the existence of opposite side hip fracture (46). Future work with radiographs that emphasizes bone geometry, a less studied determinant of bone strength, rather than bone density, is likely to be fruitful.

Quantitative Computed Tomography (QCT)

X-RAY BASED

Computed tomography (CT) can be made quantitative for bone by including appropriate standards in the scanning field (38,47,48). This is done for the spine with a phantom with several potassium phosphate standards that subtend the lumbar region. The Hounsfield number for any region is converted to one that represents BMD by comparison to the standard. Since standard CT tomes isolate the vertebral spongiosa, QCT can give information on a region that contains only cancellous bone. It discriminates osteopenic subjects as well as other techniques (19). It can also be used to find treatment effects and subgroups (49). Specialized QCT applications have begun to make possible some studies of structure (50). In vitro QCT methods can discern trabecular structure, but only at a high radiation flux (51,52).

Quantitative CT is an excellent technique that in recent years has become less frequently used for bone mass determination. Although the ready availability of dual energy x-ray absorptiometry (DXA) equipment outside departments of radiology has played a major role in this downturn, other factors have also contributed. Scanner time is often rightly reserved for applications that rely on CT's unique ability to assess in vivo morphology of diseases where it can make a noninvasive, definitive diagnosis. QCT bone mass examinations deliver a radiation dose of 2 to 3 mR, about one hundred times that of a DXA scan. A more subtle reason for QCT's declining use for bone mass measurement is the correct perception that isolating on cancellous bone gives little advantage for diagnosing or following the treatment of osteoporosis.

[125]I BASED

A technique that combines the best of ^{125}I absorptiometry (see below) with QCT for detailed, high-precision measurements of cancellous bone in limbs is

^{125}I-QCT (53,54). ^{125}I-QCT gives excellent precision in measuring separately both cancellous and cortical bone of limbs. It has never been applied in a large retrospective or prospective study of fracture risk prediction, but has been used to detect osteopenic limbs in patients with spinal cord injury (55) and changes in bone mass following treatment of osteopenia (56). The poor availability of equipment during the past decade has slowed research that would disclose the utility of this technology.

Absorptiometry

Absorptiometric techniques are based on analyzing the ability of a skeletal region to absorb photon energy. The first absorptiometric method was tested in the early 1960s and used clinically by the late 1960s. As the need for axial measurement grew, advanced methods evolved in the 1970s and came into widespread clinical use by the mid-1980s. The standardization and commercial sale of this equipment and the parallel development of desktop computers capable of handling the computational and data storage requirements of scanned images have also played major roles in the successful application of this technology. The radiation dose from a single examination is less than one tenth that delivered by a chest x-ray. DXA is today's method of choice for bone mass evaluation. A short review of past and current popular densitometry techniques that use absorptiometry follows.

SINGLE PHOTON ABSORPTIOMETRY (SPA)

Single photon absorptiometry is the oldest technique (57,58). An ^{125}I source (29 keV) and detector are mounted on a computer-controlled, movable scanning arm. The bone site, usually the forearm or heel, is immersed in water and interposed between the photon source and the detector. Photons pass through the bone site and transmitted photons are collected by the detector. As the scanning arm traverses the bone and surrounding soft tissue, differential photon transmission is sampled at multiple points along the path. In the forearm, profiles of photon intensity along the scan path are taken beginning either at one third the distance from the styloid process to the olecranon (one-third site) or at the point where the ulna and radius join (distal site). Multiple passes occur at set intervals, making a rectilinear scan. Computer postprocessing of scan data smooths edge and beam hardening artifacts and makes the appropriate comparison to scanned standards that creates an index of bone mineral content (BMC). Scans typically last 5 to 10 minutes. BMC and bone width (BW) are derived from a scan. The BMD (BMC/BW) is usually reported.

The forearm is the site most frequently measured. In the forearm, the one-third site is taken to represent cortical bone, whereas the distal site is taken to represent cancellous bone. In reality, both have appreciable fractions of cortical bone, but the distal site contains ten times more cancellous bone (3). Measuring either site provides a reliable assessment of future fracture risk (32,33,35). In the heel, the calcaneus is measured. Comparable risk assessment calculations can be made from measurements of the calcaneus as are made on forearm data (9,59). Calcaneus measurements reflect physical activity, as well as metabolic and genetic factors.

Limitations: Because of the low energy of ^{125}I photons, SPA is only useful on bone surrounded by minimal soft tissue, as in the limbs. Scans of the major osteoporotic fracture sites, like the spine and hip, are impossible. No commercially available SPA instrument allows integral assessment of BMC of a bone region. The imaging software for SPA systems is generally less sophisticated than for two energy systems, causing poorer imaging and subsequent diminished capability for analyzing scans.

DUAL PHOTON ABSORPTIOMETRY (DPA)

To facilitate the direct evaluation of bone regions likely to experience fracture, dual photon absorptiometry appeared in the mid-1970s (60,61). With higher energy photons than SPA, and two of them, conferring the ability to evaluate a three-phase (muscle, bone, and fat) system, it was the earliest widely available means to study integral BMC of both axial sites and the whole body. The patient was placed supine on a table and scanned in the anteroposterior projection (AP PA). Usual sites included the lumbar spine (L-2 to L-4) and the hip. A source delivering two photons of differing energy and a detector were mounted on a movable scanning arm. Sources included ^{241}Am and ^{137}Cs together, and ^{153}Gd (100 keV and 44 keV). Sampling at intervals as close as 0.5 mm bidirectionally occurred, making a rectilinear scan that integrated the mineral content of a region. BMC and projected area on a two-dimensional scan were combined to give BMD, a two-dimensional density somewhat normalized for bone size variation. Scans of the lumbar spine and hip typically lasted 20 minutes each. Instruments were widely available through the middle and late 1980s. Although DPA was a successful technique (62,63), it has now been completely replaced by DXA, which is discussed below.

Limitations: The problems with DPA included necessity for annual source replacement (due to isotope decay), poor isotope availability and high cost, and lengthy scan times. Because DPA seemed always to be evolving, software changes were frequent and occasional hardware changes generally altered machine performance. Early systems were based on inadequate first-generation microcomputers.

DUAL ENERGY X-RAY

Dual energy x-ray (DXA) or quantitative digital radiography (QDR) shares many principles with DPA (64–66). The main change is the substitution of an x-ray tube for the isotope source, creating a 1000-fold increase in photon flux. The photons are of two energies (140 and 70 keV), generated by filtration or rapid switching during x-ray generation. The increased photon flux is used to (1) sample more closely spaced points during the scan, (2) sample each point with improved counting statistics, and (3) decrease scan time. All improve the precision of axial site scanning. More frequent sampling with better counting statistics improves precision in the expected ways. Shorter scan times provide hidden benefits by improving the possibility that a patient can remain perfectly still throughout a scan, a welcome improvement especially for hip scans.

▶ 55

The accuracy of DXA is within 4% to 8% (39,67). It is at least as good as SPA in discriminating patients with osteoporotic fractures (68). It provides essential information that improves hip fracture risk prediction compared to that given by SPA or DPA (69–71) and provides new information on the nature of hip fractures. Hip fracture patients have moderately lower hip BMD than spinal osteoporotic persons (72). Subjects suffering trochanteric fractures have lower hip BMD than those suffering cervical fractures (73). More cases of osteopenia are revealed when scans of both the spine and hip are done (70).

Issues in the Every Day Use of DXA— *Routine precision without machine alterations:* When compared on an absolute basis to most laboratory tests and other noninvasive bone evaluation methods, DXA has excellent precision (Table 3-1). Compared to the changes it seeks to detect, it is not good enough because it is not yet possible to monitor changes in individuals. Meaningful changes in bone occur over many months or a few years, not days or weeks. Annual rates of bone loss are usually 1% or less in healthy men and women (74,75). Annual rates of change with current treatments are only 3% to 5% (76–78). Although screening is only slightly affected by precision, observing groups of patients or individuals on treatment is influenced heavily by long-term precision.

The ultimate goal for determining DXA precision in clinical studies is measurement over extended intervals of spine, hip, forearm, or whole body BMD from a group of living, nonchanging, osteopenic, older individuals. Because bone loss is considered a certain feature in older persons (79), the necessary study of DXA precision simply cannot happen. It is likely that *all* existing reports of precision are too optimistic in their description of long-term precision for DXA in aged osteopenic subjects. A clear understanding of the difficulties in determining long-term precision for application of DXA will help the reader properly monitor claims of precision.

Phantoms are often used, but even when of proper construction, they only evaluate machine stability. Stepwedge phantoms or aluminum bars that present sharp demarcation of edges on scans are not adequate. Subtle shifts in counting statistics due to source aging, collimation changes, and updated (improved) software algorithms are most likely to be expressed at the bone-soft tissue interface. The edge detection algorithms used for finding bone edges are not well tested by such sharp demarcations. The uniform and dense nature of the aluminum also does not properly duplicate the mineral distribution of intra-bony regions.

Anthropomorphic phantoms exist with bone edges, interstices, and amounts of mineral that approximate bone sites of interest in the osteopenic subject. Such phantoms are usually embedded in plastic and idealized with well-delineated intervertebral discs. Positioning on the scanner table is made easy by markings, allowing faithful alignment of the phantom axis with the long axis of the table. The exact starting point for the scan is marked on the plastic, making possible truly identical scan time after time. For DXA, the precision error is frequently 0.5% under these circumstances (80,81), when software, hardware, and sources are constant, an appreciable improvement over the 1 + % often found with DPA (82–87).

However, phantoms cannot mimic a number of the real world problems inherent in daily DXA work. These include: (1) repositioning (including parallelism with long axis of table and choice of starting point relative to bony site), (2) variation in soft tissue composition, (3) weight changes, (4) thickness changes, (5) variation in intestinal contents, and (6) true changes in mineral content of bone regions. To combat this, young, healthy, normal people are often used for precision studies. They are chosen because they are available and their bone density is steady over a few months. Recent data indicate that BMC in third decade women is rising slowly, perhaps making them a poor choice for long-term precision studies (88). Their BMC is high and their intervertebral disc regions are well defined when compared to older osteopenic subjects.

Considering the real world problems of DXA, it is not surprising on a theoretical basis that measurements on young normal people show longer term precision error of 1% in the lumbar spine, about twice that in phantoms (80,81,89–91). One report suggests that this is correct (92). Although no long-term precision studies of older, osteopenic subjects exist or seem likely, their lower bone mass, coupled with increased likelihood of interference from osteophytes, suggests a real world best-case precision error for lumbar spine BMD measurements in subjects from an age range likely to be used in studies of osteoporosis of about 2%.

Relative precision within the skeleton: In individuals in whom a 1% precision error is reported for the lumbar spine BMD, precision errors of 0.5% for whole body BMC, and 1.5% to 2.5% for BMD of the several regions of the proximal femur are reported. The excellent precision for whole body is due mostly to the large BMC (2500 g) of the whole skeleton. The worse precision for the hip region is most likely related to (1) difficulties in repositioning the hip with respect to the axis of a previous scan (80,81,84,93), (2) the lower BMC of hip regions than in spine and whole body, and (3) subtle difficulties for the patient to maintain the toe inward, optimal position for hip DXA.

▶ 57

Machine change effects on precision: Switching technologies, sources (or x-ray tubes), software versions, hardware (eg, collimator), or instruments always create changes. These problems are seldom described in published literature. Because of the excellent precision of the instruments, it is usually possible to identify baseline shifts of less than 1% (84,94). Although these changes are of no clinical significance for screening, they are important for longitudinal studies that follow the time course of bone mass. Subjects on such studies should be maintained on the same piece of equipment without software or hardware change for the duration of any study, to avoid the inevitable loss of precision that comes with a shifting baseline.

The BMD of both phantoms (82,95) and human beings (83,96) rises 1% to 3% and precision declines (95–97), the degradation being greater with greater subject thickness, as the ^{153}Gd source of DPA systems ages. This floating baseline can be accommodated by software and attention to standardization procedures (97). The influence of source age, particularly as regards the aging of x-ray tubes in DXA equipment, merits study. Software changes (85), improvements such as automatic comparison (98), and collimation make significant differences (97).

Osteophytes and endplate sclerosis: The lumbar spine has osteophytes and endplate sclerosis in 10% to 15% of individuals above age 65 (99,100). Osteophytes and endplate sclerosis can contain enough mineral to increase the apparent anteroposterior BMD (APBMD) of the lumbar spine (62,101–106). In a normal population, undetected osteophytes cause an underestimation of the number of cases with low bone density (102). In individuals, undetected osteophytes cause underestimation of the fracture risk inferred from AP lumbar BMD measurements. When they overlie disc spaces, they obscure certain identification of vertebrae. Osteophytes and endplate sclerosis are thus complications that should be checked in older patients with osteoarthritis, a history of low back pain, or documented disc disease, in whom a correct interpretation of BMD is needed. Lateral projection DXA is a newer method that can avoid this complication.

Aortic calcification: This is another potential confounding factor in antero-posterior DXA (APDXA). However, the amount of mineral usually found in calcified vasculature is so small that it does not affect the proper interpretation of APDXA values (34,63,102–108).

Vertebral deformities: Although the lumbar spine is not the chief site of vertebral deformities associated with spinal osteoporosis, their occurrence is reasonably frequent (26). Lateral spine films, not APDXA, are used to diagnose vertebral deformity. BMD is usually high in deformed vertebrae (29). To include a fractured vertebra unknowingly in a risk assessment would paradoxically underestimate risk of fracture. Thus, an individual vertebra that seems unusually short or dense relative to its neighbors on APDXA should be examined in a lateral spine film for deformity.

Fat in marrow and surrounding soft tissue: Variations in fat content of the tissue surrounding the bone of interest (eg, spine or hip) affect BMD. DXA is most certain to be valid when fat content of the surrounding tissue is constant and uniform. Inhomogeneous fat distribution, as routinely exists (109), creates inaccuracies in BMC. Relative increases in fat content in tissue surrounding the measured site artificially increase BMC (110). The meaning for clinical trials using BMD as an outcome variable is that data from subjects experiencing extreme weight changes should be scrutinized carefully.

Newer Applications of DXA—*Lateral DXA:* APDXA, which combines whole vertebrae in one measurement, can be supplemented with lateral projection DXA (LDXA) (89–91,111,112), that separates the vertebral body from the posterior elements. Positioning is crucial to successful LDXA. On conventional APDXA equipment, the patient is placed in the lateral decubitus position with knees and hips in flexion, stabilized with a positioning device. The patient may also be placed in the usual APDXA position on a scanner that allows the arm to collect data with the beam directed horizontally. In either case, the patient's arms should be raised above and in front of the head to limit interference from the ribs with imaging of L-2 (90). The scan should be done in high-resolution mode because of the increased thickness of soft tissue encountered by the beam.

Lateral DXA has produced some promising data. The rate of bone loss in the vertebral body isolated by lateral measurement is nearly twice that measured by APDXA (89–91). However, in practice, past application of LDXA has encountered problems. Except for one study (91), three vertebrae are never available for analysis. In fact, without proper attention, only one vertebrae is available in one third of subjects (89,90,111,112), severely affecting precision, because of low BMC. Precision for one vertebral body was 5.4%; for two vertebral bodies it was 1.6% to 3.8% (89,90,111,112). The proper precision for lateral scanning also seems related to a more difficult positioning method, resulting in poorer precision in reproducing the projection angle. Furthermore, the ability to differentiate osteoporotic from normal subjects is not significantly enhanced (91).

Lateral DXA is a technique with promise. It offers the chance to exclude osteophytes and focus on the vertebral body. If done with care and with the patient positioned in the conventional position of the APDXA scan (as is possible on newer equipment with rotatable arms), the greater differences detected may overcome the poorer precision to give it utility in longitudinal studies. Its capacity to differentiate osteoporotic subjects or to improve fracture risk prediction remains unproven.

▶ 59

Forearm DXA: DXA is well-suited for measuring forearm mineral content, an improvement over SPA. DXA radiation exposure is markedly lower than SPA (113). Forearm DXA forms an image of the whole distal forearm, allowing more precise placement of regions of interest than in SPA. When equal care is used in positioning in DXA and SPA, better precision in the ultradistal region, although not in the cortical regions (113), occurs with DXA. The precision error is generally lower than 1% (114,115). Although a strong correlation exists between SPA and DXA forearm BMD measurements (R≥.9 [113,116]), systematic differences between the two techniques prevent interconversion (114,116,117). The most severe impediment to using forearm DXA will be the huge normative data base of fracture risk prediction that has been accumulated for SPA (32–35). Difficulties in acquiring ^{125}I sources for SPA devices may eventually make continued maintenance of SPA instruments difficult. New screening and longitudinal studies of forearm mineral content should use DXA, but longitudinal studies started with SPA should continue with SPA because of the potential loss of sensitivity.

Clinical Limitations: These techniques cannot by themselves be used to detect conditions of defective matrix mineralization because their output expresses information only about mineral (and not matrix) quantity. Morphologic features on radiographs, biochemical measurements, histologic studies with fluorochrome labeling, and clinical history remain the best methods for identifying such conditions. DXA does poorly at identifying crush fractures and diagnosing osteoporosis.

Novel DXA Applications That Extend Its Value: DXA has proved a valuable adjunct in the management of hip prosthesis placement. It measures mineral in the femoral shaft surrounding the prosthesis with precision errors of less than 5% (118–121). In time, such technology may prove useful in detecting periprosthetic changes that signal impending failure in time for effective countermeasures to be undertaken.

The morphologic information provided in DXA scans has been used to improve the understanding of the factors that predict hip fracture. In women, trochanteric fractures are more likely related to osteopenia than are cervical fractures (73). Several studies indicate that geometric properties of the hip and proximal femur influence hip fracture incidence. Such features include shape and moment of inertia of the femoral neck (122,123) and length and angulation of the femoral neck (46,124).

Although DXA was originally conceived for human studies, it has proven useful in small and large animal studies (125–129). Its principal application in rats is in postmortem studies (130), but it is workable for longitudinal studies of living rats (125). Despite the small amount of mineral, the precision error is about 3% (125,130). SPA has also been applied successfully (131,132), but the specialized software supplied by major DXA manufacturers has made it the preferred technology today.

Geometry, Structure, and Fatigue Damage Evaluation

The dependence of bone strength on three factors—mass, geometry, and quality—was mentioned earlier. The inability of bone mass measurement to assess the latter two was mentioned with an implication that it was important to pursue new methodologies. Some promising efforts using ultrasound devices have been made, but the technology needs more work before it can become acceptable.

Ultrasound

The transmission of ultrasound through bone depends on mass, structure, and quality (133). Commercial instruments that transmit, record, and analyze ultrasound attenuation and velocity have recently become available. This new technology is much less well developed than densitometry, but it provides new opportunities. This fully portable machinery is without radiation exposure and is useful in population-based studies. Sending and receiving probes are applied closely to bones with little overlying soft tissue, like the calcaneus or patella. Microcomputer controlling software routines analyze the output for attenuation or velocity. These devices have recently been shown to supplement information provided by DXA.

Broadband attenuation recording provides similar discrimination ability with moderate correlation (R = 0.6 to 0.75) to that given by densitometry (134–141). It has been applied in some clinical studies (142). Measurement of velocity has also been done, finding different sets of persons with documented osteoporosis (143–144). The incomplete correlation of ultrasound to BMD suggests that ultrasound measures properties of bone besides mass. The repeated failure of attempts to tie ultrasound attenuation and velocity closely to BMD measurements may be better viewed not as failures, but as *successes* for ultrasound, precisely because it is detecting something other than bone mass that is indicative of fracture. Because ultrasound is routinely used commercially to measure fatigue damage of engineering materials (20), it might be inferred that it can do the same for bone.

▶61

Because of the necessity for close application of the ultrasound probes to bone with minimal overlying soft tissue, ultrasound is limited to peripheral skeletal sites. Insofar as the ability to know the condition of axial bone by direct measurement has proven advantageous for BMD (69), this equipment may be limited. Whether ultrasound assesses nonbone mass–related defects in the osteoporotic skeleton remains to be determined.

The Future for Clinical Assessment of Bone Strength

Osteoporosis is a disease of fractures that demonstrate low bone strength. Bone strength is determined by mass, geometry, and quality. Today's most popularly applied techniques assess bone mass well, but they do little to approach the other aspects of strength. The orderly evolution of bone mass measurement

TABLE 3-1 Comparison of Clinical Tools for Measuring Bone Mass and Quality in Elderly Individuals

Technique	Site(s)	Accuracy (%)	Precision (%)	Radiation Dose (rem)	Duration of Exam (min)
SPA	Forearm, calcaneus	5	2	.01	15
DPA	Spine, whole body, hip	3–5	3	.005	25
DXA	Forearm, spine, whole body, hip	3–5	1.5–2	.002	5–7
^{125}I-QCT	Forearm, tibia	3	0.5	.001	5
QCT	Spine	5–20	1.5	2	10
Ultrasound	Patella, calcaneus	x	3	0	5

DPA, dual photon absorptiometry; **DXA,** dual energy x-ray absorptiometry; **QCT,** quantitative computed tomography; **SPA,** single photon absorptiometry instruments has been driven by both the perceived needs of the field and several competitive manufacturers. This has left the field with DXA, a precise and useful technique. DXA can be used for both axial and peripheral bone sites to determine risk of future fracture and monitor longitudinal studies of groups of patients. DXA cannot diagnose osteoporosis or follow changes of less than 5% in individual subjects. Many clinical and preclinical applications for DXA exist, and new ones are always evolving. Ultrasound instruments seem able to give a more general evaluation of bone quality, but are in need of more testing. A new generation of CT-like instruments based on DXA technology is now emerging. With a higher energy x-ray tube, tighter collimation, and C arms, these instruments seem likely to provide a mix of diagnostic and densitometric abilities not now available.

References

1. Marshall JH, Liniecki J, Lloyd EL, et al. Alkaline earth metabolism in adult man. In: ICRP Publication 20. Oxford, England: Pergamon Press, 1972:34–51.

2. Johnson LC. Composition of trabecular and cortical bone in humans. In: Frost HM, ed. Bone biodynamics. Boston: Little, Brown, 1964:543–654.

3. Schlenker RA, VonSeggen WW. The distribution of cortical and trabecular bone mass along the lengths of the radius and ulna and the implications for in vivo bone mass measurements. Calcif Tissue Int 1976; 20:41–52.

4. Van Berkum FNR, Birkenhäger JC, Van Veen LCP, et al. Noninvasive axial and peripheral assessment of bone mineral content: a comparison between osteoporotic women and normal subjects. J Bone Miner Res 1989;4:679–685.

5. Sandor T, Felsenberg D, Kalender WA, Clain A, Brown E. Compact and trabecular components of the spine using quantitative computed tomography. Calcif Tissue Int 1992;50:502–506.

6. Nottestad SY, Baumel JJ, Kimmel DB, Recker RR, Heaney RP. The proportion of trabecular bone in human vertrbrae. J Bone Miner Res 1987;2:221–230.

7. Jones CD, Laval-Jeanet AM, Laval-Jeanet MH, Genant HK. Importance of measurement of spongious vertebral bone mineral density in the assessment of osteoporosis. Bone 1987;8:201–206.

8. Louis O, Van Den Winkel P, Covens P, Schoutens A, Osteaux M. Dual-energy x-ray absorptiometry of lumbar vertebrae: relative contribution of body and posterior elements and accuracy in relation with neutron activation analysis. Bone 1992;13: 317–320.

9. Vogel JM, Wasnich RD, Ross PD. The clinical relevance of calcaneus bone mineral measurements: a review. Bone Miner 1988; 5:35–58.

10. DeBisschop E, Luypaert R, Louis O, Osteaux M. Fat fraction of lumbar bone marrow using in vivo proton nuclear magnetic resonance spectroscopy. Bone 1993; 14:133–136.

11. Need AG, Horowitz M, Walker CJ, Chatterton BE, Chapman IC, Nordin BEC. Cross-over study of fat-corrected forearm mineral content during nandrolone decanoate therapy for osteoporosis. Bone 1989;10:3–6.

12. Dunnill MS, Anderson JA, Whitehead R. Quantitative histologic studies on age changes in bone. Pathol Bacteriol 1967; 94:275–291.

13. Mazess RB. Errors in measuring trabecular bone by computed tomography

due to marrow and bone composition. Calcif Tissue Int 1983;35:148–152.

14. Mazess RB. Fracture risk: a role for compact bone. Calcif Tissue Int 1990;47: 191–193.

15. Avioli LV. Significance of osteoporosis: a growing international health care problem. Calcif Tissue Int 1991;49:S5–S7.

16. Cummings SR, Kelsey JL, Nevitt MC, O'Dowd KJ. Epidemiology of osteoporosis and osteoporotic fractures. Epidemiol Rev 1985;7:178–208.

17. Bone densitometry and clinical decision-making in osteoporosis. Ann Intern Med 1988;108:293–294. Editorial.

18. Riggs BL, Wahner HW, Dunn WL, Mazess RB, Offord KP, Melton LJ. Differential changes in bone mineral density of the appendicular and axial skeleton with aging. J Clin Invest 1981;67:328–335.

19. Genant HK, Ettinger B, Cann CE, Reiser U, Gordan GS, Kolb FO. Osteoporosis: assessment by quantitative computed tomography. Orthop Clin North Am 1985;16:557–568.

20. Avallone EA, Baumeister T III. Mark's standard handbook for mechanical engineers. New York: McGraw-Hill, 1987:36–51.

21. Strong AB. Fundamentals of composites manufacturing: materials, methods, and applications. Dearborn, Mich. Society of Mechanical Engineering, 1989.

22. Kleerekoper M, Nelson DA, Peterson EL, Tilley BC. Outcome variables in osteoporosis trials. Bone 1992;13:S29–S34.

23. Saville PD, Nilsson BER. Height and weight in symptomatic postmenopausal osteoporosis. Clin Orth Rel Res 1967;45:49–54.

24. Gallagher JC, Hedlund LR, Stoner S, Meeger C. Vertebral morphometry: normative data. Bone Miner 1988;4:189–196.

25. Hedlund LR, Gallagher JC. Vertebral morphometry in diagnosis of spinal fractures. Bone Miner 1988;5:59–67.

26. Hedlund LR, Gallagher JC, Meeger C, Stoner S. Change in vertebral shape in spinal osteoporosis. Calcif Tissue Int 1989; 44:168–172.

27. Minne HW, Leidig G, Wuster C, et al. A newly developed spine deformity index (SDI) to quantitate vertebral crush fractures in patients with osteoporosis. Bone Miner 1988;3:335–349.

28. Smith-Bindman R, Steiger P, Cummings SR, Genant HK. The index of radiographic area (IRA): a new approach to estimating the severity of vertebral deformity. Bone Miner 1991;13:137–150.

29. Ryan PJ, Evans P, Blake GM, Fogelman I. The effect of vertebral collapse on spinal bone mineral density measurements in osteoporosis. Bone Miner 1992;18:267–272.

30. Wasnich RD. Bone mass measurements in diagnosis and assessment of therapy. Am J Med 1992;91(Suppl 5B):54S–588.

31. Stegman MR, Recker RR, Davies KM, Ryan RA, Heaney RP. Fracture risk as determined by prospective study designs. Osteoporosis Int 1992;2:290–297.

32. Hui SL, Slemenda CW, Johnston CC Jr. Baseline measurement of bone mass predicts fracture in white women. Ann Intern Med 1989;111:355–361.

33. Gärdsell P, Johnell O, Nilsson BE. Predicting fractures in women by using forearm bone densitometry. Calcif Tissue Int 1989;45:235–242.

34. Ross PD, Wasnich RD, Vogel JM. Detection of prefracture spinal osteoporosis using bone mineral absorptiometry. J Bone Miner Res 1988;3:1–11.

35. Gärdsell P, Johnell O, Nilsson BE. The predictive value of bone loss for fragility fractures in women: a longitudinal study over fifteen years. Calcif Tissue Int 1991; 49:90–94.

36. Black DM, Cummings SR, Genant HK, Nevitt MC, Palermo L, Browner W. Axial and appendicular bone density predict fractures in older women. J Bone Miner Res 1992;7:633–638.

37. Kleerekoper M, Villanueva AR, Stanciu J, Rao DS, Parfitt AM. The role of three dimensional trabecular microstructure in the pathogenesis of vertebral compression fractures. Calcif Tissue Int 1985; 37:594–597.

38. Genant HK, Block JE, Steiger P, Gluer CC, Ettinger B, Harris ST. Appropriate use of bone densitometry. Radiology 1989;170:817–822.

39. Genant HK, Faulkner KG, Gluer CC, Engelke K. Bone densitometry: current assessment. Osteoporosis Int 1993; (Suppl 1):S91–S97.

40. Johnston CC, Slemenda CW, Melton LJ. Clinical use of bone densitometry. N Engl J Med 1991;324:1105–1109.

41. Fogelman I, Ryan P. Measurement of bone mass. Bone 1992;13:S23–S28.

42. Meema HE, Meema S. Cortical bone mineral density versus cortical thickness in the diagnosis of osteoporosis: a roentgenologic densitometric study. J Am Geriatr Soc 1969;17:120–141.

43. Lappe JM, Heaney RP, Recker RR, Ryan RA. Radiogrammetry as a method to predict osteoporosis fractures. J Bone Miner Res 1992;7(Suppl 947):S327.

44. Fox KM, Tobin JD, Plato CC. Longitudinal study of bone loss in the second metacarpal. Calcif Tissue Int 1986;39:218–225.

45. Orvieto R, Leichter I, Rachmilewitz, Margulies JY. Bone density, mineral content, and cortical index in patients with thalassemia major and the correlation to their bone fractures, blood transfusions, and treatment with desferroxamine. Calcif Tissue Int 1992;50:397–399.

46. Gluer CC, Cummings SR, Pressman A, et al. Prediction of hip fractures from pelvic radiographs: the study of osteoporotic fractures. J Bone Miner Research 1994 (in press).

47. Cann CE, Genant HK, Kolb FO, Ettinger B. Quantitative computed tomography for prediction of vertebral fracture risk. Bone 1985;6:1–7.

48. Genant HK. Quantitative computed tomography: update 1987. Calcif Tissue Int 1987;41:179–186.

49. Ettinger B, Genant HK, Cann CE. Long-term estrogen replacement therapy prevents bone loss and fractures. Ann Intern Med 1985;102:319–324.

50. Cody DD, Flynn MJ. A technique for measuring regional bone mineral density in human lumbar vertebral bodies. Med Phys 1989;16:766–772.

51. Kuhn JL, Goldstein SA, Feldkamp LA, Goulet RW, Jesion G. Evaluation of a microcomputed tomography system to study trabecular bone structure. J Orthop Res 1990;8:833–842.

52. Kinney JH, Nichols MC. X-ray tomographic microscopy (XTM) using synchrotron radiation. Ann Rev Mat Sci 1992;22:121–152.

53. Ruegsegger P, Dambacher M. Clinical application of peripheral computed tomography. In: Frame B, Potts JT, eds. Clinical Disorders of bone and mineral metabolism. Amsterdam: Excerpta Medica, 1983;48–51.

54. Hangartner TN, Overton TR. Quantitative measurement of bone density using gamma-ray computed tomography. J Comput Assist Tomogr 1982;1156–1162.

55. Hangartner T. The OsteoQuant: an isotope based CT scanner for precise measurement of bone density. J Comput Assist Tomogr 1993;17:798–805.

56. Ruegsegger P, Dambacher MA, Ruegsegger E, Fischer JA, Anliker M. Bone loss in premenopausal and postmenopausal women. A cross-sectional and logitudinal study using quantitative computed tomography. J Bone Joint Surg 1984;66A:1015–1023.

57. Cameron JR, Sorenson J. Measurement of bone mineral in vivo: an improved method. Science 1963;142:230–232.

58. Christiansen C, Rödbro P, Jensen H. Bone mineral content in the forearm measured by photon absorptiometry. Scand J Clin Lab Invest 1975;35:323–330.

59. Lancaster EK, Evans RA, Kos S, Hills E, Dunstan CR, Wong SYP. Measurement of bone in the os calcis: a clincial evaluation J Bone Miner Res 1989;4:507–514.

60. Roos BO, Skoldborn H. Dual photon absorptiometry in lumbar vertebrae. I. Theory and method. Acta Radiol 1974;13:266–280.

61. Roos BO. Dual photon absorptiometry in lumbar vertebrae. II. Precision and reproducibility. Acta Radiol 1975;14:291–303.

62. Krolner B. Berthelsen B, Nielsen SP. Assessment of vertebral osteopenia. Acta Radiol Diagn 1982;23:517–521.

63. Pouilles JM, Tremollieres F, Louvet JP, Fournie B, Morlock G, Ribot C. Sensi-

64 ◄

tivity of dual photon absorptiometry in spinal osteoporosis. Calcif Tissue Int 1988; 43:329–334.

64. Sartoris D, Resnick D. Dual-energy radiographic absorptiometry for bone densitometry: current status and perspective. Am J Roentgenol 1989;152:241–246.

65. Cullum ID, Ell PJ, Ryder JP. X-ray dual photon absorptiometry: a new method for the measurement of bone density. Br J Radiol 1989;587–592.

66. Hansen MA, Hassager C, Overgaard K, Marslew U, Riis BJ, Christiansen C. Dual energy x-ray absorptiometry: a precise method of measuring bone mineral density in the lumbar spine. J Nucl Med 1990;31:1156–1162.

67. Ho C, Kim R, Schaffler M, Sartoris D. Accuracy of dual-energy radiographic absorptiometry of the lumbar spine. Radiology 1990;176:171–173.

68. Overgaard K, Hansen MA, Riis BJ, Christiansen C. Discriminatory ability of bone mass measurements (SPA and DXA) for fractures in elderly postmenopausal women. Calcif Tissue Int 1992;50:30–35.

69. Cummings SR, Black DM, Nevitt MC, et al. Bone density at various sites for prediction of hip fractures. Lancet 1993; 341:72–75.

70. Pouilles JM, Tremollieres F, Ribot C. Spine and femur densitometry at the menopause: are both sites necessary in the assessment of the risk of osteoporosis? Calcif Tissue Int 1993;52:344–347.

71. Melton LJ, Atkinson EJ, O'Fallon WM, Wahner HW, Riggs BL. Long-term fracture prediction by bone mineral assessed at different skeletal sites. J Bone Miner Res 1993;8:1227–1233.

72. Libanati CR, Schulz EE, Shook JE, Bock M, Baylink DJ. Hip mineral density in females with a recent hip fracture. J Clin Endocrinal Metab 1992;74:351–356.

73. Karlsson MK, Johnell O, Nilsson BE, Sernbo I, Obrant KJ. Bone mineral mass in hip fracutre patients. Bone 1993; 14:161–165.

74. Rodin A, Murby B, Smith MA, et al. Premenopausal bone loss in the lumbar spine and femoral neck: a study of 225 Caucasian women. Bone 1990;11:1–5.

75. Elders PJM, Netelenbos JC, Lips P, et al. Calcium supplementation reduces vertebral bone loss in perimenopausal women: a controlled trial in 248 women between 46 and 55 years of age. J Clin Endocrinol Metab 1991;73:533–540.

76. Passeri M, Baroni MC, Pedrazzoni M, et al. Intermittent treatment with intravenous 4-amino-1-hydroxybutylidene-1,1-bisphosphonate (AHBuBP) in the therapy of postmenopausal osteoporosis. Bone Miner 1991;15:237–248.

77. Storm T, Thamsborg G, Steiniche T, Genant HK, Sorensen OH. Effect of intermittent cyclical etidronate therapy on bone mass and fracture rate in women with postmenopausal osteoporosis. N Engl J Med 1990;322:1265–1271.

78. Watts NB, Harris ST, Genant HK, et al. Intermittent cyclical etidronate treatment of postmenopausal osteoporosis. N Engl J Med 1990;323:73–79.

79. Parfitt AM. Dietary risk factors for age-related bone loss and fractures. Lancet 1983;2:1181–1185.

80. Johnson J, Dawson-Hughes B. Precision and stability of dual-energy x-ray absorptiometry measurements. Calcif Tissue Int 1991;49:174–178.

81. Mazess R, Chesnut CH, McClung M, Genant H. Enhanced precision with dual energy x-ray absorptiometry. Calcif Tissue Int 1992;51:14–17.

82. Leblanc AD, Evans HJ, Marsh C, Schneider V, Johnson PC, Jhingran SG. Precision of dual photon absorptiometry measurements. J Nucl Med 1986;27:1362–1365.

83. Shipp CC, Berger PS, Deehr MS, Dawson-Hughes B. Precision of dual photon absorptiometry. Calcif Tissue Int 1988;42:287–292.

84. Lees B, Stevenson JC. An evaluation of dual-energy x-ray absorptiometry and comparison with dual photon absorptiometry. Osteoporosis Int 1992;2:146–152.

85. Kelly TL, Slovik DM, Schoenfeld DA, Neer RM. Quantitative digital radiography versus dual photon absorptiometry of the lumbar spine. J Clin Endocrinol Metab 1988;67:839–847.

86. Strause L, Bracker M, Saltman P, Sartoris D, Kerr E. A comparison of quan-

titative dual energy radiographic absorptiometry and dual photon absorptiometry of the lumbar spine in postmenopausal women. Calcif Tissue Int 1989;45:288–291.

87. Gluer CC, Steiger P, Selvidge R, Ellisesen-Klieforth K, Hayashi C, Genant HK. Comparative assessment of dual photon absorptiometry and dual energy radiography. Radiology 1990;174:223–228.

88. Davies KM, Recker RR, Hinders S, Stegman MR, Heaney RP, Kimmel DB. Third decade bone gain in women. JAMA 1993;268:2403–2408.

89. Rupich RC, Pacifici R, Griffin M, Vered I, Susman N, Avioli LV. Lateral dual energy radiography, a new method for measuring vertebral bone density: a preliminary study. J Clin Endocrinol Metab 1990;70:1768–1770.

90. Slosman DO, Rizzoli R, Donath A, Bonjour JPH. Vertebral bone mineral density measured laterally by dual-energy x-ray absorptiometry. Osteoporosis Int 1990;1:23–29.

91. Uebelhart D, Duboeuf F, Meunier PJ, Delmas PD. Lateral dual photon absorptiometry: a new technique to measure bone density at the lumbar spine. J Bone Miner Res 1990;5:525–531.

92. Orwoll ES, Oviatt SK. The nafarelin/bone study group. 1991 logitudinal precision of dual-energy x-ray absorptiometry (DXA) in a multicenter study. J Bone Miner Res 1991;6:191–198.

93. Wilson CR, Fogelman I, Blake GM, Rodein A. The effect of positioning on dual energy x-ray bone densitometry of the proximal femur. Bone Miner 1991;13: 69–76.

94. Faulkner KG, Gluer CC, Estilo M, Genant HK. Cross calibration of DXA equipment; upgrading from a Hologic QDR 1000/W to a QDR 2000. Calcif Tissue Int 1993;52:79–84.

95. Lindsay R, Fey C, Haboubi A. Dual photon absorptiometric measurements of bone mineral density increase with source life. Calcif Tissue Int 1987;41:293–294.

96. Ross PD, Wasnich RD, Vogel JM. Precision error in dual photon absorptiometry related to source age. Radiology 1988;166:523–527.

97. Dawson-Hughes B, Deehr MS, Berger PS, Dallal GE, Sadowski LJ. Correction of the effects of source, source strength, and soft-tissue thickness on spine dual-photon absorptiometry measurements. Calcif Tissue Int 1989;44:251–257.

98. Verheli LF, Blokland JAK, Papapoulos SE, Bijvoet OLM, Pauwels EKJ. Automated comparison of dual-photon absorptiometric studies of the lumbar spine. J Bone Miner Res 1991;6:575–581.

99. Kellgren JH, Lawrence JS. Osteoarthrosis and disk degeneration in an urban population. Ann Rheum Dis 1958;17: 388–397.

100. Lawrence JS. Generalized osteoarthrosis in a population sample. Am J Epidemiol 1969;90:381–389.

101. Hopkins A, Zylstra S, Hreshchyshyn MM, Anbar M. Normal and abnormal features of the lumbar spine observed in dual energy absorptiometry scans. Clin Nucl Med 1989;14:410–414.

102. Orwoll ES, Oviatt SK, Mann T. The impact of osteophytic and vascular calcifications on vertebral mineral density measurements in men. J Clin Endocrinol Metab 1990;70:1202–1207.

103. Bjarnason K, Overgaard K, Christiansen C. DXA of the lumbar spine vertebral endplate sclerosis may severely confound both anterior and lateral measurements. J Bone Miner Res 1993;8(Suppl 1):S344 (#911).

104. Reid IR, Evans MC, Ames R, Wattie DJ. The influence of osteophytes and aortic calcification on spinal mineral density in postmenopausal women. J Clin Endocrinol Metab 1991;72:1372–1374.

105. Drinka PJ, DeSmet AA, Bauwens SF, Rogot A. The effect of overlying calcification on lumbar bone densitometry. Calcif Tissue Int 1992;50:507–510.

106. Cann CE, Rutt BK, Genant HK. Effect of extraosseous calcification on vertebral mineral measurement. Calcif Tissue Int 1983;35:667.

107. Frohn J, Wilken T, Jeibmann J, Falk S, Stutte H-J, Hor G. Influence of aortic sclerosis on spinal BMC measurements by dual photon absorptiometry. Osteoporosis Int 1991;1:198.

108. Frye MA, Melton LJ, Bryant SC, et al. Osteoporosis and calcification of the aorta. Bone Miner 1992;19:185–194.

109. Farrell TJ, Webber CE. The error due to fat inhomogeneity in lumbar spine bone mineral measurements. Clin Phys Physiol Meas 1989;10:57–64.

110. Hangartner TN, Johnston CC. Influence of fat on bone measurements with dual-energy absorptiometry. Bone Miner 1990;9:71–82.

111. Larnach TA, Boyd SJ, Smart RC, Butler SP, Rohl PG, Diamond TH. Reproducibility of lateral spine scans using dual energy x-ray absorptiometry. Calcif Tissue Int 1992;51:255–258.

112. Mazess RB, Gifford CA, Bisek JP, Barden HS, Hanson JA. DXA measurement of spine density in the lateral projection. I: Methodology. Calcif Tissue Int 1991;49:235–239.

113. Nieves JW, Cosman F, Mars C, Lindsay R. Comparative assessment of bone mineral density of the forearm using single photon and dual x-ray absorptiometry. Calcif Tissue Int 1992;51:352–355.

114. Nelson D, Feingold M, Mascha E, Kleerekoper M. Comparison of single-photon and dual-energy x-ray absorptiometry of the radius. Bone Miner 1992;18:77–83.

115. Sievanen H, Kannus P, Oja P, Vuori I. Precision of dual energy x-ray absorptiometry in the upper extremities. Bone Miner 1993;20:235–243.

116. Weinstein RS, New KD, Sappington LJ. Dual-energy x-ray absorptiometry versus single photon absorptiometry of the radius. Calcif Tissue Int 1991;49:313–316.

117. Larcos G, Wahner HW. An evaluation of forearm bone mineral measurement with dual-energy x-ray absorptiometry. J Nucl Med 1991;32:2101–2106.

118. Kiratli BJ, Heiner JP, McBeath AA, Wilson MA. Determination of bone mineral density by dual x-ray absorptiometry in patients with uncemented total hip arthroplasty. J Orthop Res 1992;10:836–844.

119. Scott DF, Jaffe F, Jaffe W. DXA analysis of femoral remodeling observed with uncemented prosthesis of different designs. J Bone Miner Res 1993;8(Suppl 1):S347 (#922).

120. Hyman JE, Bouxsein ML, Reilly DT, Hayes WC. DXA precisely measures bone mineral density around uncemented and cemented proximal femoral prostheses in vitro. J Bone Miner Res 1993;8(Suppl 1):S350 (#932).

121. Trevisan C, Bigoni M, Cherubini R, Steiger P, Randelli G, Ortolani S. DXA for the evaluation of bone density from the proximal femur after total hip arthroplasty: analysis protocols and reproducibility. Calcif Tissue Int 1993;53:158–161.

122. Bohr HH, Schaadt OP. Structural changes of the femoral shaft with age measured by dual photon absorptiometry. Bone Miner 1990;11:57–362.

123. Beck TJ, Ruff CB, Scott WW, Plato CC, Tobin JD, Quan CA. Sex differences in geometry of the femoral neck with aging: a structural analysis of bone mineral data. Calcif Tissue Int 1992;50:24–29.

124. Faulkner K, Cummings SR, Black D, Palermo L, Gluer CC, Genant HK. Simple measurement of femoral geometry predicts hip fracture: the study of osteoporotic fractures. J Bone Miner Res 1993;8:1211–1218.

125. Amman P, Rizzoli R, Slosman D, Bonjour JP. Sequential and precise in vivo measurement of bone mineral density in rats using dual energy x-ray absorptiometry. J Bone Miner Res 1992;7:311–317.

126. Griffin MG, Kimble R, Hopfer W, Pacifici R. DXA of the rat: accuracy, precision, and measurement of bone loss. J Bone Miner Res 1993;8:795–800.

127. Drezner MK, Nesbitt T. Role of calcitriol in prevention of osteoporosis: Part I. Metabolism 1990;39(Suppl 1):18–23.

128. Mann DR, Gould KG, Collins DC. A potential primate model for bone loss resulting from medical oophorectomy or menopause. J Clin Endocrinol Metab 1990;71:105–110.

129. Jayo MJ, Rankin SE, Weaver DS, Carlson CS, Clarkson TB. Accuracy and precision of lumbar bone mineral content by DXA in live female monkeys. Calcif Tissue Int 1991;49:438–440.

130. Kimmel DB, Wronski TJ. Non-destructive measurement of bone mineral in femurs from ovariectomized rats. Calcif Tissue Int 1990;46:101–110.

131. Kiebzak GM, Smith R, Howe JC, Sacktor B. Bone mineral content in the senescent rat femur: an assessment using single photon absorptiometry. J Bone Miner Res 1988;3:311–317.

132. Awbrey BJ, Hagaman JR, Lester GE, Talmage RV. In vivo bone mineral analysis throughout skeletal growth in rats: differences due to sex or vitamin D deficiency. J Orthop Res 1985;3:456–463.

133. McCloskey EV, Murray SA, Charlesworth D, et al. Assessment of broadband ultrasound attenuation in the os calcis in vitro. Clin Sci 1990;78:221–225.

134. Baran DT, Kelly AM, Karellas A, et al. Ultrasound attenuation of the os calcis in women with osteoporosis and hip fractures. Calcif Tissue Int 1988;43:138–142.

135. Waud CE, Lew R, Baran DT. The relationship between ultrasound and densitometric measurements of bone mass at the calcaneus in women. Calcif Tissue Int 1992; 51:415–418.

136. Herd RJM, Ramalingham T, Ryan PJ, Fogelman I, Blake GM. Measurements of broadband ultrasonic attenuation in the calcaneus in premenopausal and postmenopausal women. Osteoporosis Int 1992;2: 247–251.

137. Damilakis JE, Dretakis E, Gourtsoyiannis NC. Ultrasound attenuation of the calcaneus in the female population: normative data. Calcif Tissue Int 1992;51: 180–183.

138. Palacios S, Menendez C, Calderon J, Rubio S. Spine and femur density and broadband ultrasound attenuation of the calcaneus in normal Spanish women. Calcif Tissue Int 1993;52:99–102.

139. Baran DT, McCarthy CK, Leahey D, Lew R. Broadband ultrasound attenuation of the calcaneus predicts lumbar and femoral neck density in Caucasian women: a preliminary study. Osteoporosis Int 1991;1:110–113.

140. Agren M, Karellas A, Leahey D, Marks S, Baran D. Ultrasound attenuation of the calcaneus: a sensitive and specific discriminator of osteopenia in postmenopausal women. Calcif Tissue Int 1991;48: 240–244.

141. McCloskey EV, Murray SA, Miller C, et al. Broadband ultrasound attenuation in the os calcis: relationship to bone mineral at other skeletal sites. Clin Sci 1990;78:227–233.

142. Jones PRM, Hardman AE, Hudson A, Norgan NG. Influence of brisk walking on the broadband ultrasonic attenuation of the calcaneus in previously sedentary women aged 30–61 years. Calcif Tissue Int 1991;49:112–115.

143. Heaney RP, Avioli LV, Chesnut CH, Lappe J, Recker RR, Brandenburger GH. Osteoporotic bone fragility: detection by ultrasound transmission velocity. JAMA 1989;261:2986–2990.

144. Miller CG, Herd RJM, Ramalingam T, Fogelman I, Blake GM. Ultrasonic velocity measurements through the calcaneus: which velocity should be measured? Osteoporosis Int 1993;3:31–35.

4 ▶ Bone Acquisition in Childhood and Adolescence

▶ ▶ ▶ Laura Bachrach

Senile osteoporosis is a paediatric disease.
—Charles E. Dent (1)

Osteoporosis, for which there is no "cure," is well recognized as a major health problem for the elderly (2,3). At best, current therapy slows the rate of further bone loss or results in small increases in bone mineral. This failure to "cure" osteoporosis emphasizes the need to prevent its occurrence. Bone density and fracture risk in later years are determined by the peak bone mass achieved and the subsequent rate of bone loss during adult life. Thus, the goals of an osteoporosis prevention program are to maximize bone mineral acquisition and minimize subsequent losses. Achievement of these goals requires increased understanding of the process of normal bone mineral accretion in childhood and the determinants of bone loss.

In general, the acquisition of bone mineral parallels skeletal growth in healthy children. Bone mass increases rapidly during infancy, slowly throughout childhood, and substantially again at puberty (4–14). Adolescence is a particularly critical period for bone mineral accretion because at least half the adult bone mass is acquired during the teen years. Genetics, nutrition, sex steroids, and exercise appear to influence the bone mineral status of children, although the relative contribution of each of these factors remains controversial.

Bone mineral reaches a maximum by early adulthood and this peak bone mass serves as the "bone bank" for the remainder of adult life. Thereafter, there are inevitable "withdrawals" from this "account" as secondary bone loss occurs with aging, declining sex steroid levels, and superimposed illness. Continued loss of bone mineral may result in significantly reduced bone mass, a condition termed *osteopenia.* Further decreases may lead to *osteoporosis,* a disruption of normal bone architecture sufficient to produce atraumatic fractures. Although osteoporosis generally presents in the elderly, children and adolescents with chronic illness, malnutrition, or metabolic disorders may also develop significant deficits in bone mineral. Anorexia nervosa, exercise-associated amenor-rhea, delayed puberty, and cystic fibrosis have all been associated with osteopenia in young patients (15–20). The reversibility of these deficits in bone mineral remains uncertain, making early identification and treatment important.

In summary, the bone mineral "well-being" of children and adolescents should be considered a legitimate concern for the pediatrician. As Charles Dent noted 20 years ago, senile osteoporosis has its roots in childhood (1) and pre-vention should begin during the first two decades of life. Childhood and ado-lescence are critical periods for amassing bone mineral, and optimizing bone accretion at this time may delay or prevent the development of symptomatic bone deficits. The goal in counselling healthy children should be to encourage life-style habits that foster bone mineral acquisition. In addition, young patients at risk for early osteoporosis should be identified and appropriate measures taken to augment bone accretion. This chapter reviews patterns of normal bone acquisition throughout childhood and adolescence and the risk factors for os-teopenia in younger patients. The contributions of genetics, nutrition, sex ste-roids, and exercise as determinants of bone mass are considered.

Assessment of Bone Mineral Status

The noninvasive methods available to measure bone mass have been reviewed in detail (21,22). Single photon absorptiometry (SPA) is used to evaluate bone mass in the appendicular skeleton, most commonly at the mid-radius. SPA is rapid and readily available but assesses primarily cortical bone, which predom-inates at these sites. Bone mass is expressed as bone mineral content (BMC), the total grams of bone mineral within a given area of bone, or as bone mineral den-sity (BMD), the BMC normalized for the projected area (in g/cm^2).

Quantitative computerized tomography (QCT) can provide accurate measurements of trabecular bone within lumbar vertebrae; estimates of the cor-tical bone shell can also be derived using this technique. Bone mass is expressed as milligrams of mineral equivalent per cubic centimeter with this technique. Unfortunately, the radiation exposure associated with QCT makes it unaccept-able for repeated use in young subjects.

Dual photon absorptiometry (DPA) and dual energy x-ray absorptio-metry (DXA) can be used to evaluate both the axial skeleton (spine and hip) and the appendicular skeleton (whole body). The bone mineral data derived from DPA and DXA reflect the contribution of both trabecular and cortical bone at axial sites and predominantly cortical bone for the whole body. As with SPA, bone mass data are expressed as BMC and BMD. The speed, precision, and low radiation exposure associated with DXA make it the preferred technique for evaluating bone mineral in children and adolescents.

These techniques are considerably more sensitive than standard radiographs for detecting subtle deficits in bone mineral. Furthermore, repeated measurements provide quantitative data on the progression or reversibility of osteopenia with time and treatment. Bone mineral measurements are also useful for estimating fracture risk because the bone mass at a given skeletal site is related to bone strength. It is estimated that for each standard deviation that BMD falls below predicted mean values for age and sex, the risk of subsequent fracture increases by two- to threefold (23).

The differences among these bone measurement methods must be considered when interpreting published data. Systematic differences between measurements derived from SPA, DPA, DXA, and QTC preclude their interchangeable use. In fact, densitometric results from DPA or DXA equipment from different manufacturers are sufficiently different to prevent their direct comparison. It is also important to consider the relative contribution of cortical versus trabecular bone mass at the site studied because trabecular bone turnover is considerably more rapid than cortical bone. Thus, changes in bone mass may be detected more readily in the lumbar spine than at the mid–radius because of the greater trabecular bone content.

Interpretation of Bone Mineral Status

The assessment of bone mineral in children is considerably more challenging than in adults because of the major changes in bone size that occur during skeletal growth. These changes in bone dimensions confound the interpretation of bone mineral when expressed in conventional terms of BMC or BMD. Neither expression of bone mass accounts for changes in bone *thickness*. Because bone thickness is proportional to its other dimensions, these measures may overestimate the bone mineral in larger bones and underestimate the bone mineral in smaller bones (Fig. 4-1). To detect changes in bone mineral *properties* as distinct from changes in bone *size* requires a new estimate of bone mineral, which is normalized to a derived bone volume.

Two models have recently been developed to approximate *volumetric* bone density using DPA and DXA densitometry data (24,25). The BMC at a given site is corrected for a reference bone volume (V*) which is derived from scaling equations based on bone geometry at that site. These expressions must be viewed as only approximations of true volumetric bone density because bone volume is not measured directly. However, since these estimates minimize the

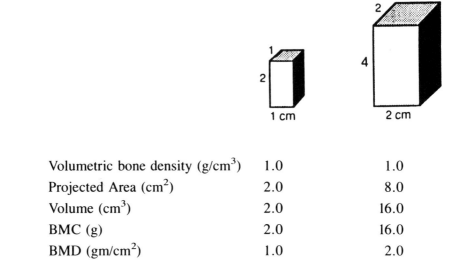

Volumetric bone density (g/cm^3)	1.0	1.0
Projected Area (cm^2)	2.0	8.0
Volume (cm^3)	2.0	16.0
BMC (g)	2.0	16.0
BMD (gm/cm^2)	1.0	2.0

FIGURE 4-1 Effect of bone size on commonly measured bone mineral parameters. Bone densitometry identifies the projected area, which is equal to the area on the front face of the bone. The bone mineral content (BMC) is the total amount of bone mineral (g) in the sample. The bone mineral density (BMD) is calculated as BMC divided by the projected area. Both bone samples have identical volumetric densities; however, the BMD of the larger sample is twice that of the smaller sample. (*Reprinted by permission from Carter DR, Bouxsein ML, Marcus R. New approaches for interpreting projected bone densitometry data. J Bone Miner Res 1992;7:137–145.*)

influence of bone geometry, they represent a reasonable approach for comparing the bone mineral status of bones of differing size. Volumetric bone density models may be particularly useful when evaluating the bone mineral status of growing children when bone size changes dramatically.

To estimate the bone mineral apparent density (BMAD) of the lumbar spine, Carter and colleagues (24) assumed vertebral body thickness to be proportional to its height and width. Thickness of the bone would, therefore, be proportional to the square root of the width times length (which is equivalent to the projected area or A_p measured during densitometry). Therefore, lumbar spine BMAD was calculated using the following formula:

$$\text{BMAD (L}_{2-4}) = \text{BMC} \div A_p^{3/2}$$

Other formulae have been developed to approximate the volume of the femoral neck, mid-radius, and whole body based on geometry of bone in these regions (14).

By contrast, Kroger and coworkers proposed that the geometry of the vertebral column approximates a cylinder (25). BMD for the lumbar spine corrected for volume was estimated as:

$$\text{Spine BMD}_{corr} = \text{BMC} \div \text{Volume} = \text{BMD} \times [4 \div (\pi \times \text{width})]$$

The formulae proposed by Kroger result in systematically lower estimates of the volumetric bone densities than those derived with the Carter formulae. However, both models address the problem of comparing the mineral status in bones of differing size and help to distinguish between bone expansion and gains in bone mineral properties during skeletal growth.

Normative Studies

The growing interest in bone mineral accretion is reflected in the recent proliferation of studies in healthy children and adolescents. This research has helped to define the tempo of bone mineral acquisition and the clinical correlates of bone mass. It is evident from these studies that normative values will be influenced by age, sex, pubertal stage, and body mass as well as by the technique used to determine bone mass. These factors must be considered to interpret accurately the results of bone densitometry in pediatric patients.

Gains in bone mineral occur normally throughout the period of skeletal growth. The rates of bone accretion are greatest in infancy and adolescence, coinciding with the most rapid gains in bone growth. Acquisition of bone mineral plateaus as full pubertal development and final adult height are reached, although the precise timing of peak bone mass remains controversial. In fact, much of the increase in bone mineral can be explained by the expansion of bone volume during skeletal growth. However, the bone mineral per unit volume is also increased at some skeletal sites during adolescence, indicating gains in the mineral *property* of bone as well.

In healthy prepubertal children, gains in skeletal mass are gradual. Early studies demonstrated a steady increase in forearm bone mass with age (4,5,7). More recently, gains in lumbar spine, femur, and whole body bone mineral during childhood have been examined by DPA (9,11,13,14,26,27,51) and DXA (8,10,12,14,25,28). These studies indicated that bone mass increased with age, height, and weight. By contrast, trabecular bone mass in the vertebral spine, as measured by QCT, was unchanged throughout childhood until the onset of puberty (6). These discrepant results may be explained in part by differences in densitometric techniques. DPA and DXA reflect the trabecular and cortical bone mineral whereas QTC measures solely trabecular bone. Furthermore, BMC and BMD measurements by DPA and DXA are influenced by skeletal size to a greater extent than QTC measurements of bone mass.

Bone accretion increases dramatically during puberty. Longitudinal data indicate that girls gain bone mineral most rapidly between the ages of 11 and 14, whereas gains are greatest between 13 and 17 years in boys (28). Net bone min-

TABLE 4-1 Univariate Logarithmic Regressions for Bone Mineral

	r^2		
	BMC	BMD	BMAD
Lumbar spine			
Age	0.684*	0.597*	0.351*
Tanner score	0.739*	0.658*	0.400*
Wt	0.724*	0.609*	0.328*
Ht	0.843*	0.733*	0.424*
Femoral neck			
Age	0.430*	0.430*	0.018
Tanner score	0.547*	0.495*	0.244
Wt	0.602*	0.482*	0.003
Ht	0.727*	0.573*	0.005
Whole body			
Age	0.724*	0.715*	0.004
Tanner score	0.792*	0.709*	0.049
Wt	0.872*	0.714*	0.149
Ht	0.864*	0.702*	0.073
Mid-radius			
Age	0.664*	0.737*	0.304*
Tanner score	0.839*	0.716*	0.230*
Wt	0.647*	0.563*	0.100
Ht	0.746*	0.729*	0.206

*$P < 0.0001$
BMC, bone mineral content; **BMD,** bone mineral density;
BMAD, bone mineral apparent density
(Reprinted by permission from Katzman DR, Bachrach LK,
Carter DR, Marcus R. Clinical and anthropometric correlates
of bone mineral acquisition in healthy adolescent girls. J
Clin Endocrinol Metab 1991;73:1332–1339.)

eral accretion then slows dramatically as sexual maturity and final adult height are attained. Cross-sectional studies have shown a plateau in forearm bone mass at approximately 20 years in women and at 25 years in men (5). Hip, spine, and whole body BMC and BMD appear to plateau by age 16 in females and by age 20 in males (8,10–12,14,25,27) in most studies. This pattern of bone mineral accretion has been confirmed in a recent longitudinal study (28). Females had no significant gains in femoral or spine bone mass between 17 and 20 years, whereas males had small, but significant, increments in lumbar spine and femoral shaft BMD but not femoral neck bone mass until age 20.

How much of these gains in bone mass can be explained by increases in bone size during these periods of dramatic skeletal growth? This question has been addressed by two studies applying expressions of volumetric bone mass. Katzman and colleagues analyzed the bone mineral status of 45 healthy girls, aged 9 to 21 years, using DXA (14). Measurements of lumbar spine, femoral neck, and whole body were expressed as BMC, BMD, and BMAD, and were correlated with several anthropometric variables (Table 4-1). A hierarchy of relationships emerged in which BMC was most strongly correlated, BMD was correlated to an intermediate degree, and BMAD correlated only modestly or without significance to age, weight, height, or body mass index. Thus, most of the age-related changes reflected increasing bone size, rather than greater mineralization of bone matrix. Using the observed correlations, it appeared that 99% of the pubertal gains in whole body bone mineral could be accounted for by bone expansion rather than by an increase in bone mineral per unit volume. At the femoral neck, 96% of the gains appeared due to bone growth. By contrast, only 55% of the change in mid-radial and 50% of the change in lumbar spine bone mineral could be accounted for by expansion of bone volume; the remainder was postulated to reflect enhanced bone mineral property.

▶ 75

Kroger and colleagues also concluded that much of the gain in bone mineral during adolescence resulted from bone expansion (25). The same hierarchy of relationships was noted between age and body size variables and the three expressions of bone mass; correlation coefficients were highest for BMC, slightly lower for BMD, and markedly decreased for BMD_{corr}, the estimated volumetric bone mineral density. Thus, when corrected for changes in bone volume, bone mineral properties at the spine increased slowly through childhood and adolescence but were unchanged at the femoral neck.

Peak Bone Mass

The age at which peak bone mass is attained remains disputed. Several cross-sectional studies have demonstrated a plateau in bone accretion by late adolescence (6,8,11–14,25,27). Femoral neck and lumbar spine bone mass at this time is similar to adult levels, resulting in speculation that bone mass is at or near maximal levels by the end of the second decade (6,12,31). However, other studies have shown gains in bone mass in early adulthood (4,32,33). Healthy women followed longitudinally increased their bone mass up to age 29 (32,33). The amount of bone mineral gained varied by skeletal site, with changes of 4.8% per decade in forearm bone mineral, 6.8% in vertebral bone density, and 12.5% for whole body (33). By contrast, Barden and Mazess observed no increase in lumbar spine BMD among women ages 20 to 39 years studied longitudinally (34). Even if bone mineral increases into early adulthood, it must be emphasized that the gains in the third decade are clearly small when compared with the dramatic mineral accretion of adolescence.

Correlates of Bone Accretion

More than half of the variance in adult bone mass can be attributed to heredity, while nongenetic factors such as physical activity, diet, body mass, sex hormone status, calcium balance, and medications contribute to the remainder (35–38). These factors influence bone mass in children and adolescents as well, although the independent contribution of each remains unknown.

Genetic/Ethnic Determinants

Genetic and ethnic factors are generally viewed as the most important determinants of peak bone mass (35,38–42). However, the mechanism(s) by which genetic factors govern bone mass remains speculative. Inherited similarities in bone size, body composition, and endocrine function likely explain much of the genetic similarities. However, the common environment shared by families and ethnic groups may also contribute to similarities in bone mass.

GENETIC STUDIES

The genetic influence on adult bone density has been confirmed by considerable research (35). An estimated 46% to 80% of the total variance in adult bone mass is attributed to genetic determinants (36,38). The bone mineral status of parents and that of their offspring are highly correlated, whether comparisons are made between mother-daughter pairs (35,40), fathers and sons (38), or both parents and their children (38). Twin studies indicate that the bone mineral status of monozygotic is more similar than that of dizygotic pairs (35,39,41). Heritable factors are proposed to influence both the level of peak bone mass and the subsequent rate of bone loss (40,43).

Similarities in body (and bone) size may explain some differences in bone mass. Furthermore, families share a common environment that may be even more similar in monozygotic twins. Common life-style habits including physical activity, calcium intake, and smoking or alcohol use may contribute to familial resemblance in bone mass. In some follow-up studies, the variance in bone mass among monozygotic twins is similar to that of dizygotic twin pairs, suggesting that genetic determinants play a greater role during childhood and early adulthood, whereas environmental factors exert a greater influence on bone mineral in adulthood (35).

RACIAL/ETHNIC DIFFERENCES

Racial or ethnic differences in adult bone mass and fracture risk have been observed in a number of studies. African-American women are reported to have a greater BMD and a lower incidence of osteoporosis than Caucasian women (44,45); the bone mass of Asian and Hispanic adults has been shown to be less than that in Caucasians (35,46). Several factors complicate any study of ethnic differences. Defining racial or ethnic groups is difficult because ethnic identity may be determined as much by social and cultural factors as by inheritance. Furthermore, diet, activity levels, or other life-style variables are likely to be similar within a given ethnic group. Thus, a combination of genetic and environmental factors may contribute to ethnic differences in bone mass. This complex topic has been reviewed in detail (35,47), and will be discussed only briefly here.

Little is known about ethnic influences on bone mineral acquisition during childhood and adolescence because most recent normative studies in children have been limited to Caucasian subjects. Forty years ago, Trotter and Hixon compared the skeletal weight per unit volume of cadavers from African-Americans and Caucasians; from infancy through adulthood, African-American males and females had denser bones than did Caucasians (48). This racial influence on bone mass has been confirmed by some (7,49–51) but not all (10,27,52) subsequent studies using noninvasive measurement techniques. Mean cortical bone of African-American children exceeds that of Caucasian children in early childhood (7) and adolescence in the United States (7,49,51) but not in South Africa (52). By contrast, comparisons of axial bone density are conflicting. Two studies observed no racial differences in the vertebral bone density of subjects between ages 1 and 19 years (10,27), whereas two others reported that African-American children and teens had significantly greater BMD at the lumbar spine (49,51), trochanter (49), and femoral neck (49) than age-matched Caucasian boys and girls. Most recently Gilsanz and colleagues observed no racial differences in QTC measurements of vertebral bone mass until late puberty, when African-American adolescent girls gained significantly more trabecular bone than Caucasian girls; this resulted in differences in peak bone mass (50). These disparate results may reflect technical differences between DPA (49) and DXA (10) versus QCT (50). Alternatively, the differences may reflect small sample size or geographical diversity.

Data on the skeletal mass of children from other ethnic groups are even more limited. One recent study by McCormick and colleagues observed the vertebral bone density of Hispanic and Caucasian children to be similar (51). Noninvasive studies of bone mass in Caucasian and Asian youth have not been reported.

Comparisons of bone mass between ethnic groups are potentially confounded by differences in body size. As discussed above, conventional expressions of bone mineral may overestimate the bone mineral of larger bones and underestimate the bone mineral of smaller bones. Most studies have addressed the problem of racial differences in body mass by correcting bone mineral data for height or weight. Estimates of volumetric bone mineral (24,25) may prove helpful in determining if racial differences in bone mass represent true differences in bone mineral properties.

If ethnic differences in bone mineral property per se are confirmed, what factor(s) mediates these differences? Studies of bone metabolism indicate a slower rate of bone turnover in African-Americans than Caucasians, which may result in preservation of bone mineral (53). Alternatively, the greater bone mass in African-Americans could be mediated by increased production of factors that influence bone formation and resorption, such as insulin-like growth factor-I, lymphokines, or cytokines (54). In addition, distinctive diet, activity patterns, or other life-style variables may contribute to differences between ethnic groups. Further studies are needed to evaluate the contribution of race and ethnicity to bone mineral acquistion and peak bone mass.

78 ◄

Gender

The influence of gender on bone mineral status remains unsettled. From early childhood, there is evidence that boys have greater radius bone mass than girls (7,9). Although prepubertal boys and girls have similar vertebral spine and femoral neck bone mass in most studies (6,8,10–12,25,51), Thomas and colleagues observed femoral neck, Ward's triangle, and greater trochanter BMD to be greater in young boys (27).

Gender differences have been reported more commonly during adolescence. In the early teen years, vertebral bone mineral has been found to be greater in girls than boys in most (8,12,25,51) but not all (6) studies. In part, this gender-related difference may be explained by the tempo of puberty, which is begun and completed earlier in girls. In one study, replotting bone mineral data by pubertal stage instead of by age eliminated sex differences in vertebral spine bone BMD (Figure 4-2); however, boys had significantly greater femoral neck and shaft BMD as well as lumbar spine BMC after correcting for puberty (12).

Gender differences in skeletal mass persist through late adolescence. Males have greater bone density than females at the mid- and distal radius (5), the femoral neck, and the femoral shaft (12,25). However, vertebral spine BMD has been found to be greater in females than males in some studies (25,51), whereas other studies indicate no significant sex differences at this site (6,10–12,27). Sex differences in adult peak bone mass have also been observed. In a study of adult dizygotic twins (mean age 37 years) of differing within-pair sex, Kelly found males to have higher BMD at the radius, whereas females had greater lumbar spine BMD (55). Femoral neck BMD values were similar for men and women; however, when these values were corrected for differences in BMI, women had significantly greater bone mass than their male co-twins at the hip as well.

Osteoporosis

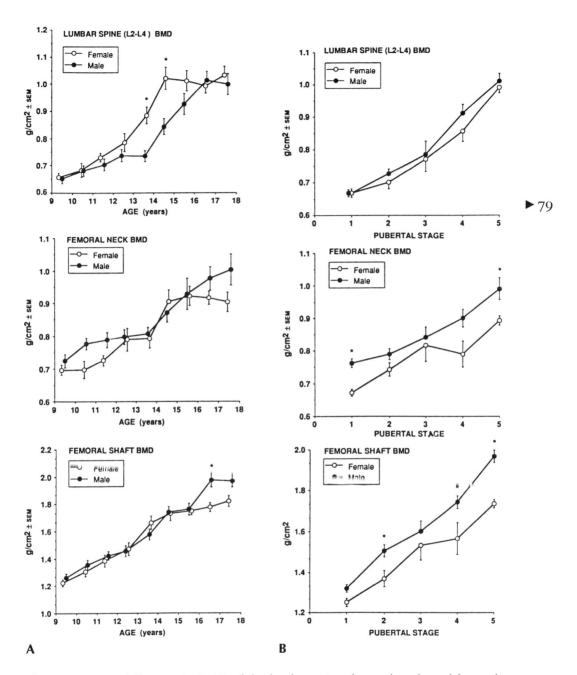

Figure 4-2 Sex difference in BMD of the lumbar spine, femoral neck, and femoral spine. BMD results for males and females are plotted by age (A) and by pubertal stage (B). *P < 0.05 according to Bonferroni's method for multiple comparisons. (*Reprinted by permission from Bonjour J-P, Theintz G, Buchs B, Slosman D, Rizzoli R. Critical years and stages of puberty for spinal and femoral bone mass accumulation during adolescence. J Clin Endocrinol Metab 1991;73:555–563.*)

Any comparison of bone mineral status by gender is potentially confounded by differences in bone size. It is to be expected that the BMC, and to a lesser extent BMD, would be greater in males as a reflection of greater body size. However, gender differences have been observed even when bone mass has been corrected for bone volume (25), suggesting that males and females may differ in bone mineral property at the hip and spine. Kroger and coworkers found that females had greater vertebral bone mass while males had significantly greater femoral neck bone mass (25). By contrast, Gilsanz and colleagues observed no sex difference in vertebral trabecular bone mass as measured by QTC, a technique that is not influenced by bone size (6). Further research on gender-related differences in bone mass is needed to resolve the contribution of gender to peak bone mass.

Environmental Influences

Although genetic factors determine the limits of peak bone mass, environmental factors can modify the outcome. Body mass, calcium nutriture, activity level, endocrine status, drug exposure, and chronic illness will determine whether the genetic potential for peak bone mass is achieved.

BODY MASS

In nearly all studies of young, healthy subjects, body mass has been a significant predictor of bone mass. Whether expressed as weight, height, body surface area, or body mass index (weight/height^2), body size has been shown to correlate with BMC and BMD of both the axial (8–10,12,14,26,28) and appendicular (9,14,15) skeleton. The relationship between body mass and bone mass will be influenced by the term used to express bone mineral. BMC is most affected by bone size, BMD to an intermediate degree, and BMAD or other volumetric expressions least of all. Thus, body mass variables correlate most highly with BMC and least strongly with BMAD (14).

The relationship between body mass and bone mineral status may not be solely an artifact of the terms used to estimate bone mass. Increased body mass increases the mechanical load on the skeleton, which may directly contribute to bone mineral accretion. Furthermore, body mass reflects overall nutritional status. As discussed below, low body mass appears to be an important risk factor for osteopenia in children and young adults.

SEX STEROIDS

Bone accretion increases dramatically during adolescence, coinciding with the onset of puberty in both boys and girls. Since the pubertal growth spurt occurs simultaneously with the rise in sex steroids, it is difficult to separate the contributions of body mass and hormones to bone mineral gains. However, pubertal stage has been shown to predict bone mineral status independently of body mass, supporting an independent effect of sex steroids on bone mineral accretion during adolescence (6,8,10–13).

Although pubertal stage correlates well with bone mineral status in adolescents, the predictive value of sex steroid levels has proven to be variable. Dhuper and colleagues observed that clinical measures of estrogen sufficiency in adolescent girls correlated well with BMD, but that serum estradiol, luteinizing hormone (LH), follicle-stimulating hormone (FSH), prolactin, and dehydroepiandrosterone sulfate (DHEAS) levels did not (17). Other studies have found a significant correlation between estrogen (56) or androgen levels (17,56,57) and bone density in young females. Thus, a combination of clinical and laboratory assessments may be needed to fully explore the relationship between bone density and sex steroids.

▶ 81

DIETARY CALCIUM

The importance of calcium nutriture to bone health remains controversial, but a growing literature supports its link to bone mass. Of 43 studies published since 1988, 26 found a significant link between calcium intake and bone mass, bone loss, or fractures (58). Retrospective studies have shown a correlation between reported milk intake in childhood and bone mass in later life (59–61). Furthermore, peak bone mass is lower and the fracture incidence higher in geographical areas of low dietary calcium intake when compared to regions with normal intake (61). From a meta-analysis of the literature to date, calcium intake accounts for a measurable amount of the variability in adult bone mass (62). Approximately 15% of the variance in the bone mineral status of postmenopausal women can be explained by calcium nutriture (37).

Calcium balance at any age reflects calcium intake, absorption, and excretion. In healthy children, calcium intake and vitamin D are the major determinants of calcium balance (30). Calcium requirements are maximal during infancy and adolescence, when skeletal growth is most rapid. To meet these needs, calcium retention during puberty must be twice the childhood rate (63). Paradoxically, urinary calcium losses increase during adolescence, reducing net calcium retention at a period of greatest need (63). The current recommended daily allowance for calcium intake is 800 mg for ages 1 to 10 years and 1200 mg from ages 11 to 24 years (64). However, based on calcium balance studies, this recommendation may be too low and Heaney has proposed that the optimal daily calcium requirement for adolescents may approximate 1600 mg (63). Unfortunately, as calcium requirements reach their peak because of skeletal growth, adolescents tend to reduce their dietary calcium. In fact, the calcium intake of American adolescents typically falls well below the dietary recommendations for calcium (14,65,66). In one study, only 15% of the girls and 53% of the boys over age 11 met the recommended dietary allowance for calcium (67).

If calcium intake is low, optimal bone accretion may not occur. Studies have demonstrated a correlation between reported calcium intake and bone mineral in children (67) and young adults (68), whereas other have not (8,14). These differences may be explained by inherent inaccuracies of dietary recall or by sample sizes that are inadequate to detect a small contribution of calcium to bone mass. If variation in calcium balance accounts for only 15% to 20% of the variability in bone mass (37), this effect may be obscured by more dramatic changes in body mass and pubertal development. To complicate the analysis further, calcium intake may be linked to other environmental and behavioral patterns that influence bone mass and confound the results. For example, teens with high activity levels may have greater dietary calcium intake than their more sedentary peers.

The limited data from intervention studies also support the influence of calcium intake on bone mass in healthy children. Matkovic and coworkers reported greater gains in bone mineral in 20 adolescent girls who received calcium supplementation than in 8 nonsupplemented controls although these differences were not statistically different (69). In a 3-year study of 45 identical twin pairs, Johnston and colleagues found that subjects receiving daily calcium supplements of 700 mg had greater increases in bone mineral than their placebo-treated twins (70). However, gains in bone mass with calcium supplementation were significant only in those children who remained prepubertal throughout the study (Table 1). This observation may indicate that supplementation must be given early to be effective; alternatively, the supplemental dose may have been inadequate in the adolescent subjects or the influence of calcium overshadowed by changes in bone mass associated with pubertal growth and development. Regardless, this study has important implications because calcium supplementation appeared beneficial in these well-nourished children already receiving close to the recommended daily allowance of calcium.

Whether gains in bone mass with calcium supplementation are sustained remains a concern. Fehily and colleagues compared the bone mineral status of 371 young adults (ages 20–23 years) who had participated 14 years earlier in a 2-year milk supplementation trial (71). No significant differences were observed in forearm bone mineral between the intervention and control groups. Further studies are needed to determine the critical timing and dosage of calcium supplementation and the duration required to influence adult bone mass.

TABLE 4-2 Difference in Bone Mineral Density between the Calcium-Supplement and Placebo Groups, According to Pubertal Status

Site	Prepubertal Twins (22 Pairs)	Pubertal or Postpubertal Twins (23 Pairs)
	% difference (95% confidence interval)	
Midshaft radius	5.1 (1.5-8.7)	−0.1 (−3.0-2.9)
Distal radius	3.8 (1.4-6.2)	2.9 (−0.7-6.5)
Lumbar spine	2.8 (1.1-4.5)	−1.0 (−3.2-1.2)
Femoral neck	1.2 (−1.6-4.0)	−0.4 (−3.4-2.5)
Ward's triangle	2.9 (−0.1-5.9)	−0.4 (−3.7-2.9)
Greater trochanter	3.5 (−0.2-7.1)	0.2 (−3.6-4.1)
Average	2.9 (0.9-4.9)	0.3 (−1.6-2.2)

▶ 83

(Reprinted by permission of the New England Journal of Medicine from Johnston CC, Miller JZ, Slemenda CW, et al. Calcium supplementation and increases in bone mineral density in children. N Engl J Med 1992;327:82–87.)

Other nutrients may also influence bone mineral acquisition but have received far less attention. One study found no correlation between calcium and bone mass but observed the ratio of calcium/protein to be predictive of bone mineral status (33). Dhuper and colleagues observed that high fiber intake was negatively correlated with bone mass (17), perhaps reflecting the effects of fiber on calcium absorption and balance (72,73) and sex steroid levels (74). Further studies of dietary fiber, protein, phosphorus, and trace minerals are needed to determine their contribution to bone mineral status.

EXERCISE

Despite the widespread belief that weight-bearing activity promotes bone mineral, this has been difficult to prove quantitatively. In laboratory animals, bone mass has been shown to increase with mechanical loading on the skeleton and to decline rapidly with inactivity (75). Furthermore, elite athletes have significantly greater bone mass than sedentary controls (76,77). However, the impact of more moderate exercise on bone mineral status is less well established. Exercise history has correlated with bone mass in some studies (25,33,68,71,78). Slemenda and colleagues observed a positive correlation between weight-bearing activities and BMD in the radius, spine, and hip, which persisted after correction for age and gender effects (78). From their data, the authors estimated that more active children might gain 5% to 10% more bone mass through adolescence than less active peers. Other studies have failed to find a correlation between activity levels and skeletal mass at any site (10,14,79). These discrepancies may reflect the variety of questionnaires and activity diaries used to estimate activity patterns, as well as the errors of self-reported recall. Furthermore, most studies examined only recreational activity, overlooking the possible contribution of skeletal loading from nonrecreational activities (such as lifting, climbing stairs). As with calcium nutriture, the independent contribution of activity to bone mass may be small in comparison to the influence of body mass, hormonal status, or other variables. For adolescent girls, dramatic changes in bone mass with growth and puberty may have obscured a lesser effect of exercise (14).

Even well-controlled prospective studies have led to conflicting conclusions about the impact of exercise on adult bone mass. Snow-Harter and colleagues observed small but significant gains in bone mineral in a group of college women after 8 months of resistance training or running; control subjects who maintained their habitual activity showed no gains in bone mineral during this period (79). Training increased vertebral but not femoral neck bone mass, perhaps reflecting the greater contribution of trabecular bone in the spine. Studies in older premenopausal women found that weight training resulted in insignificant gains (80) or measurable loss (81) of vertebral bone mineral. It is evident that more research is needed to resolve questions concerning the type and intensity of activity needed to enhance bone mass and whether the response is influenced by age.

Interaction of Variables

In summary, the achievement of peak bone mass is analogous to attainment of final adult height; the genetic potential for skeletal mass is predetermined but the peak bone mass actually attained will be influenced by environmental variables such as nutrition, physical activity, and endocrine function (36). In assessing the influence of nature versus nurture, Kelly has proposed that life-style factors such as calcium intake and activity have the greatest impact on individuals with the greatest genetic potential (36). However, for individuals dealt a family history of osteoporosis, maximizing skeletal mass through diet and activity may be critical to delay or prevent fractures.

Acquisitional Osteopenia

Although osteoporosis is predominantly an affliction of the elderly, significant deficits in bone mineral can develop in childhood and adolescence. Osteoporosis has been observed as early as the neonatal period, particularly in the premature infant. Risk factors for bone mineral deficits in infancy include younger gestational age, chronic diuretic use, prolonged parenteral feeding, and chronic pulmonary disease (82). Fortunately, premature infants with an uncomplicated neonatal course generally recover from this deficit, achieving a normal BMC by 6 to 12 months of age (83). Osteoporosis of prematurity has been reviewed (82) and is not discussed further in this chapter. Genetic disorders causing osteoporosis such as osteogenesis imperfecta (84) and lysinuric protein intolerance (85) are also not discussed.

Beyond infancy, risk factors for osteopenia include malnutrition, low body weight, hormone deficiencies, and chronic illness. These factors are associated with reduced bone mass, although it is unknown how much of the deficit results from reduced bone formation versus accelerated bone loss. Because adolescence is a critical period for amassing bone, the impact of illness at this time may be profound and potentially prolonged.

Delayed Puberty

Delayed sexual maturation predisposes to osteopenia that may persist into adulthood. Warren and colleagues observed significantly more fractures and scoliosis in female ballet dancers with late menarche than those who progressed normally through puberty (18). The greater the delay in menses, the more likely these disorders were to occur. Although bone mass was not formally assessed in this study, the stress fractures were assumed to reflect inadequate bone mineral, and the scoliosis was attributed to delayed epiphyseal closure and reduced spine stability. Estrogen deficiency was presumed to contribute to osteopenia, but nutritional factors were also implicated because these girls were underweight and had inadequate calcium and vitamin D intake. The reversibility of the deficits in bone mass was not addressed in this cross-sectional study.

Delayed puberty in boys has also been associated with bone mineral deficits (19). Finkelstein and colleagues examined the bone mineral status of young men whose puberty had begun after age 15. Peak bone mass was significantly lower in these men when compared to controls without a history of delayed puberty; nearly half had forearm or vertebral bone densities 1 SD or more below the normal mean. Because these subjects were otherwise healthy, delayed puberty was the only identified risk factor for osteopenia. These data suggest that even transient sex steroid deficiency during adolescence may result in sustained deficits in bone mass.

Other studies also underscore the importance of pubertal timing for peak bone mass. Males with idiopathic hypogonadotropic hypogonadism are osteopenic as adolescents and achieve low peak bone mass as adults despite sex steroid replacement (86). It is possible that some factor(s) associated with hypogonadism per se contributes to osteopenia in these patients. Alternatively, earlier replacement of sex steroids might be necessary to prevent persistent deficits in bone mass. Further research is needed to define the optimal time to initiate hormone therapy for all forms of delayed puberty.

Anorexia Nervosa

Anorexia nervosa is a psychiatric disorder characterized by low body weight, an intense fear of weight gain, and amenorrhea (87). This eating disorder presents most commonly in middle to late adolescence, when major gains in bone mineral are expected. Bone accretion may be interrupted and bone loss accelerated by the estrogen deficiency, malnutrition, low body mass, and hypercortisolism associated with anorexia nervosa.

Despite the fact that anorexia nervosa typically presents in adolescence, the sequelae of this disorder have been studied primarily in adult patients. Osteoporosis and pathologic fractures are established complications of chronic anorexia nervosa in adult women (88–92). With treatment, these deficits appear to be at least partially reversible. Charig and Fletcher observed that bone mass was improved in patients who gained weight but had not resumed menses; the bone mineral status of women who recovered both weight and menstrual function was normal (93). Other studies have observed persistent deficits in bone mass despite apparent recovery. Our own group observed that lumbar spine bone density remained more than 2 SD below normal in 3 of 9 weight-rehabilitated women (94). Similarly, Rigotti noted that radius bone mineral was not significantly improved by weight gain, calcium supplements, exercise, resumption of menses, or estrogen therapy in 27 women at varying stages of recovery from anorexia nervosa (95). These women continued to have an increased rate of non-spine fractures as well.

Considerably less is known about the impact of anorexia nervosa on bone mass during adolescence. Most data on younger patients consists of case reports of pathologic fractures or studies in which data from adolescent patients and older women have been combined (89–91,96). Our group compared 18 teens with anorexia nervosa (mean age 16.6 years) to healthy controls of similar age and observed significant deficits in bone mineral (97). Girls with anorexia nervosa had deficits of 20% to 25% in mean lumbar spine and whole body bone densities when compared with normals; mid-radius bone mineral was not significantly reduced for age. Two thirds of the patients had marked osteopenia with bone densities at or below −2 SD and half of these had been ill for less than 1.5 years. This may indicate that osteopenia occurs more rapidly in younger patients with eating disorders or that the illness had gone unrecognized for a longer period. Body mass, age at onset, and duration of anorexia nervosa predicted bone mineral status; calcium intake and reported activity levels were not significantly correlated with bone mineral density at any site.

Osteoporosis

Although this study indicated that adolescents with anorexia nervosa face a significant risk of osteopenia, several questions remain unanswered. Did the deficit in bone mineral result from decreased bone accretion, accelerated bone loss, or both? Was the osteopenia reversible with recovery? To address these issues, 15 of the 18 patients described above were restudied one year later (94). Change in bone density was highly correlated with change in body mass, and skeletal mass improved in girls who gained weight but had not resumed menses. Patients who failed to gain weight had unchanged or even decreased bone mineral. Despite gains in bone mass at follow-up, mean bone density in these patients was −1 to −1.5 SD below normal for age at the spine and whole body, respectively, raising concerns that some deficits may not be fully reversible. ▶87

Treatment of osteopenia associated with anorexia nervosa includes weight rehabilitation. Nutritional support is a safe and rational therapy because bone density increases with weight gain, even before the return of menses (93,94). It is also prudent to ensure adequate daily calcium (1200 mg/d) despite difficulties in demonstrating a relationship between calcium intake and bone mass in this disorder (92,97).

The role of exercise and sex steroids in treating osteopenia in this disorder is more controversial. Seeman and colleagues observed that young women with anorexia nervosa who had received with oral contraceptives had significantly greater spine bone density than patients who had not been given estrogen, although both groups remained significantly below normal for age. No protective effect of estrogen was detected at the femoral neck (92). Whether earlier intervention or a higher replacement dose would improve outcome remains unanswered. Little is known about the effect of estrogen therapy on adolescent patients. However, a 10% gain in spine bone density was observed in a single patient following treatment with oral contraceptives despite ongoing weight loss (94). Estrogen is contraindicated in young patients with open epiphyses because the therapeutic dose required to prevent bone loss in adults will accelerate skeletal maturation, thus compromising final adult height (98).

The potential benefits of exercise in anorexia nervosa must be weighed against the risks of pathologic fractures, prolonged amenorrhea, and slower weight rehabilitation. Some studies have shown a protective effect of activity both at weight-bearing (92,99) and non−weight-bearing sites (88), whereas others have failed to confirm this benefit (96,97).

Exercise-Induced Amenorrhea

Intense physical training increases the risk of osteoporosis and fractures in men (100) and women (101–104). These complications have been studied most extensively in amenorrheic adult athletes. Cann and coworkers reported significant reductions in lumbar spine bone density in physically active amenorrheic women when compared with sedentary eumenorrheic controls (103). Subsequently, Drinkwater and colleagues (104) and Marcus and coworkers (101) observed that amenorrheic athletes had significantly lower vertebral bone density than eumenorrheic athletes. Intensive exercise appeared to have a less deleterious effect on the appendicular skeleton; radial BMD has been consistently normal (101,104) but some deficits have been observed in other cortical sites (105). The greater loss of axial bone mass has also been confirmed in a study of adolescent athletes (17).

Three patterns of reproductive dysfunction have been associated with intensive exercise. Delayed puberty and primary amenorrhea may occur when the activity is begun before puberty, and menarche may be delayed by as much as 5 months for each year of training (106,107). Even without premenarchal training, however, there is a high incidence of delayed menarche in endurance runners, perhaps reflecting a selection factor for girls with a young adolescent physique (108). When intensive activity is initiated after menarche, secondary oligomenorrhea or amenorrhea occurs in as many as 5% to 50% of women (108). Milder disturbances in the menstrual cycle, such as shortened luteal phases, may occur more frequently but elude clinical detection (109). In most cases, disturbances in reproductive function can be reversed within 2 to 6 months if physical activity is reduced (110) and bone mineral status improves in adults with return of menses (111). The reversibility of osteopenia in adolescent athletes has not been adequately determined. Theintz and colleagues have observed that linear bone growth is compromised in adolescent gymnasts who fail to exhibit a pubertal growth spurt; final height predictions are reduced in these girls (112). Whether permanent deficits in bone mass accompany this abnormality in linear growth is a concern (113).

Although sex steroid deficiency likely contributes to exercise-associated osteopenia, poor nutrition has also been implicated. Not uncommonly, athletes limit their intake of calories, fat, protein, and calcium (108). Malnutrition increases the risk of reproductive dysfunction (114) and reduced body mass may contribute directly to osteopenia. Stress fractures in dancers with marginal nutrition precede apparent changes in bone density, suggesting that a decline in the quality of bone mineral may develop before detectable changes in bone mass (115). Increased production of endogenous opioids or glucocorticoids has also been proposed to contribute to osteopenia in athletes (116).

Although less is known about the impact of exercise-induced menstrual dysfunction in adolescents, strenuous training in teens must be viewed as a risk for osteopenia if associated with delayed puberty or amenorrhea. This has prompted a series of recommendations by the Committee on Sports Medicine of the American Academy of Pediatrics (117). A complete evaluation, including physical examination and nutritional assessment, is indicated for adolescents with delayed menarche or secondary amenorrhea. In addition, thyroxine, thyroid-stimulating hormone (TSH), prolactin, estradiol, LH, and FSH should be measured to evaluate thyroid and ovarian function and to rule out hyperprolactinemia; a pregnancy test should be performed in sexually active teens. Additional studies may be appropriate including a bone age examination to assess the extent of delay in skeletal and pubertal maturation and bone densitometry to determine if significant osteopenia has developed.

Treatment guidelines for amenorrheic athletes have been outlined by the American Academy of Pediatrics (117). These include ensuring adequate daily protein and calcium intake. Estrogen replacement was not advised for amenorrheic athletes within 3 years of menarche. For amenorrheic athletes over age 16, sex hormone therapy with low-dose oral contraceptives was considered "reasonable." Unfortunately, no prospective studies assess the efficacy of estrogen replacement in amenorrheic athletes. One retrospective study has suggested that the risk of stress fractures may be diminished with oral contraceptive use (102), but controlled prospective trials are needed to determine if estrogen can reverse osteopenia associated with intensive exercise. Until studies are performed, estrogen therapy may be reserved for teens seeking contraception. Ensuring that athletes improve their nutrition and diminish the intensity of exercise may prove to be a safer and more effective alternative to hormone therapy.

▶ 89

Turner Syndrome

Females with Turner syndrome are another population at risk for osteopenia because of estrogen deficiency. This syndrome, caused by absence or deletion of the second X chromosome, is associated with short stature, diverse anatomic abnormalities and primary ovarian failure (118). Without treatment, most patients with Turner syndrome have low to undetectable estrogen levels throughout adolescence. Unlike girls with anorexia nervosa, patients with Turner syndrome have normal to increased weight-to-height ratios. Therefore, bone mineral studies in these patients provide insight into impact of estrogen deficiency on adolescent bone accretion without the confounding variable of low body mass.

Osteopenia has been described commonly in adults with Turner syndrome. Initial studies demonstrated that the bone mineral content of the calcaneus or radius was markedly reduced in some, but not all, patients (119–121). Sex steroid replacement has been shown to ameliorate this osteopenia. The mean vertebral BMC of women receiving estrogen treatment was 2.3 SD below expected as compared with a mean of −4.5 SD in untreated Turner patients (122). Vertebral bone mineral has been shown to correlate with the duration of estrogen replacement in these patients (123). Despite the reported osteopenia, none of these studies of Turner women has observed an increased incidence of pathologic fractures.

Data on the bone mineral status of children and adolescents with Turner syndrome are inconsistent. Using conventional radiographs, the vertebrae and carpal bones of these patients frequently have a coarse trabecular pattern and reduced cortical thickness (124). Significant deficits of the mid-radius BMC and BMD have been observed using SPA (121,125). DPA measurements of spine BMD have been reported as normal in younger teens with Turner syndrome (125,126), whereas patients 14 years or older have been found to have a normal (125,127) or reduced spine BMD (126). These discrepancies may be explained in part by patient selection because some girls had received growth hormone or estrogen therapy while others were untreated.

None of these earlier studies addressed the problems of interpreting the bone mineral status in Turner patients in light of their short stature and delayed puberty. Girls with Turner syndrome are significantly shorter than age-matched controls and conventional expressions of bone mass likely underestimate the bone mineral properties of these smaller bones. In addition, females with Turner syndrome typically have delayed skeletal maturation with bone ages of 1 to 3 years below chronologic age. Spontaneous puberty is similarly delayed or may not occur without estrogen supplementation. Because bone mineral acquisition is normally highly correlated with pubertal development, these delays in maturation may lead to underestimation of bone mineral.

Neely and colleagues recently evaluated the bone mineral status in adolescents with Turner syndrome addressing both of these concerns (127). The bone mass of 19 adolescents with Turner syndrome was evaluated by DPA of the lumbar spine and whole body and compared with a normal female control group of the same mean age (14.3 years). Mean height and Tanner breast stage were greater in controls than in the Turner patients. Vertebral spine and whole body BMC were significantly lower in the Turner subjects than in the normal girls, but mean spine and whole body BMD was not significantly lower in the Turner population. Mean BMAD for these sites was identical in the two groups. These data suggest that the differences in bone mass between adolescents with Turner syndrome and age-matched controls can be explained largely by differences in body (and bone) size. As expected, the Turner patients had delays of 1 to 3 years in skeletal age relative to chronologic age and delayed breast development as well. When the bone mineral data of patients were evaluated relative to bone age and pubertal stage, BMD and BMAD were equal to or greater than control values.

This is not to say that sex steroid therapy is without benefit in Turner patients. As noted above, estrogen therapy in adult patients appears to improve but not normalize bone mass. Similarly, longitudinal studies in 10 adolescents indicated more rapid gains in bone mineral in Turner girls treated with estrogen than those without this supplement (125). However, this study does provide reassurance that girls with Turner syndrome treated with growth hormone maintain a normal rate of bone mineral accretion through the mid-teens without estrogen replacement. Thus, the initiation of sex steroid replacement can be determined by personal preference and growth considerations without jeopardizing skeletal health in these patients.

Cystic Fibrosis

Cystic fibrosis is an inherited multisystem disease characterized by chronic pulmonary disease and failure of the exocrine pancreas. With recent advances in medical care, the expected life span of these patients increased from a median age of 10 years in 1968 to more than 30 years in 1988 (128). However, survival to adulthood has been shadowed by the emergence of serious medical complications including diabetes (129), infertility (130), and osteopenia (131–133).

Deficits in bone mineral are detectable from early childhood in cystic fibrosis. Decreased cortical bone has been observed using conventional x-ray (133) and SPA (133,134) in all but one study (135). Gibbons and colleagues found deficits in trabecular bone mass as measured by QTC in a group of 57 cystic fibrosis patients (20). Mean vertebral bone density was 10% lower in patients than age-matched healthy controls and 14% had bone densities at or below -2 SD. The severity of osteopenia was correlated with disease severity and nutritional status.

Osteopenia and osteoporosis have also been observed in adults with cystic fibrosis. Stead and coworkers observed a significant reduction in mid-radius bone mass (131) and our group noted significant deficits in vertebral, hip, and whole body bone mineral (132). Since the patients with cystic fibrosis were smaller than healthy controls, comparisons of BMC and BMD were potentially misleading. However, estimates of volumetric BMAD were also significantly reduced in the patients when compared with controls. Thus, the deficit in bone mineral could not be explained by the reduced body and bone size of these patients. Three of these young adults had experienced atraumatic rib or hip fractures, indicating that bone fragility was increased.

The determinants of osteopenia in cystic fibrosis have not been fully defined, although several potential risk factors can be identified. Disease severity has been shown to predict bone mass in pediatric patients (20) but not in young adults (132). Reduced body mass has also correlated with deficits in bone mineral (20,132). Vitamin D deficiency has been linked with osteopenia (131,132) and inadequate calcium nutriture may also be a factor. Delayed puberty and hypogonadism, commonly seen in cystic fibrosis patients, may also contribute to osteopenia in adolescents and adults, although this has not been shown definitively (132). Chronic glucocorticoid therapy is an additional risk factor but no significant correlation between steroid use and bone mineral has been shown to date (132). Similarly, the contribution of physical activity (or inactivity) in cystic fibrosis has not been adequately assessed.

Since the etiology of osteopenia in cystic fibrosis is incompletely understood, optimal therapy has not been determined. However, it appears rational and without risk to optimize the nutritional status of patients both to increase body mass and to ensure adequate protein, calcium, and phosphorus intake. Vitamin D supplementation should be provided at a dose sufficient to achieve normal serum 25-hydroxyvitamin D levels. Testosterone therapy should be considered in hypogonadal men and in boys with significantly delayed puberty (136). Sex steroid replacement may also be indicated for amenorrheic women if such therapy is tolerated without exacerbating pulmonary symptoms (137). The efficacy of other antiresorptive agents such as calcitonin or bisphosphonates has not been studied systematically. As with all forms of osteoporosis, strategies to prevent osteopenia may prove more effective than efforts to reverse established deficits. Therefore, the bone mineral status should be evaluated from childhood in patients with cystic fibrosis.

Other Endocrine Disorders

Endocrine disorders other than hypogonadism have been linked with osteopenia. Growth hormone deficiency and diabetes mellitus have been linked with osteopenia in children; the effects of hyperthyroidism and hyperprolactinemia on bone mass have been evaluated predominantly in adult patients. The impact of these endocrinopathies on bone accretion and bone loss in childhood and adolescence is reviewed briefly.

GROWTH HORMONE DEFICIENCY

Growth hormone and the insulin-like growth factors (IGFs) are important regulators of bone growth and remodeling (138). Not unexpectedly, growth hormone excess or deficiency alters skeletal mass. Untreated children with growth hormone deficiency have low bone mineral for age (139–141). Some of this osteopenia can be explained by delayed skeletal maturation, but bone mass remains significantly reduced even when corrected for bone age (139,141). Deficits of cortical bone of the appendicular skeleton are greater than those of the spine and hip. This osteopenia is thought to be due to direct effects of growth hormone/IGF-I on both bone cells and vitamin D metabolism. Bio-chemical markers of bone formation are reduced in untreated patients, supporting the view that bone cell activity is reduced in growth hormone/IGF-I deficiency (137,139). Renal hydroxylation of 25-hydroxyvitamin to the active 1,25-dihydroxyvitamin D form is also reduced in growth hormone deficiency (141,142).

Skeletal mass increases with growth hormone (hGH) therapy if given at an adequate dose and frequency. Although thrice weekly injections of hGH (0.3 IU/kg/wk) stimulated linear growth, this treatment regimen failed to result in significant gains in bone mineral of the radius, ulna, and humerus (139); with higher doses of hGH (0.5 to 0.6 IU/kg/wk) given at a frequency of 6 times per week, bone accretion increased (140,141). Whether bone mass can be fully restored to normal remains controversial. Saggese and colleagues reported complete recovery of bone mass in nearly half of the 26 children studied after only a year of hGH therapy (141). However, a study of 30 adults with growth hormone deficiency since childhood noted persistent deficits in bone mass despite hGH therapy (143). Since the rate of bone loss was not increased in these young adults, osteopenia was attributed to inadequate bone mineral accretion during childhood and adolescence. The deficit in peak bone mass could be due to inadequate dosing, since most of the subjects had been treated with a thrice weekly hGH regimen. Alternatively, other pituitary hormone deficiencies present in most of the patients may have contributed to reduced bone mass. However, future research should examine peak bone mass achieved with adequate growth hormone dosing and address the need for ongoing hGH therapy to optimize and maintain peak bone mass after linear growth is complete.

DIABETES MELLITUS

The association between diabetes mellitus and osteopenia was first noted more than 30 years ago (144), but the frequency and pathogenesis of bone mineral deficits in diabetics remain controversial. Decreased cortical bone mineral has been observed both in children and adolescents with insulin-dependent diabetes mellitus (IDDM); forearm bone mass was reduced for age in as many as 25% of these patients (145–147). Deficits were more common in males and were unrelated to duration of illness in most studies. The osteopenia could not be explained by the delayed skeletal maturation associated with IDDM since bone mass remained low after correction for bone age.

In contrast to these studies of the appendicular skeleton, Ponder and colleagues observed lumbar spine BMD to be normal in 56 children with IDDM (148). Boys who had IDDM for more than one year had significantly reduced weight and height for age, but BMD corrected for height was normal. Duration of IDDM and current metabolic control were not significantly correlated with lumbar BMD. Further longitudinal studies are needed to clarify the relative risk and clinical correlates of osteopenia in IDDM.

HYPERTHYROIDISM

Thyroid hormone excess increases bone resorption and may result in significant loss of trabecular bone (149). The accelerated bone resorption associated with thyrotoxicosis raises serum calcium and phosphorus concentrations, in turn suppressing parathyroid hormone levels and reducing the conversion of 25-hydroxyvitamin D to 1,25-dihydroxyvitamin D. As a result, intestinal calcium absorption is reduced and urinary calcium loss is increased. The risk of osteoporosis increases with the severity and duration of hyperthyroidism and the presence of other risk factors, such as estrogen deficiency.

Bone loss was first described in adults with Graves' disease and other forms of endogenous hyperthyroidism (150). More recent studies have shown that excessive thyroxine replacement, sufficient to suppress serum TSH, may produce similar deficits in bone mineral (149). Little is known about the impact of thyroid hormone excess in childhood. Children with congenital hypothyroidism warrant particular attention because relatively large doses of thyroxine are prescribed from birth in these patients to ensure normal intellectual development (151). Until further research is completed, it appears prudent to avoid supraphysiologic doses of thyroxine by maintaining serum TSH levels within the normal range. Hyperthyroidism due to Graves' disease warrants prompt medical or surgical intervention to avoid potential bone loss. Bone mineral deficits are likely to be reversible in childhood and adolescence as the hyperthyroidism is corrected.

GLUCOCORTICOID EXCESS

Osteoporosis is a well-established complication of glucocorticoid excess in children as well as adults (152). Glucocorticoids act directly to inhibit bone formation and indirectly increase bone resorption activity by altering calcium homeostasis. Steroids inhibit intestinal calcium absorption and may suppress renal tubular calcium resorption. The combination of reduced absorption and increased renal excretion may result in secondary hyperparathyroidism and increased bone resorption. The typical skeletal manifestations of glucocorticoid excess are osteopenia and osteoporosis affecting both the appendicular and axial skeleton. Avascular necrosis of the femoral head is a less common complication. Pathologic fractures occur most frequently in the ribs and vertebrae.

Although Cushing's disease and other forms of cortisol overproduction can lead to bone loss, steroid-induced osteoporosis results more commonly from prolonged glucocorticoid therapy. Bone loss may begin soon after initiation of glucocorticoid therapy, but the risk of bone disease in several studies is related to the cumulative dose of glucocorticoids used. In children treated for juvenile arthritis, vertebral fractures were observed only after a cumulative dose of greater than 5 g prednisone; once this threshold was surpassed, the risk of fracture correlated with mean daily dose of steroid (153). However, the risk of steroid-induced bone loss may also be influenced by other factors associated with the underlying disorder requiring glucocorticoid therapy. Chronic illness, decreased mobility, malnutrition, malabsorption, sex steroid deficiency, or renal dysfunction accompanying chronic diseases are likely to limit bone accretion or exacerbate bone loss.

▶ 95

No effective means of preventing or treating steroid-related bone loss has been established. Disorders of glucocorticoid overproduction, such as Cushing's disease, should be treated expeditiously, and partial recovery of bone mass can be anticipated (154). Treatment options are more limited for patients who require steroid therapy to control inflammatory disease (152). Glucocorticoid therapy should be reduced to the lowest effective dose because the risk of associated osteopenia appears to be dose-related. Whether alternate-day steroids results in less bone loss than daily dosing remains controversial. Intranasal glucocorticoids (155) and newer steroid derivatives, such as deflazacort (156,157), have shown bone-sparing effects in a small number of children and warrant further study. Daily supplements with vitamin D and calcium are reasonable to offset increased urinary calcium excretion. Inhibitors of bone loss, such as calcitonin, have been shown to improve bone mineral status in small numbers of glucocorticoid-treated children (158).

HYPERPROLACTINEMIA

Hyperprolactinemia and its complications develop typically in early adulthood (159). However, this disorder has been observed in adolescents and must be considered in the differential diagnosis of delayed puberty (160), secondary amenorrhea (161), and galactorrhea (162).

Both cortical and trabecular bone mineral are reduced with prolactin excess; thin women and those with low androgen levels appear to be at increased risk for osteoporosis (159,163,164). Deficits in skeletal mass are generally attributed to bone loss resulting from hypogonadism (159), although Schlechte and coworkers have proposed that bone mineral accretion is also inadequate (164). In some, but not all studies, bone loss is progressive over time. With drug-induced or spontaneous recovery of gonadal function, hyperprolactinemic patients show gains in bone mineral; whether bone mass can be completely restored remains controversial (163–165).

Management of adolescents with hyperprolactinemia should include bone densitometry. Bromocriptine or pergolide should be considered for hypogonadal patients although the effect of such treatment on adolescent bone mass has not been studied sytematically.

Acute Lymphoblastic Leukemia

As long-term survival from acute lymphoblastic leukemia improves, the sequelae of this common childhood malignancy are of increasing concern. Infrequently, diffuse osteopenia and vertebral fractures are present at the time of diagnosis (166). These bone lesions have been attributed to direct infiltration by leukemic cells or to tumor cell production of a humoral factors such as parathyroid hormone-related peptide, prostaglandin E, or osteoblast inhibiting factor (166).

Deficits in bone mineral may also develop following treatment for acute lymphoblastic leukemia (167,168). Lumbar spine and distal radius bone mineral may be reduced, resulting in symptomatic bone pain and pathologic fractures. The cause of osteopenia during treatment remains controversial. Chemotherapy for acute lymphoblastic leukemia includes prednisone and methotrexate, agents implicated in causing at least transient bone loss. Atkinson and colleagues observed hypocalcemia, hypomagnesemia, and suppressed levels of 1,25-dihydroxyvitamin D during chemotherapy and proposed that drug-induced alterations in mineral homeostasis contributed to decreased cortical bone mass (167). Gilsanz and coworkers observed deficits in vertebral bone mineral only in those patients who received cranial irradiation in addition to chemotherapy, suggesting these agents are not sufficient to account for trabecular bone loss (168). Alterations in mineral homeostasis observed during chemotherapy resolve and depressed osteocalcin levels rise significantly after completion of treatment (167). However, the extent to which deficits in bone mineral can be restored during remission remains unknown.

Idiopathic Juvenile Osteoporosis

As the term implies, idiopathic juvenile osteoporosis is a rare disorder of bone demineralization whose etiology is unknown. Patients present with nonspecific findings of bone pain, difficulty walking, and fractures of the long bones or vertebrae. The onset occurs typically in early puberty, coinciding with the pubertal growth spurt although the diagnosis has been made in children under the age of 5 years. Most patients recover spontaneously within 3 to 4 years. Osteopenia is evident by x-ray in most patients or by SPA in a few cases in which this technique has been applied (169).

By definition, idiopathic juvenile osteoporosis can be diagnosed only after the exclusion of other causes of childhood osteoporosis including osteogenesis imperfecta, calcium or vitamin D deficiency, malabsorption, hyperparathyroidism, hyperthyroidism, and Cushing's syndrome. No consistent biochemical abnormality has been associated with this disorder; serum calcium, phosphate, magnesium, parathyroid hormone, alkaline phosphatase, calcitonin, and 25-hydroxyvitamin D have been reported as normal (169). However, most patients demonstrate a negative calcium balance that resolves with recovery (170). Low 1,25-dihydroxyvitamin D levels have been observed in some patients (169,171) leading to the hypothesis that a partial defect in renal α-hydroxylase contributes to osteopenia. However, elevated 1,25-dihydroxyvitamin D levels have been observed in one patient in whom calcitonin deficiency was proposed to be the cause (172). Given the lack of specific clinical and laboratory findings, idiopathic juvenile osteoporosis may not represent a distinct disorder but a variety of mild defects in bone mineral acquisition.

▶ 97

There is no established therapy for idiopathic juvenile osteoporosis. For patients with low circulating levels of 1,25-dihydroxyvitamin D, calcitriol (1,25-dihydroxycholecalciferol) therapy may be beneficial. In one study, 3 patients given calcitriol were found to have normal bone mineral after a year of therapy, whereas the untreated patient showed no improvement (169). Calcitonin therapy was tried in another patient with elevated serum 1,25-dihydroxyvitamin D; this therapy failed to the improve bone mineral status (172). Fortunately, idiopathic juvenile osteoporosis appears to be a self-limited disorder that resolves with the progression of puberty, and the need for intervention is uncertain.

Bones of Today are Bones of Tomorrow

The bone mass achieved during the first two decades forms the foundation for adult bone health. To foster skeletal health, pediatricians need to encourage children and adolescents to work toward skeletal "well-being" during the first two decades. Although peak bone mass may be genetically predetermined, nutrition, activity, and hormonal status influence whether this genetic potential is reached. Many questions remain about the determinants of normal bone accretion. However, it is possible to recommend life-style practices likely to contribute to bone mass. Adequate daily intake of calories, protein, and calcium should be encouraged and a calcium supplement considered if the diet fails to provide at least the age-appropriate daily allowance. The benefits of exercise in moderation, particularly weight-bearing activities, should be stressed; children engaged in more intensive athletics should be educated about the risks of menstrual irregularities, pubertal delay, or inadequate weight gain during growth. Cigarette smoking and alcohol intake should be discouraged.

Chronic illness in the first two decades may interrupt normal bone accretion, resulting in significant bone mineral deficits. The reversibility of acquisitional osteopenia remains a concern. To monitor for skeletal deficits, bone mineral should be assessed in patients at risk, such as those with cystic fibrosis, anorexia nervosa, delayed puberty, and amenorrhea. Treatment of osteopenia should include optimizing nutrition, calcium intake, and appropriate activity. The benefits of sex steroids to augment bone mineral during adolescence is more controversial because their efficacy in preventing or reversing osteopenia in these disorders is unproven. Estrogen/progesterone or testosterone replacement should be reserved for osteopenic teens with mature epiphyses. Other therapeutic agents such calcitonin or bisphosphonates have not been adequately evaluated and their use remains experimental in this age group.

Considerably more research is needed to complete our understanding of normal bone accretion. Further longitudinal studies will be necessary to determine when peak bone mass is achieved and bone loss begins. Gender and racial differences in bone mineral acquisition should be explored in healthy Caucasian, African American, Asian, and Hispanic youth. The relative contribution of adequate nutrition, calcium, activity, and hormonal factors needs to be examined in greater detail. With improved knowledge, physicians can assume a more active and informed role in preventing brittle bones in the future.

References

1. Dent CE. The keynote address: problems in metabolic bone diesase. In: Frame B, Parfitt M, Duncan H (eds). Clinical aspects of metabolic bone disease. (Proceedings of the International Symposium on Clinical Aspects of Metabolic Bone Disease. Henry Ford Hospital, Detroit, June, 1972). Amsterdam: Excerpta Medica, 1973:1–7.

2. Riggs BL, Melton LJ III. Involutional osteoporosis. N Engl J Med 1986;314: 1676–1686.

3. Osteoporosis. In: Berg RL, Cassells JS, eds. The second fifty years: promoting health and preventing disability. Washington, DC: National Academy Press, 1990: 76–100.

4. Garn SM. The earlier gain and the later loss of cortical bone. Springfield, Ill: CC Thomas, 1970.

5. Hui SL, Johnston CC Jr, Mazess RB. Bone mass in normal children and young adults. Growth 1985;49:34–43.

6. Gilsanz V, Gibbens DT, Roe TF, et al. Vertebral bone density in children: effect of puberty. Radiology 1988;166:847–850.

7. Li J-Y, Specker BL, Ho ML, Tsang RC. Bone mineral content in black and white children 1 to 6 years of age. Am J Dis Child 1989;143:1346–1349.

8. Glastre C, Braillon P, David L, Cochat P, Meunier PJ, Delmas PD. Measurement of bone mineral content of the lumbar spine by dual energy x-ray absorptiometry in normal children: correlations with growth parameters. J Clin Endocrinol Metab 1990;70:1330–1333.

9. Miller JZ, Slemenda CW, Meaney FJ, Reister TK, Hui S, Johnston CC. The relationship of bone mineral density and anthropometric variables in healthy male and female children. Bone Miner 1991;14:137–152.

10. Southard RN, Morris JD, Mahan JD, et al. Bone mass in healthy children: measurement with quantitative DXA. Radiology 1991;179:735–738.

11. DeSchepper J, Derde MP, Van den Broeck M, Piepsz A, Jonckheer MH. Normative data for lumbar spine bone mineral content in children: influence of age, height, weight, and pubertal stage. J Nucl Med 1991;32:216–220.

12. Bonjour J-P, Theintz G, Buchs B, Slosman D, Rizzoli R. Critical years and stages of puberty for spinal and femoral bone mass accumulation during adolescence. J Clin Endocrinol Metab 1991;73:555–563.

13. Gordon CL, Halton JM, Atkinson SA, Webber CE. The contributions of growth and puberty to peak bone mass. Growth Dev Aging 1991;5:257–262.

14. Katzman DK, Bachrach LK, Carter DR, Marcus R. Clinical and anthropometric correlates of bone mineral acquisition in healthy adolescent girls. J Clin Endocrinol Metab 1991;73:1332–1339.

15. Bachrach LK, Guido D, Katzman D, Litt IF, Marcus R. Decreased bone density in adolescent girls with anorexia nervosa. Pediatrics 1990;86:440–447.

16. Lloyd T, Myers C, Buchanen JR, Demers LM. Collegiate women athletes with irregular menses during adolescence have decreased bone density. Obstet Gynecol 1988;4:639–642.

17. Dhuper S, Warren MP, Brooks-Gunn J, Fox R. Effects of hormonal status on bone density in adolescent girls. J Clin Endocrinol Metab 1990;71:1083–1088.

18. Warren MP, Brooks-Gunn J, Hamilton LH, Warren LF, Hamilton WG. Scoliosis and fractures in young ballet dancers. N Engl J Med 1986;314:1348–1353.

19. Finkelstein JS, Neer RM, Biller BMK, Crawford JD, Klibanski A. Osteopenia in men with a history of delayed puberty. N Engl J Med 1992;326:600–604.

20. Gibbens DT, Gilsanz V, Boechat MI, Dufer D, Carlson ME, Wang C-I. Osteoporosis in cystic fibrosis. J Pediatr 1988;113:295–300.

21. Wahner HW. Measurements of bone mass and bone density. Endocrinol Metab Clin North Am 1989;18:995–1012.

22. Kimmel DB. In: Marcus R, ed. Osteoporosis. Boston: Blackwell Scientific Publications, 1994:49–68.

23. Hui SL, Slemenda CS, Johnston CC Jr. Age and bone mass as predictors of fracture in a prospective study. J Clin Invest 1988;81:1804–1809.

24. Carter DR, Bouxsein ML, Marcus R. New approaches for interpreting projected bone densitometry data. J Bone Miner Res 1992;7:137–145.

25. Kroger H, Kotaniemi A, Vainio P, Alhava E. Bone densitometry of the spine and femur in children by dual-energy x-ray absorptiometry. Bone Miner 1992;17:75–85.

26. Ponder SW, McCormick DP, Fawcett D, Palmer JL, McKernan MG, Brouhard BH. Spinal bone mineral density in children ages 5.00 through 11.99 years. Am J Dis Child 1990;144:1346–1348.

27. Thomas KA, Cook SD, Bennett JT, Whitecloud TS, Rice JC. Femoral neck and lumbar spine bone mineral densities in a normal population 3–20 years of age. J Pediatr Orthop 1991;11:48–58.

28. Theintz G, Buchs B, Rizzoli R, et al. Longitudinal monitoring of bone mass accumulation in healthy adolescents: evidence for a marked reduction after 16 years of age

at the levels of lumbar spine and femoral neck in female subjects. J Clin Endocrinol Metab 1992;75:1060–1065.

29. White CM, Hergendroeger AC, Klish WJ. Bone mineral density in 15- to 21-year old eumenorrheic and amenorrheic subjects. Am J Dis Child 1992;146:31–35.

30. Matkovic V. Calcium and peak bone mass. J Intern Med 1992;231:151–160.

31. Gilsanz V, Gibbens DT, Carlson M, Boechat MI, Cann CE, Schulz EE. Peak trabecular vertebral density: a comparison of adolescent and adult females. Calcif Tissue Int 1988;43:260–262.

32. Davies KM, Recker RR, Stegman MR, Heaney RP, Kimmel DB, Leist J. Third decade bone gain in women. In: Cohn DV, Glorieux FH, Martins TJ, eds. Calcium regulation and bone metabolism. New York: Elsevier, 1990:497–501.

33. Recker RR, Davies M, Hinders SM, Heaney RP, Stegman MR, Kimmel DB. Bone gain in young adult women. JAMA 1992;268:2403–2408.

34. Barden HS, Mazess RB. Longitudinal study of bone mineral density in premenopausal women. J Bone Miner Res 1990;5(Suppl 2):S180.

35. Pollitzer WS, Anderson JJB. Ethnic and genetic differences in bone mass: a review with a hereditary vs environmental perspective. Am J Clin Nutr 1989;50:1244–1259.

36. Kelly PJ, Eisman JA, Sambrook PN. Interaction of genetic and environmental influences on peak bone density. Osteoporosis Int 1990;1:56–60.

37. Avioli LV, Heaney RP. Calcium intake and bone health. Calcif Tissue Int 1991;48:221–223. Editorial.

38. Krall EA, Dawson-Hughes B. Heritable and lifestyle determinants of bone mineral density. J Bone Miner Res 1993;8:1–9.

39. Pocock NA, Eisman JA, Hopper JL, Yeates MG, Sambrook PN, Ebert S. Genetic determinants of bone mass in adults: a twin study. J Clin Invest 1987;80:706–710.

40. Seeman E, Hopper JL, Bach LA, et al. Reduced bone mass in daughters of women with osteoporosis. N Engl J Med 1989;320:554–558.

41. Slemenda CW, Christian JC, Williams CJ, Norton JA, Johnston CC Jr. Genetic determinants of bone mass in adult women: a reevaluation of the twin model and the potential importance of gene interactions on heritability estimates. J Bone Miner Res 1991;6:561–567.

42. Ott SM. Bone density in adolescents. N Engl J Med 1991;325:1646–1647.

43. Lutz J, Tesar R. Mother-daughter pairs: spinal and femoral bone densities and dietary intakes. Am J Clin Nutr 1990;52:872–877.

44. Cohn SH, Abesamis C, Yasumura S, Aloia JF, Zanzi I, Ellis KJ. Comparative skeletal mass and radial bone mineral content in black and white women. Metabolism 1977;26:171–178.

45. Luckey MM, Meier DE, Mandeli JP, DaCosta MC, Hubbard ML, Goldsmith SJ. Radial and vertebral bone density in white and black women: evidence for racial differences in premenopausal bone homeostasis. J Clin Endocrinol Metab 1989;69:762–770.

46. Yamo K, Wasnich R, Vogel JM, Heilbrun LK. Bone mineral measurements among middle-aged and elderly Japanese residents of Hawaii. Am J Epidemiol 1984;119:751–764.

47. Villa ML. Ethnicity and skeletal health. In: Marcus R, ed. Osteoporosis. Boston: Blackwell Scientific Publications, 1994;125–145.

48. Trotter M, Hixon BB. Sequential changes in weight, density, and percentage ash weight of human skeletons from early fetal period through old age. Anat Rec 1973;179:1–18.

49. Bell NH, Shary J, Stevens J, Garza M, Gordon L, Edwards J. Demonstration that bone mass is greater in black than in white children. J Bone Miner Res 1991;7:719–723.

50. Gilsanz V, Roe TF, Mora S, Costin G, Goodman WG. Changes in vertebral bone density in black girls and white girls during childhood and puberty. N Engl J Med 1991;325:1597–1600.

51. McCormick DP, Ponder SW, Fawcett HD, Palmer JL. Spinal bone mineral density in 335 normal and obese children and adolescents: evidence for ethnic and sex differences. J Bone Miner Res 1991;6:507–513.

52. Patel DN, Pettifor JM, Becker PJ, Grieve C, Leschner K. The effect of ethnic group on appendicular bone mass in children. J Bone Miner Res 1992;7:263–272.

53. Weinstein RS, Bell NH. Diminished rates of bone formation in normal black adults. N Engl J Med 1988;319:1698–1701.

54. Bell NH. Cellular mechanisms. Am J Med 1988;84:275–282.

55. Kelly PJ, Twomey L, Sambrook PN, Eisman JA. Sex differences in peak adult bone mineral density. J Bone Miner Res 1990;5:1169–1175.

56. Buchanen JR, Myers C, Lloyd T, Leuenberger P, Demers LM. Determinants of peak trabecular bone density in women: the role of androgens, estrogen, and exercise. J Bone Miner Res 1988;3:673–680.

57. Buchanen JR, Hospodar P, Myers C, Leuenberger P, Demers LM. Effect of excess endogenous androgens on bone density in young women. J Clin Endocrinol Metab 1988;67:937–943.

58. Heaney RP. Nutritional factors in osteoporosis. Annu Rev Nutr 1993;13:287–316.

59. Sandler RB, Slemenda CW, LaPorte RE, et al. Postmenopausal bone density and milk consumption in childhood and adolescence. Am J Clin Nutr 1985;42:270–274.

60. Halioua L, Anderson JJ. Lifetime calcium intake and physical activity habits: independent and combined effects on the radial bone of healthy premenopausal Caucasian women. Am J Clin Nutr 1989;49:534–541.

61. Matkovic V, Kostial K, Simonovic I, Buzina R, Brodarec A, Nordin BEC. Bone status and fracture rates in two regions of Yugoslavia. Am J Clin Nutr 1979;32:540–549.

62. Cumming RG. Calcium intake and bone mass: a quantitative review of the evidence. Calcif Tissue Int 1990;47:194–201.

63. Heaney RP. Calcium in the prevention and treatment of osteoporosis. J Intern Med 1992;231:169–180.

64. Committeee on Dietary Allowances, Food and Nutrition Board, National Research Council. Recommended dietary allowances, 10th ed. Washington, DC: National Academy Press, 1989.

65. Carroll MD, Abraham S, Dresser CM. Dietary intake source data: United States 1976–1980. Hyattsville, MD: National Center for Health Statistics, 1983. DHHS Pub. No. (PHS) 83-1681.

66. Food and nutrient intakes of individuals in 1 day in the United States, spring 1977. Preliminary report no. 2 of the Nationwide Food Consumption Survey 1977–78. Washington, DC: Department of Agriculture, 1980.

67. Chan GM. Dietary calcium and bone mineral status of children and adolescents. Am J Dis Child 1991;145:631–634.

68. Kanders B, Dempster DW, Lindsay R. Interaction of calcium nutrition and physical activity on bone mass in young women. J Bone Miner Res 1988;3:145–149.

69. Matkovic V, Fontana D, Rominac C, Goel P, Chestnut C. Factors that influence peak bone mass formation: a study of calcium balance and the inheritance of bone mass in adolescent females. Am J Clin Nutr 1990;53:878–888.

70. Johnston CC Jr, Miller JZ, Slemenda CW, et al. Calcium supplementation and increases in bone mineral density in children. N Engl J Med 1992;327:82–87.

71. Fehily AM, Coles RJ, Evans WD, Elwood PC. Factors affecting bone density in young adults. Am J Clin Nutr 1992;56:579–586.

72. Cummings JH, Hill MJ, Jivray T, Houston H, Branch WJ, Jenkins DJA. The effect of mean protein and dietary fiber on colonic function and metabolism. Changes in bowel habits, bile acid excretion and calcium absorption. Am J Clin Nutr 1979;32:2086–2093.

73. Sandberg A, Hasselblad C, Hasselblad K, Hulten L. The effect of wheat bran on the absorption of minerals in the small intestine. Br J Nutr 1982;47:451–460.

74. Goldin BR, Adlercreutz H, Gorbach SL, et al. The relationship between estro-

gen levels and diets of Caucasian American and Oriental immigrant women. Am J Clin Nutr 1986:44:945–953.

75. Lanyon LE. Strain-related bone modeling and remodeling. Top Geriatr Rehabil 1989;4:13–24.

76. Dalen N, Olsson KE. Bone mineral content and physical activity. Acta Orthop Scand 1974;45:170–174.

77. Lane NE, Bloch DE, Jones HH, Marshall WH, Wood PD, Fries JF. Long-distance running, bone density, and osteoarthritis. JAMA 1986;255:1147–1151.

78. Slemenda CW, Miller JZ, Hui SL, Reister TK, Johnston CC Jr. Role of physical activity in the development of skeletal mass in children. J Bone Miner Res 1991;6:1227–1233.

79. Snow-Harter C, Bouxsein ML, Lewis BT, Carter DR, Marcus R. Effects of resistance and endurance exercise on bone mineral status of young women: a randomized exercise intervention trial. J Bone Miner Res 1992;7:761–769.

80. Gleeson PB, Protas EJ, LeBlance AD, Schneider VS, Evans JH. Effects of weight lifting on bone mineral density in premenopausal women. J Bone Miner Res 1990;5:153–158.

81. Rockwell J, Sorensen A, Baker S, et al. Weight training decreases vertebral bone density in premenopausal women: a prospective study. J Clin Endocrinol Metab 1990;71:988–993.

82. Bishop N. Bone disease in preterm infants. Arch Dis Child 1989;64:1403–1409.

83. Congdon PJ, Horsman A, Ryan SW, Truscott JG, Durward H. Spontaneous resolution of bone mineral depletion in preterm infants. Arch Dis Child 1990;65:1038–1042.

84. Prockop DJ. Osteogenesis imperfecta. Arthritis Rheum 1988;31:1–8.

85. Carpenter TO, Levy HL, Holtrop ME, Shih VE, Anast CS. Lysinuric protein intolerance presenting as childhood osteoporosis. N Engl J Med 1985;312:290–294.

86. Finkelstein JS, Klibanski A, Neer RM, et al. Increases in bone density during treatment of men with idiopathic hypogonadotropic hypogonadism. J Clin Endocrinol Metab 1989;69:776–783.

87. Diagnostic and statistical manual of mental disorders. 3d ed, rev. Washington, DC: American Psychiatric Association, 1987:63.

88. Rigotti NA, Nussbaum SR, Herzog DB, Neer RM. Osteoporosis in women with anorexia nervosa. N Engl J Med 1984;311:1601–1606.

89. Ayers JWT, Gidwani GP, Schmidt IMV, Gross M. Osteopenia in hypoestrogenic young women with anorexia nervosa. Fertil Steril 1984;41:224–228.

90. Brotman AW, Stern TA. Osteoporosis and pathologic fractures in anorexia nervosa. Am J Psychiatry 1985;142:495–496.

91. Biller BMK, Saxe V, Herzog DB, Rosenthal DI, Holzman S, Klibanski A. Mechanisms of osteoporosis in adult and adolescent women with anorexia nervosa. J Clin Endocrinol Metab 1989;68:548–554.

92. Seeman E, Szmukler GI, Formica C, Tsalamandris C, Mestrovic R. Osteoporosis in anorexia nervosa: the influence of peak bone density, bone loss, oral contraceptive use and exercise. J Bone Miner Res 1992;7:1467–1474.

93. Charig MJ, Fletcher EWL. Reversible bone loss in anorexia nervosa. Br Med J 1987;295:474–475.

94. Bachrach LK, Katzman DK, Litt IF, Guido D, Marcus R. Recovery from osteopenia in adolescent girls with anorexia nervosa. J Clin Endocrinol Metab 1991;72:602–606.

95. Rigotti NA, Neer RM, Skates SJ, Herzog DB, Nussbaum SR. The clinical course of osteoporosis in anorexia nervosa. A longitudinal study of cortical bone mass. JAMA 1991;265:1133–1138.

96. Raymond CA. Long-term sequelae pondered in anorexia nervosa. JAMA 1987;257:3324–3325.

97. Bachrach LK, Guido D, Katzman D, Litt IF, Marcus R. Decreased bone density in adolescent girls with anorexia nervosa. Pediatrics 1990;86:440–447.

98. Ettinger B, Genant HK, Cann CE. Postmenopausal bone loss is prevented by treatment with low-dose estrogen with calcium. Ann Intern Med 1987;106:40–45.

99. Joyce JM, Warren DL, Humphries LL, Smith AJ, Coon JS. Osteoporosis in

women with eating disorders: comparison of physical parameters, exercise and menstrual status with SPA and DPA evaluation. J Nucl Med 1990;31:325–331.

100. Bilanen JE, Blanchard MS, Rusek-Cohen E. Lower vertebral bone density in male long distance runners. Med Sci Sports Exerc 1989;21:66–70.

101. Marcus R, Cann C, Madvig P, et al. Menstrual function and bone mass in elite women distance runners. Ann Intern Med 1985;102:158–163.

102. Myburgh KH, Hutchins J, Fataar AB, Hough SF, Noakes TD. Low bone density is an etiologic factor for stress fractures in athletes. Ann Intern Med 1990;113:754–759.

103. Cann CE, Martin MC, Genant HK, Jaffe RB. Decreased spinal mineral content in amenorrheic women. JAMA 1984;251:626–629.

104. Drinkwater BL, Nilson K, Chestnut CH III, Bremner WJ, Shainholtz S, Southworth MB. Bone mineral content of amenorrheic and eumenorrheic athletes. N Engl J Med 1984;311:277–281.

105. Myburgh KH, Bachrach, LK, Lewis B, Kent K, Marcus R. Low bone mineral density at axial and appendicular sites in amenorrheic athletes. Med Sci Sports Exerc 1993;25:1197–1202.

106. Frisch RE, Wehlergan AV, McArthur JW, et al. Delayed menarche and amenorrhea of college athletes in relation to age of onset of training. JAMA 1981;246:1559–1563.

107. Warren MP. The effects of exercise on pubertal progression and reproductive function in girls. J Clin Endocrinol Metab 1980;61:1150–1157.

108. Warren MP. Amenorrhea in endurance runners. J Clin Endocrinol Metab 1992;75:1393–1397.

109. Bullen BA, Skrinar GS, Beitins IZ, Von Merging G, Turnball BA, McArthur JW. Induction of menstrual disorders by strenuous exercise in untrained women. N Engl J Med 1985;312:1349–1353.

110. Bullen BA, Warren MP, Stager JM, Ritchie-Flanagan B, Robertshaw D. Reversibility of amenorrhea in athletes. N Engl J Med 1984;310:51–52.

111. Drinkwater BL, Nilson K, Ott S, Chestnut CH III. Bone mineral density after resumption of menses in amenorrheic athletes. JAMA 1986;256:380–382.

112. Theintz GE, Howald H, Weiss U, Sizonenko PC. Evidence for a reduction in growth potential in adolescent female gymnasts. J Pediatr 1993;12:306–313.

113. Mansfield MJ, Emans SJ. Growth in female gymnasts: should training decrease in puberty? J Pediatr 1993;122:237–240.

114. Bonen A, Calcastro AN, Ling WY, Simpson AA. Profiles of selected hormones during menstrual cycles of teenage athletes. J Appl Physiol: Respir Environ Exerc Physiol 1981;50:545–551.

115. Frusztajer NT, Dhuper S, Warren MP, Brooks-Gunn J, Fox RP. The role of nutritional intake in the incidence of stress fractures in ballet dancers. Am J Clin Nutr 1990;51:779–783.

116. Ding JH, Sheckter CB, Drinkwater BL, Soules MR, Bremner WJ. High serum cortisol levels in exercise-associated amenorrhea. Ann Intern Med 1988;108:530–534.

117. Committee on Sports Medicine. Amenorrhea in adolescent athletes. Pediatrics 1989;84:394–395.

118. Rosenfeld RG, Grumbach MM, eds. Turner syndrome. New York: Marcel Dekker, 1990.

119. Risch WD, Banzer DH, Moltz L, et al. Bone mineral content in patients with gonadal dysgenesis. Am J Radiol 1976;126:1302–1309.

120. Smith MA, Wilson J, Pricer WH. Bone demineralisation in patients with Turner's syndrome. J Med Genet 1982;19:100–103.

121. Shore RM, Chesney RW, Mazess RB, Rose PG, Bargman GJ. Skeletal demineralization in Turner's syndrome. Calcif Tissue Int 1982;34:519–522.

122. Stepan JJ, Musilova J, Pacovsky V. Bone demineralization, biochemical indices of bone remodeling, and estrogen replacement therapy in adults with Turner's syndrome. J Bone Miner Res 1989;4:193–198.

123. Naeraa RW, Brixen K, Hansen RM, et al. Skeletal size and bone mineral content in Turner's syndrome: relation to karyo-

type, estrogen treatment, physical fitness, and bone turnover. Calcif Tissue Int 49:77–83.

124. Barr DGO. Bone deficiency in Turner's syndrome measured by metacarpal dimensions. Arch Dis Child 1974;49:821–822.

125. Ross JL, Long LM, Feuillan P, Cassorla F, Cutler GB. Normal bone density of the wrist and spine and increased wrist fractures in girls with Turner's syndrome. J Clin Endocrinol Metab 1991;73:355–369.

126. Rubin KR. Osteoporosis in Turner syndrome. In: Rosenfeld RG, Grumbach MM, eds. Turner syndrome. New York: Marcel Dekker, 1990:301–317.

127. Neely EK, Marcus R, Rosenfeld RG, Bachrach LK. Turner syndrome adolescents receiving growth hormone are not osteopenic. J Clin Endocrinol Metab 1993;76:861–866.

128. Corey M, McLaughlin FJ, Williams M, Levison H. A comparison of survival, growth, and pulmonary function in patients with cystic fibrosis in Boston and Toronto. J Clin Epidemiol 1988;41:583–591.

129. Finkelstein SM, Wielinski CL, Elliot GR, et al. Diabetes mellitus associated with cystic fibrosis. J Pediatr 1988;112:373–377.

130. Denning CR, Sommers SC, Quigley HJ Jr. Infertility in male patients with cystic fibrosis. Pediatrics 1968;41:1–17.

131. Stead RJ, Houlder S, Agnew J, et al. Vitamin D and parathyroid hormone and bone mineralisation in adults with cystic fibrosis. Thorax 1988;43:190–194.

132. Bachrach LK, Loutit CW, Moss RB, Marcus R. Osteoporosis in adults with cystic fibrosis. Am J Med 1994;96:27–34.

133. Mischler EH, Chesney PJ, Chesney RW, Mazess RB. Demineralization in cystic fibrosis. Am J Dis Child 1979;133:632–635.

134. Hahn TJ, Squires AE, Halstead LR, Strominger DB. Reduced serum 25-hydroxyvitamin D concentration and disordered mineral metabolism in patients with cystic fibrosis. J Pediatr 1979;94:38–42.

135. Solomons NW, Wagonfeld JB, Rieger C, et al. Some biochemical indices of nutrition in treated cystic fibrosis patients. Am J Clin Nutr 1981;34:462–474.

136. Landon C, Rosenfeld RG. Short stature and pubertal delay in male adolescents with cystic fibrosis. Am J Dis Child 1984;138:388–391.

137. Juniper EF, Kline PA, Roberts RS, Hargreave FE, Daniel EE. Airway responsiveness to methacholine during the natural menstrual cycle and the effect of oral contraceptives. Am Rev Respir Dis 1987;135:1039–1042.

138. Raisz LG. Local and systemic factors in the pathogenesis of osteoporosis. N Engl J Med 1988;318:818–828.

139. Shore RM, Chesney RW, Mazess RB, Rose PG, Bargman GJ. Bone mineral status in growth hormone deficiency. J Pediatr 1980;96:393–396.

140. Zambone G, Antoniazzi R, Radetti G, Musumeci C, Tato L. Effects of two different regimens of recombinant human growth hormone therapy on the bone mineral density of patients with growth hormone deficiency. J Pediatr 1991;119:483–485.

141. Saggese G, Baroncelli BI, Bertelloni S, Cinquanta L, Di Nero G. Effects of long-term treatment with growth hormone on bone and mineral metabolism in children with growth hormone deficiency. J. Pediatr 1993;122:37–45.

142. Harbison MD, Gertner JM. Permissive action of growth hormone on the renal response to dietary phosphorus deprivation. J Clin Endocrinol Metab 1990;70:1035–1040.

143. Kaufman J-M, Taelman P, Vermeulen A, Vandeweghe M. Bone mineral status in growth hormone-deficient males with isolated and multiple pituitary deficiencies of childhood onset. J Clin Endocrinol Metab 1992;74:118–123.

144. Albright R, Reifenstein EC. Parathyroid glands and metabolic bone disease: selected studies. Baltimore: Williams & Wilkins, 1948:150.

145. Santiago JV, McAlister WH, Ratzan SK, et al. Decreased cortical thickness and osteopenia in children with diabetes mellitus. J Clin Endocrinol Metab 1977;45:845–848.

146. Rosenbloom AL, Lezotte DC, Weber FT, et al. Diminution of bone mass in

childhood diabetes. Diabetes 1977;26: 1052–1055.

147. Shore RM, Chesney RW, Mazess RB, Rose PG, Bargman GJ. Osteopenia in juvenile diabetes. Calcif Tissue Int 1981;33:455–457.

148. Ponder SW, McCormick DP, Fawcett D, et al. Bone mineral density of the lumbar vertebrae in children and adolescents with insulin-dependent diabetes mellitus. J Pediatr 1992;120:541–545.

149. Wartofsky L. Osteoporosis and therapy with thyroid hormone. The Endocrinologist 1991;1:57–61.

150. Meunier PJ, Bianchi GGS, Edouard CM, Bernard JC, Courprou P, Vignou GE. Bone manifestations of thyrotoxicosis. Orthop Clin North Am 1972;3:745–774.

151. Heyerdahl S, Kase BF, Lie SO. Intellectual development in children with congenital hypothyroidism in relation to recommended thyroxine treatment. J Pediatr 1991;118:850–857.

152. Lukert BP, Raisz LG. Glucocorticoid-induced osteoporosis: pathogenesis and management. Ann Intern Med 1990; 112:352–364.

153. Varanos S, Ansell BM, Reeve J. Vertebral collapse in juvenile chronic arthritis: its relationship with glucocorticoid therapy. Calcif Tissue Int 1987;41:75–78.

154. Pocock NA, Eisman JA, Dunstan CR, et al. Recovery from steroid-induced osteoporosis. Ann Intern Med 1987; 107:319–323.

155. Konig P, Hillman L, Cervantes C, et al. Bone metabolism in children with asthma treated with inhaled beclomethasone dipropionate. J Pediatr 1993;122:219–226.

156. Balsan S, Steru D, Bourdeau A, et al. Effects of long-term maintenance therapy with a new glucocorticoid, deflazacort, on mineral metabolism and statural growth. Calcif Tissue Int 1987;40:303–309.

157. Loftus J, All R, Hesp R, et al. Randomized, double-blind trial of deflazacort versus prednisone in juvenile chronic (or rheumatoid) arthritis: a relatively bone-sparing effect of deflazacort. Pediatrics 1991;88:428–436.

158. Nishioka T, Kurayama H, Yasuda T, Udagawa J, Matsumura C, Niimi H. Nasal administration of salmon calcitonin for prevention of glucocorticoid-induced osteoporosis in children with nephrosis. J Pediatr 1991;118:703–707.

159. Wardlaw SL, Bilezikian JP. Hyperprolactinemia and osteopenia. J Clin Endocrinol Metab 1992;75:690–691. Editorial.

160. Patton ML, Woolf PD. Hyperprolactinemia and delayed puberty: a report of three cases in their response to therapy. Pediatrics 1983;71:572–575.

161. Ridgeway EW, Emans SJ, Fisher EG, et al. Prolactinomas causing primary and secondary amenorrhea in adolescents. J Adolesc Health Care 1982;3:148.

162. Rohn RD. Galactorrhea in the adolescent. Sexually Active Teenagers 1988;2: 21–33.

163. Biller BMK, Baum HBA, Rosenthal DI, et al. Progressive trabecular osteopenia in women with hyperprolactinemic amenorrhea. J Clin Endocrinol Metab 1992;75:692–697.

164. Schlechte J, Walkner L, Kathol M. A longitudinal analysis of premenopausal bone loss in healthy women and women with hyperprolactinemia. J Clin Endocrinol Metab 1992;75:698–703.

165. Klibanski A, Greenspan SL. Increase in bone mass after treatment of hyperprolactinemic women. J Clin Endocrinol Metab 1986;315:542–546.

166. Samuda GM, Cheng MY, Yeung CY. Back pain and vertebral compression: an uncommon presentation of childhood acute lymphoblastic leukemia. J Pediatr Orthop 1987;7:175–178.

167. Atkinson SA, Fraher L, Gundberg CM, Andrew M, Pai M, Barr RD. Mineral homeostasis and bone mass in children treated for acute lymphoblastic leukemia. J Pediatr 1989;114:793–800.

168. Gilsanz V, Carlson ME, Rose TF, Ortega JA. Osteoporosis after cranial irradiation for acute lymphoblastic leukemia. J Pediatr 1990;117:238–244.

169. Saggese G, Bertelloni S, Baroncelli GI, Perri G, Calderazzi A. Mineral metabolism and calcitriol therapy in idiopathic ju-

venile osteoporosis. Am J Dis Child 1991; 145:457–462.

170. Jowsey J, Johnson KA. Juvenile osteoporosis: bone findings in seven patients. J Pediatr 1972;81:511–517.

171. Marder HK, Tsang RC, Jug G, Crawford AC. Calcitriol deficiency in idio-pathic juvenile osteoporosis. Am J Dis Child 1982;136:914–917.

172. Jackson EC, Strife F, Tsang RC, Marder HK. Effect of calcitonin replacement therapy in idiopathic juvenile osteoporosis. Am J Dis Child 1988;142:1237–1239.

Osteoporosis

5 ▸ Adult Bone Loss

▶ ▶ ▶ Charles W. Slemenda

Peak bone mass, defined here as the maximum skeletal mineral content achieved by an individual, is thought to occur near age 30 (1), although some have argued that peak mass occurs earlier, near the end of adolescence (2; see Chapter 4). For clinical purposes the mean bone mass of people between 25 and 30 years of age would undoubtedly serve as an adequate reference. Beyond this point there is a period of varying length during which skeletal mass is relatively stable, after which bone loss gradually diminishes skeletal integrity. This bone loss proceeds at varying rates throughout the rest of life, and in women is probably most rapid in the period of time immediately following menopause. Men also experience bone loss but this has been less well studied than that of women (see Chapter 7). This review examines adult bone loss in several ways. First, when does it begin and at what rates does it proceed between peak mass and the end of life? Second, what factors influence rates of loss? Third, how does loss influence fracture susceptibility? Fourth, should we attempt to measure loss clinically, and how might these data be used? And finally, can rates of bone loss be altered, pharmacologically or otherwise?

When Does Bone Loss Begin?

For the purposes of this discussion *bone loss* is defined as the diminution of skeletal mineral detectable by densitometric measurements. Before considering bone loss, it is necessary to specify the sites being considered. Bone mass data on the radius have been available for more than 20 years, whereas measurements of the spine have been made for about 10 years in most centers, and data on the hip have been available for an even shorter period. Data on metacarpal (primarily cortical) bone have been available longer than for any of these other sites, and although there are extensive cross-sectional data, few longitudinal studies have been published (3). Thus, there is less certainty regarding bone loss from the hip, arguably the most important skeletal site in terms of osteoporotic fractures. Also, most studies have included only Caucasian women, reflecting their very high risk of osteoporotic fractures, and therefore data on bone loss in men and in other racial groups are sparse.

The Radius

Studies have generally shown little or no radial bone loss in women prior to the sharp decline in ovarian function that precedes clinical menopause (4). In some women who continue to menstruate, albeit irregularly, radial bone loss can be demonstrated in those with elevated concentrations of follicle-stimulating hormone and diminished estrogen concentrations (4). In the years immediately following the complete cessation of menses, radial bone loss is more rapid than during any other period of life (4,5). In the next few years radial bone loss begins to slow, and then continues for many years at a more or less steady rate. It has been reported that radial loss may actually stop completely very late in life (3,6) when periosteal apposition of bone finally exceeds endosteal resorption. Thus, for the radius and *perhaps* for other primarily cortical bone sites (the shafts of the bones of the arms and legs), bone loss in women is most substantial around the menopause and continues at diminishing rates for at least 30 years.

In men from the mid-40s to about age 60 there is radial bone loss at a rate of about 6% per decade (7,8), a rate slightly greater than half that of similarly aged women. Whether this loss is steady or fluctuates over this period will require further study. Longitudinal data for men beyond age 65 have not been published, but cross-sectional data indicate that bone loss probably continues into the ninth decade of life.

The Spine

As with the radius, bone loss from the spine is most rapid in the years immediately surrounding menopause and then is less pronounced as years go by. There are, however, several differences between the radius and spine in both the timing and magnitude of bone loss. There have been reports of bone loss from the spine in premenopausal women (9), although we and others have failed to observe such effects (4). In addition, the rates of bone loss from the spine are generally greater than the rates from other sites, at least in response to menopausal estrogen deficiency. The trabecular bone of the spine may also be more sensitive to many other influences on bone loss, as will be discussed later.

This issue, however, also requires consideration of the techniques used for assessing bone loss. Two primary methods are used clinically—photon absorptiometry ([PA]; the source of photons being either a radioisotope or an x-ray tube), and computed tomography (CT). PA measures the entire vertebral body and anything else that lies between the photon source and the detector (eg, the posterior elements of the spine), whereas CT can be used either for the entire vertebral body or for some region (eg, the trabecular interior). Additionally, CT generally excludes the posterior elements of vertebral bodies, which cannot be done using PA. For these reasons, rates of bone loss estimated by CT can frequently be much higher, perhaps 6% to 8% per year or more, than those obtained using PA. Predominantly trabecular bone appears to be more sensitive to some causes of bone loss (eg, estrogen deficiency) than cortical bone. This will be discussed in greater detail later.

Although studies of spinal bone loss in the very old have not been frequently done, nor are there many reports of spinal bone loss in men, it would seem that in both groups rates of loss from the spine are less than in younger, menopausal women.

▶ 109

The Hip

Although hip fractures are the most devastating and costly of fragility-related fractures, less is known about bone loss from the hip than from other sites. This is because measurements of bone mass in the hip were most recently developed and because the precision of these measurements is somewhat poorer than that of other skeletal sites. (Reasons for poorer precision in this area relate to several factors, among them the smaller area being scanned and the difficulty in ensuring that the axis of the femoral neck lies perpendicular to the path of the photons). Further complicating this problem are difficulties in defining the hip. All manufacturers of PA equipment have software that defines a region as "femoral neck," but the algorithms for selection of the femoral neck differ substantially. As a result, rates of femoral neck bone loss from one manufacturer's equipment may reflect changes at a different site from that of another manufacturer. Similar problems arise with the definition of Ward's triangle and trochanteric or intertrochanteric regions.

These technical complications aside, the greatest uncertainties in estimates of bone loss from the hip arise due to the relatively short follow-up in the few longitudinal studies that have been done. As with the spine, premenopausal bone loss from the hip has been reported (10). And again, bone loss is accelerated in menopausal women. A recent report in a small group of elderly women showed annual rates of bone loss from the hip, which varied widely from region to region, with no loss from the femoral neck to 4% loss from the trochanter (11). Whether such patterns reflect scan technology or true biologic variability will require further studies. In this center we have been unable to demonstrate significant rates of bone loss from the femoral neck in premenopausal women (11); however, a small group of women with evidence of probable anovulatory cycles (defined as the absence of a progesterone spike in the luteal phase) did have significantly more negative slopes of bone mass over a period of 3 years than women with apparently normal cycles.

Summary

Bone loss in most women probably does not begin until the decline of ovarian function that precedes clinical menopause. After this time, bone loss continues throughout life, slowing (probably exponentially) in the radius. The rates of bone loss among very old women, especially from the hip, are not well described as yet, and will require further study, although it can safely be said that diminished mobility would probably accelerate negative changes in the hip. Premenopausal bone loss almost certainly occurs in some women, but this is not likely a generalized phenomenon. Women with premature ovarian failure, anovulatory cycles, and other problems associated with diminished concentrations of sex steroids are the most likely candidates for this early loss of skeletal mineral.

What Factors Influence Rates of Bone Loss?

Genetics

Influences on rates of bone loss may be divided into endogenous and environmental, although it will be shown that this division may be more arbitrary than is at first appreciated. Numerous studies have shown that bone mass, even among older people, is strongly influenced by genetics (12–15). However, it remains to be shown that there are genetic influences on bone *loss*. The focus must be on loss rather than rates of change because increases in bone mass must presumably be strongly influenced by genetics, given the strong heritability estimates for peak bone mass. Genetic studies of bone loss in women have not been published, although several reports touch on this area. Kelly and colleagues have published data showing genetic effects on both serum concentrations of osteocalcin, a marker of skeletal turnover, and change in bone mass (16,17). However, the changes in bone mass observed in this study were predominantly *increases* in bone mass (22 of 30 members of monozygotic pairs and 18 of 32 members of dizygotic pairs), as would be expected given the high heritability estimates for premenopausal subjects in other studies (13,18).

Differences in bone mass between members of identical twin pairs increase significantly with aging (19). Because such differences can arise due only to environmental influences, this suggests that nongenetic factors play an increasingly important role in bone loss. It has also been shown, however, that serum concentrations of osteocalcin are influenced by genetic factors (16), and others have shown strong correlations between osteocalcin concentrations and bone loss around menopause (4), leaving open the possibility that in women some genetic effects on bone loss will eventually be detected.

One long-term study of genetic influences on bone loss in men has been completed (7,14). Intraclass correlations in bone loss between members of monozygotic twin pairs were around 0.6, slightly but not significantly greater than the correlations in dizygotic pairs (r = 0.4 to 0.5). A second study in these same men found that monozygotic pairs also had significantly more similar self-selected environments (eg, smoking, drinking, and exercise patterns) than dizygotic pairs. Adjustments for these environmental influences on bone loss lowered the correlations in both types of pairs to 0.4. A finding of significant but nearly identical correlations in monozygotic and dizygotic pairs indicates strong common environmental, but no genetic, influences on bone loss in these men. These studies alone are not adequate to rule out the possibility of some genetic influence on bone loss in men, given the limited size of the study sample, but they do indicate that if genetic factors play a role, it is probably much smaller than that for the development of peak mass. It should be noted that although men and women probably share most influences on bone loss, the effects of menopause in women are the single most important element, and it remains to be shown whether or not this is under genetic control, or whether the female skeleton's response to estrogen deficiency is influenced by genetic factors. Long-term studies of menopausal women who are losing bone mass will be necessary to address this question.

▶ 111

One further note regarding environmental and genetic influences on rates of bone loss should be made. In the study of men described above, environmental influences on bone loss were significantly more similar among members of monozygotic than members of dizygotic pairs (18). Numerous other studies have also found strong evidence for familial and presumably genetic influences on patterns of behavior, including the use of tobacco and alcohol, and perhaps physical activity. If these behaviors are partially genetically determined, then their influences on bone loss may also be considered to result partially from genetic influences, albeit indirect ones. The difficulty in separating genetic and environmental influences on bone loss (and bone mass) is a problem that will not easily be solved.

Hormones

Aside from severe restrictions in activity (eg, prolonged bed rest, paralysis), disturbances in normal gonadal function are the most important causes of adult bone loss. Even before peak bone mass is achieved, amenorrhea associated with athletic activity (20), eating disorders (21), and other factors frequently result in bone loss, although there are exceptions (22). It is also worthy of note that late onset of menarche can result in lowered premenopausal bone mass (23), suggesting that estrogen deficiency may not only cause bone loss but also diminish mineral accretion in the growing skeleton. Recent prospective data on growing children show more than a doubling of the rate of mineral accretion in the spines of children entering puberty, in contrast to relatively small changes in the growth of the radius (24). These data together emphasize the importance of estrogens and perhaps androgens even before bone loss begins.

At menopause, bone loss is accelerated in virtually all women and is associated with both endogenous estrogen and testosterone concentrations (4). The mechanism of estrogen action on bone is unclear, but estrogen receptors have been found in cultured cells (25; see Chapters 2 and 10) and it is likely that there is at least some direct action of estrogen on bone cells. Trabecular bone may be more sensitive to the actions of estrogens, given the greater rates of loss observed in the spine at the time of menopause (5).

The role of androgens in bone loss in women is less clear, but estrogen-deficient premenopausal women with higher than normal androgen concentrations do not appear to lose bone, despite amenorrhea (26). Moreover, hirsute women (with higher androgen concentrations) who continue to cycle have significantly higher than normal bone mass (27). In addition to the report mentioned above, postmenopausal women with the highest testosterone concentrations have been shown to lose bone at slower rates than other women. Thus, androgens appear beneficial, probably both in the development of peak mass and in the prevention of loss. There may also be beneficial skeletal effects of therapeutic doses of testosterone in men. Hypogonadal men using a testosterone substitute in doses adequate to normalize testosterone concentrations had significant improvements both in markers of skeletal turnover and in bone mass (28).

Thus, sex steroids, across the entire range of concentrations from very low or absent to therapeutic levels, appear to have important effects on skeletal turnover and both bone growth and loss. Among the modifiable influences affecting the skeleton, the maintenance or restoration of appropriate serum concentrations of sex steroids appears to offer the strongest point of intervention to prevent bone loss and osteoporosis.

Among other hormones that might affect rates of bone loss, parathyroid hormone and vitamin D are the most directly related to calcium metabolism and have the most established relationships to alterations in skeletal integrity. Hyperparathyroidism, although frequently without detrimental skeletal effects, can be associated with excessive bone loss that is reversible with parathyroidectomy (29). The extent to which bone loss varies with parathyroid hormone concentrations within the normal range is not known.

Osteoporosis

Physical Activity

It is well established that immobilization causes rapid bone loss (30), and it appears that extremely intense activities (eg, professional-level athletics) result in greater than normal bone mass at the skeletal sites stressed by these activities (22,31). However, these extremes affect only a very small fraction of adults, most of whom are sedentary or have modest activity levels. What is the role of physical activity within the more normal range occupied by most adults?

Some observational studies in older women have shown that more active women have somewhat slower rates of bone loss (32), although many studies have failed to observe such effects. In this area, negative studies may result not only from the absence of an effect, but also from the difficulty in accurately assessing physical activity, particularly in primarily sedentary groups (33). In one long-term study of bone loss in men intense physical activity was also associated with slower bone loss, even though the activity levels were quite low (approximately 2 hours a week in intense activities) (7).

▶ 113

The most convincing data supporting the role of activity in the prevention of bone loss come from intervention studies. Randomized activity trials are difficult to do in any area, but at least one has shown women randomized to an activity group had significantly slower rates of bone loss than controls (34). The benefit is probably limited to those sites stressed by the activity used. Clinical trials in exercise remain among the most difficult to complete, due largely to noncompliance with recommended activity programs, and perhaps to a lesser degree to the currently poor understanding of the type, frequency, and intensity of exercise necessary to achieve skeletal effects (35).

Numerous questions remain to be answered regarding the utility of physical activity in the prevention of bone loss. How intense must the activity be? Studies have failed to show beneficial effects of walking programs (36,37), although arguments could be made that these studies were either too small (36) or measured the wrong skeletal sites (37). In any case, it remains to be shown that walking is an effective way to prevent bone loss. (It should be noted that the ultimate prevention of fractures may depend not only on the preservation of bone mass but perhaps also on the maintenance of muscle function, the prevention of falls, and other factors that may be positively affected by regular walking.) Similarly, swimming has not been shown to be beneficial, probably because of the absence of weight-bearing during this activity. At the opposite extreme, even among populations demonstrating benefits of intense physical activity, there appear to be levels (perhaps 20 hours a week or more) at which detrimental skeletal effects occur (22). Between these extremes little is known regarding either the quantity or type of activity necessary to prevent or slow bone loss.

What is certain regarding the role of exercise in bone loss is that: (1) more weight-bearing activity appears to be better than less; (2) greatly diminished activity will cause substantial and rapid bone loss; and (3) excessive activity that results in oligomenorrhea or amenorrhea in younger women causes detrimental changes in bone mass similar to those observed at menopause.

Tobacco and Alcohol Use

These behaviors are more common and more intense in older men, making the study of their effects on bone loss easier in this group than in women. However, smoking clearly has detrimental skeletal effects. Studies have shown that female smokers have lower bone mass (38), higher rates of vertebral fracture (39), and greater rates of bone loss shortly after the menopause (40). Smoking has been shown to alter the metabolism of estrogen so as to reduce its biologic effectiveness (41), but it is not clear that the mechanism of smoking's effect on skeletal tissue involves estrogen at all. In men, for example, one-pack-per-day smokers lost bone at about twice the rate of nonsmokers over a period of 16 years (7), and it seems unlikely that estrogen effects would be involved here. However, effects on androgens or direct effects on bone seem possible. Smoking is also associated with lower body weight, which in turn is associated with lower bone mass, but the negative effects of smoking appear to be independent of body weight (38,40).

Alcohol consumption at modest levels (1.5 drinks per day) has been associated with bone loss in men, independent of smoking effects (7). Numerous studies in women have failed to find associations between alcohol consumption and bone loss. This, however, may reflect the modest levels of consumption by the women in these studies. Alcoholism is clearly associated with fracture risk, but the reasons for this association could include falling, nutritional deficiencies, and numerous other factors unrelated to bone loss (42).

Tobacco and alcohol consumption are related behaviors, occurring more frequently together than expected by chance, being strongly addictive in some people, and showing genetic influences on both the choice and intensity of these behaviors. In regression analyses, however, they appear to have independent effects on bone loss (7).

The magnitude of bone loss caused by tobacco and alcohol use is difficult to estimate precisely. However, in the study of middle-aged men those who both smoked (more than 10 cigarettes per day) and drank (more than 1.5 drinks per day) lost bone at about twice the rate of abstainers from both behaviors. This would result in bone mass lowered by an additional 10% (about one standard deviation) after 20 years. In menopausal women long-term heavier (more than 15 cigarettes per day) smokers had spine bone mass about 0.08 g/cm² lower than nonsmokers; this is just under a 10% difference. The effect size from these studies is, therefore, fairly consistent, and suggests a substantial long-term negative effect on bone mass. Of course, those who smoke and drink heavily will be underrepresented in the older segments of the population due to higher death rates, and, thus, the effects of these behaviors on fracture rates may be more difficult to demonstrate. Recently, however, it has been reported that smoking doubles the risk of hip fracture, independent of bone mass (43), suggesting that the effects of smoking may extend beyond its detrimental influence on skeletal mass. Because of the high prevalence of both smoking and drinking, even small relative risks would translate into high attributable risks, and, therefore, further study into these influences is important.

▶ 115

Medications

Numerous drugs have been suggested to affect skeletal mass. Most prominently, long-term corticosteroid therapy has been associated with reduced bone mass and has been considered by experts as one of the four clear indications (along with estrogen deficiency, spinal crush fractures, and hyperparathyroidism) justifying diagnostic bone mass measurements (44). The extent to which such therapy can be adjusted obviously depends on the patient's health, but in cases where reductions in steroid dose are possible this should be considered. This may be an especially important consideration in the treatment of juvenile rheumatoid arthritis, due to the possibility of interfering with normal skeletal development during a period of rapid growth. However, the substitution of newer treatments for corticosteroids may not ensure amelioration of detrimental skeletal effects. Many of these drugs, (eg, methotrexate and hydroxychloroquine) have not been studied with respect to skeletal effects, and should not be assumed to be benign.

Thyroid medications have also been implicated in bone loss (45). There is some dispute whether or not the adverse skeletal effects relate to over-treatment, which is a relatively common occurrence.

Among other drugs suspected of causing bone loss are anticonvulsants. Anticonvulsant use has been associated with detrimental skeletal effects in long-term users (46). However, the extent to which modifications in this therapy are possible is not clear.

Drugs not originally developed to prevent bone loss may possibly have beneficial skeletal effects. Thiazide diuretics have been reported to be associated with higher bone mass, presumably by preventing bone loss, although not all investigators have found such effects. Curiously, tamoxifen, which somehow interferes with estrogen binding to its receptor, appears to prevent bone loss in postmenopausal women. Again, however, reports are conflicting in this regard.

A clinical trial is now underway testing the long-term effects of tamoxifen in both pre- and postmenopausal women. It is plausible but unproven that tamoxifen may fail to show beneficial effects or may actually be detrimental in estrogen-replete women (ie, normally cycling, premenopausal), due to its estrogen receptor-blocking effects.

Drugs being used therapeutically to prevent bone loss or treat osteoporosis are considered below.

Diseases

A number of diseases are associated with increased rates of bone loss. To discuss all such conditions would be beyond the scope of this chapter, but several of the more common conditions and their effects are listed below.

Asymptomatic hyperparathyroidism is perhaps the most common of these conditions. Commonly detected during routine biochemical screening tests, hyperparathyroidism may be completely without adverse effects, but excessive bone loss is a possible sequel (44), which may be obviated by surgery (29,44). This was considered by an expert panel of the National Osteoporosis Foundation to be one of four clinical indications for bone mass measurements.

Many conditions, including Graves' disease, rheumatoid arthritis, Cushing disease and others, have been associated with reduced bone mass. However, the extent to which treatment of these diseases should be altered by the presence of low bone mass is uncertain. For example, should patients with rheumatoid arthritis be switched from corticosteroids to other therapies (eg, hydroxychloroquine, methotrexate) to prevent bone loss, and what are the consequences of these alternative treatments? Clearly, more study is required.

Does Bone Loss Influence Fracture Susceptibility?

The obvious answer to this question is yes, but it is a more complex question than it first seems. Insofar as bone loss leads to lower bone mass and reduced bone mass leads to fracture, this must be true. Because bone mass at age 50 explains approximately 65% of the variability in bone mass at age 70, bone loss (and measurement error) must account for the other 35%. Obviously, the contribution of bone loss continues to increase with increasing age. It remains to be shown, however, that measuring bone loss can help in the prediction of fractures. In fact, in those few studies with long-term data, measurement of bone loss has not been a significant predictor of incident fractures. This is probably due to several factors discussed in more detail below. Briefly, short-term measurements of bone loss may not correlate strongly with longer-term loss, both because of biologic variability in bone loss and because of errors in estimating it (47).

A second issue is whether more rapid bone loss causes structural skeletal damage beyond that attributable to the loss of mass. For example, does rapid loss lead to perforation rather than just thinning of trabecular plates, thereby producing a weaker structure? Direct evidence for such an effect is lacking, but some data are worth examining in this regard. Ross and colleagues have shown that the presence of a previous fracture (in the spine or elsewhere), independent of bone mass, predicts fracture incidence in the spine (48). This suggests that there is a factor in addition to bone mass that contributes to fracture risk in some individuals. Many possibilities exist to explain this observation, including the introduction of instability in the spinal geometry, or the presence of general structural differences in the microarchitecture of the skeleton. Whether or not this element is some structural characteristic that might be affected by bone loss remains to be determined. Additionally, Christiansen has reported that measurements of markers of both bone turnover and loss in menopausal women are associated with incident spine fractures, independent of bone mass, suggesting again that rates of loss may somehow contribute independently to spine fragility (49).

The biologic contribution of bone loss to skeletal fragility cannot be denied, but the utility of measurements of bone loss to estimate this contribution remain somewhat less certain.

The Clinical Measurement of Bone Loss—Methods and Utility

The measurement of bone mass has now progressed to the point that it is considered routine and of excellent precision. Although many issues remain, including cross-calibration of instruments from different manufacturers, assignment of fracture risk based on different sites, and the ideal timing of these measurements, there is little doubt that a single measurement of bone mass can provide a useful estimate of fracture risk, including fracture risk for specific sites, such as the hip. Recently, a paper has been published showing a relative risk for hip fracture of 2.7 per SD change in femoral neck bone mass (50). These are the strongest data, thus far, showing the value of bone mass measurements.

The measurement of bone loss, however, is much more difficult. Whereas the measurement of mass (or areal density) has a precision on the order of 0.7% to 2.0% (compared with a SD in the adult population of 10% to 16% for most sites), the precision of loss measurements is a much larger fraction of the SD of rates of loss. This leads to a much greater chance for misclassification when attempting to rank people in terms of bone loss, as compared with rankings done on the basis of bone mass. Further complicating this problem are elements which contribute to biological variability in bone loss. For example, some women may lose 3% to 5% of bone mass each year for 2 to 3 years and then later slow to less than 0.5% per year. The period of rapid loss usually occurs near menopause, but for some women it is much later. The correlation between rates of loss in consecutive 5-year periods is only about 0.2 (47), suggesting a relatively weak relationship between measured rates of loss over even fairly short periods of time. Thus, the justification for measuring bone loss must be other than attempting long-term predictions of future bone mass. To place this in better perspective, the value of estimates of bone loss for fracture prediction would require that these estimates contribute information beyond that provided by the last bone mass measurement used in the calculation of rates of loss. This is a stringent but reasonable criterion for assessing the value of measurements of loss in fracture prediction.

Monitoring either the effectiveness of various therapies or short-term bone loss in certain medical conditions (eg, asymptomatic hyperparathyroidism) appear to be the most appropriate indications for measuring bone loss clinically. The National Osteoporosis Foundation Scientific Advisory Board recommendations (published in 1989) refrained from recommending the measurement of bone loss for any indication, although these were considered in detail under "Other potential indications," in that document. Since its publication, however, the precision of x-ray-based absorptiometry systems has greatly improved the possibilities in this area.

Several approaches will improve the precision of estimates of bone loss. As mentioned above, the use of more precise systems is critical. Sites with measurement errors much greater than 1% (ie, the coefficient of variation of repeated measurements within an individual) will require measurement intervals of 3 or more years to achieve good precision in bone loss assessment. Secondly, measurements should be made at the site of greatest clinical interest if acceptable precision is possible; correlations among skeletal sites are modest (in the neighborhood of 0.5) and do not permit extrapolation of estimates from one site to others. Third, two measurements made at each visit will improve the precision of that estimate of bone mass, and hence the estimates of loss between measurements. Fourth, the longer the interval between measurements the better. With this last recommendation some caution is required. If the goal of the measurements is to estimate the effectiveness of a therapy, a wait of 2 years might allow the patient to suffer unacceptable bone loss. A compromise might be to measure markers of bone turnover in the very short term to establish that the therapy has succeeded at the biochemical level (perhaps accepting reduced levels of markers of turnover as evidence), and then to measure the skeleton at some longer interval. This is not, however, a proven effective strategy.

As an example, consider a therapy to which 85% of patients have a positive clinical response (ie, bone loss is stopped). If nonresponders are menopausal women losing 3% of vertebral bone mass per year (and 3% loss per year is considered the cut-off for nonresponse), and intervals between measurements are 2 years with an instrument with 1% measurement error, then 84% of nonresponders would be correctly identified, and virtually none of the responders would be misclassified. Two years may be an unacceptable interval for some patients and their physicians, but generally the bone loss over 2 years would not be so great as to preclude this being a reasonable strategy. It should also be noted that if the therapy being tested causes some short-term gain in bone mass, or if more than one measurement at each time point is used, then these calculations are conservative (ie, misclassification would be even less).

How Can Rates of Bone Loss Be Altered?

In menopausal women the most common and effective approach to the prevention of bone loss is estrogen replacement therapy (ERT). It is now common to add a progestin to this hormone replacement therapy (HRT) so as to reduce the risk of endometrial cancer, but estrogen alone is adequate to stop bone loss for long periods of time (51–53). The effectiveness of long-term ERT in fracture prevention is certain, with 25% to 50% reductions in fracture incidence normally observed (54). ERT has both additional risks and benefits. Among the risks are an increase in endometrial cancer incidence (but not mortality) (55) and the possibility of a small increase in breast cancer (again, perhaps without an increase in mortality) (56). This last issue remains controversial and is the focus of ongoing study. Additionally, it appears that therapeutic estrogens reduce the risk of cardiovascular disease (57). Although these additional risks and benefits are not directly related to bone loss, they do influence the proportion of women offered and accepting ERT/HRT. Clarification of the magnitude of these other risks and benefits will ultimately help menopausal women and their physicians make better informed choices regarding ERT/HRT for the prevention of bone loss.

Because of these questions regarding ERT/HRT, several bone-specific agents have been developed. Both calcitonin and bisphosphonates have been shown to prevent bone loss (58,59), and studies examining their effects on fracture incidence are underway. The need to demonstrate effective fracture prevention, particularly with respect to hip fractures, will require many years of observation. The prevention of bone loss and the prevention of fractures would be parallel if normal bone was formed during therapy, but questions regarding this issue have been raised as a result of clinical trials examining the utility of fluoride therapy (60,61). As has been long observed, fluoride increased bone mass in predominantly trabecular bone, but fracture rates were significantly higher in the fluoride group than among those receiving placebo (60). This suggests that the bone formed during therapy may not have been as strong as normal bone. This may relate to the changes in the apatite crystal during fluoride therapy, or it may be due to some more subtle process, but this will require further study.

With respect to calcitonin and bisphosphonates, there seems little chance that abnormal bone is formed. Each of these therapies halts bone loss by slowing the bone remodeling rate; bisphosphonates achieve this by binding, apparently permanently, to bone. Because of this, there is some question regarding the long-term effects of bisphosphonates on skeletal strength, although no evidence exists to suggest that bone is weakened by this therapy. Although bisphosphonates are not yet approved by the Food and Drug Administration, calcitonin (subcutaneous injection) has been. Nasal administration of calcitonin is under study.

Further comments regarding exposure to fluoride are required, although it seems clear that bone loss from the spine is actually reversed, and bone loss from the hip is not increased. Several recent studies have suggested that even low exposures to fluoride may result in increased fracture frequency (62,63). These ecologic studies have shown that communities with fluoridated water (about 1 mg fluoride/L) have higher rates of hip fractures than those without. Communities with higher natural levels of fluoride (4–8 mg fluoride/L) in their water also appear to have higher fracture rates (64), again without excessive bone loss. The levels of fluoride consumed in these communities depend on how much water is ingested, but probably range from about 3 to 15 mg/d, in contrast to the 30 mg/d in the clinical trials cited above. Whether there is an effective therapeutic range for fluoride remains to be shown.

Calcium supplementation has been shown both to increase the rate of gain in bone mass in children (65) and to slow bone loss in older people (66). The effects of calcium during periods of rapid bone loss have been intermediate between placebo and estrogen in studies where these have been compared (66). Other have found benefits only in those with low calcium intakes (67) and not at all skeletal sites (66,67). Calcium deficiency plays only a minor role in menopausal bone loss, but is probably more important among the elderly. It has been suggested that 1500 mg or more per day may be necessary to prevent bone loss in the very old (68), although others have disputed this. The efficacy of calcium in slowing (but not completely preventing) bone loss in the very old seems established.

Vitamin D also offers promise in the prevention of bone loss in older people. Perhaps most importantly, calcium and vitamin D used together have been shown to reduce hip fracture incidence and to slow bone loss (69), although the effects on bone loss were inconsistent and varied widely according to skeletal site. For example, at the femoral neck, the site that would logically have shown good results (given the fracture findings), neither placebo nor treatment group lost bone. Although intuitively one would attribute the effects on fracture incidence to preservation of bone mass, there are other possibilities. For example, vitamin D might also have effects on reversing muscle weakness in people with vitamin D deficiencies, and perhaps preventing falls. Of course from a practical perspective the effectiveness of these treatments together is the critical element.

▶ 121

As mentioned above, the value of exercise in the prevention of bone loss requires further study. The duration, type, and intensity necessary to prevent bone loss remain to be determined, although it is certain that activity is necessary to maintain skeletal integrity. No specific exercise regiments can, as yet, be recommended, but weight-bearing appears to be necessary. Swimming and walking, though widely recommended, do not seem to confer skeletal benefits, although it is plausible that in completely sedentary populations walking might be of some benefit. It should also be recognized that exercise might have benefits in terms of fracture prevention through mechanisms not involving bone mass (eg, reductions in the severity of frequency of falls).

References

1. Recker RR, Davies KM, Hinders SM, Heaney RP, Stegman MR, Kimmel DB. Bone gain in young adult women. JAMA 1992;268:2403–2408.

2. Theintz G, Buchs B, Rizzoli R, et al. Longitudinal monitoring of bone mass accumulation in adolescents: evidence for a marked reduction after 16 years of age at the levels of lumbar spine and femoral neck in female subjects. J Clin Endocrinol Metab 1992;75:1060–1065.

3. Garn SM. The earlier gain and the later loss of cortical bone. Springfield, Ill: Charles C Thomas, 1970.

4. Slemenda CW, Hui SL, Longcope CL, Johnston CC. Sex steroids and bone mass: a study of changes about the time of menopause. J Clin Invest 1987;80:1261–1269.

5. Harris S, Dawson-Hughes B. Rates of change in bone mineral density of the spine, heel, femoral neck and radius in healthy, postmenopausal women. Bone Miner 1992; 17:87–92.

6. Hui SL, Wiske PS, Norton JA, Johnston CC. A prospective study of change in bone mass with age in postmenopausal women. J Chron Dis 1982;35:715–720.

7. Slemenda CW, Christian JC, Reed T, Reister TK, Williams CJ, Johnston CC. Long-term bone loss in men: effects of genetic and environmental factors. Ann Intern Med 1992;117:286–291.

8. Orwoll ES, Oviatt SK, McClung MR, Deftos LJ, Sexton G. The rate of bone mineral loss in normal men and the effects of calcium and cholecalciferol supplementation. Ann Intern Med 1990;112:29–34.

9. Buchanan JR, Myers C, Lloyd T, Greer RB. Early vertebral trabecular bone loss in normal premenopausal women. J Bone Miner Res 1988;3:583–587.

10. Riggs BL, Wahner HW, Seeman E, et al. Changes in bone mineral density of the proximal femur and spine with aging. J Clin Invest 1982;70:716–723.

11. Johnston CC, Slemenda CW, Longcope C. The role of androgens in skeletal integrity in women. Presented at the 4th International Symposium on Osteoporosis. Abstract #722, 1993.

12. Smith DM, Nance WE, Kang KW, Christian JC, Johnston CC. Genetic factors in determining bone mass. J Clin Invest 1973;52:2800–2808.

13. Pocock NA, Eisman JA, Hopper JL, Yeates MG, Sambrook PN, Eben S. Genetic determinants of bone mass in adults: a twin study. J Clin Invest 1987;80: 706–710.

14. Christian JC, Yu P-L, Slemenda CW, Johnston CC. Heritability of bone mass: a longitudinal study in aging male twins. Am J Hum Genet 1989;44:429–433.

15. Krall EA, Dawson-Hughes B. Heritable and life style determinants of bone mineral density. J Bone Miner Res 1993; 8:1–9.

16. Kelly PJ, Hopper JL, McCaskill GT, Pocock NA, Sambrook PN, Eisman JA. Genetic factors in bone turnover. J Clin Endocrinol Metab 1991;72:808–813.

17. Kelly PJ, Nguyen T, Hopper J, Pocock N, Sambrook P, Eisman J. Changes in axial bone density with age: a twin study. J Bone Miner Res 1993;8:11–17.

18. Slemenda CW, Christian JC, Williams CJ, Norton JA, Johnston CC. Genetic determinants of bone mass in adult women: a reevaluation of the twin model and the potential importance of gene interaction on heritability estimates. J Bone Miner Res 1991;6:561–567.

19. Slemenda CW, Christian JC, Williams CJ, Johnston CC. The changing relative importance of genetics and environment in adult women. In: Cohn DV, Glorieux FH, Martin TJ, eds. Calcium regulation and bone metabolism. Amsterdam: Elsevier Science Publishers (Biomedical Division), 1990:491–496.

20. Drinkwater BL, Nilson K, Ott S, et al. Bone mineral content of amenorrheic and eumenorrheic athletes. N Engl J Med 1984;311:277–281.

21. Seeman E, Szmulkler GI, Formica C, Tsalamandis C, Mestrovic R. Osteoporosis in anorexia nervosa: the influence of peak bone density, bone loss, oral contraceptive use and exercise. J Bone Miner Res 1992;7:1467–1474.

22. Slemenda CW, Johnston CC. High intensity activities in young women: site specific bone mass effects among female figure skaters. Bone Miner 1993;20: 125–132.

23. Armamento-Villereal R, Villereal D, Avioli L, Civitelli R. Estrogen status and heredity are major determinants of premenopausal bone mass. J Clin Invest 1992;90:2464–2471.

24. Slemenda CW, Reister TK, Miller JZ, Hui SL, Johnston CC. Influences on bone growth in children and adolescents: evidence for varying effects of sexual maturation and activity. (Under review).

25. Eriksen EF, Colvard DS, Berg NJ, et al. Evidence of estrogen receptors in normal human osteoblast-like cells. Science 1988;241:84–86.

26. Buchanan JR, Hospodar P, Myers C, Leuenberger P, Demers LM. Effects of excess endogenous androgens on bone density in young women. J Clin Endocrinol Metab 1988;67:937–943.

27. Dixon JE, Rodin A, Murby B, Chapman MG, Fogelman I. Bone mass in hirsute women with androgen excess. Clin Endocrinol 1989;30:271–277.

28. Devogelear JP, DeCooman S, Nagant de Deuxchaisnes C. Low bone mass in hypogonadal males. Effect of testosterone substitution therapy, a densitometric study. Maturitas 1992;15:17–23.

29. Copley JB, Hui SL, Leapman S, Slemenda CW, Johnston CC. Longitudinal study of bone mass in end-stage renal dis-

ease patients: effects of parathyroidectomy for renal osteodystrophy. J Bone Miner Res 1993;8:415–422.

30. Prince RL, Price RI, Ho S. Forearm bone loss in hemiplegia: a model for the study of immobilization osteoporosis. J Bone Miner Res 1988;3:305–310.

31. Huddleston AL, Rockwell D, Kuland D, Harrison RB. Bone mass in lifetime tennis athletes. JAMA 1980;244:1107–1109.

32. Nelson ME, Meredith CN, Dawson-Hughes B, Evans WJ. Hormone and bone mineral status in endurance trained and sedentary postmenopausal women. J Clin Endocrinol Metab 1988;66:927–933.

33. LaPorte RE, Kuller LH, Kupfer DJ, McPartland RJ, Matthews G, Casperson C. An objective measure of physical activity for epidemiologic research. Am J Epidemiol 1979;109:158–168.

34. Chow R, Harrison HE, Notarius C. Effect of two randomized exercise programs on bone mass of healthy postmenopausal women. Br Med J 1987;295:1441–1444.

35. Forwood MR, Burr D. Physical activity and bone mass: exercises in futility? J Bone Miner Res 1993;21:89–112.

36. Cavanaugh DJ, Cann CE. Brisk walking does not stop bone loss in postmenopausal women. Bone 1988;9:210–214.

37. Sandler RB, Slemenda CW, LaPorte RE, et al. Postmenopausal bone density and milk consumption in childhood and adolescence. Am J Clin Nutr 1985;42:270–274.

38. Slemenda CW, Hui SL, Longcope C, Johnston CC. Cigarette smoking, obesity and bone mass. J Bone Miner Res 1989; 4:737–741.

39. Daniell HW. Osteoporosis of the slender smoker. Arch Intern Med 1976; 136:298–304.

40. Krall EA, Dawson-Hughes B. Smoking and bone loss among postmenopausal women. J Bone Miner Res 1991; 6:331–338.

41. Michnovicz JJ, Hershkopf RJ, Naganuma H, Bradlow HL, Fishman J. Increased 2-hydroxylation of estradiol as a possible mechanism for the anti-estrogenic effect of cigarette smoking. N Engl J Med 1986;315:1305–1309.

42. Bikle DD, Genant HK, Cann CE, Recker RR, Halloran BP, Strewler GJ. Bone disease in alcohol abuse. Ann Intern Med 1985;103:42–48.

43. Cummings SR. Risk factors for fractures: new findings, new concepts, new questions. Presented at the 4th International Symposium on Osteoporosis. Abstract #15, 1993.

44. Johnston CC, Melton LJ, Lindsay R, Eddy DM. Clinical indications for bone mass measurements. J Bone Miner Res 1989;4(Suppl 2):1–28.

45. Fallon MD, Perry HM, Bergfeld M, et al. Exogenous hyperthyroidism with osteoporosis. Arch Intern Med 1983;143:442–444.

46. Weinstein RS, Bryce GF, Sappington LJ, King DW, Gallager BB. Decreased serum ionized calcium and normal vitamin D metabolite levels with anti-convulsant treatment. J Clin Endocrinol Metab 1984; 48:1003–1009.

47. Hui SL, Slemenda CW, Johnston CC. The contribution of bone loss to postmenopausal osteoporosis. Osteoporosis Int 1990;1:30–34.

48. Ross PD, David JW, Epstein RS, Wasnich RD. Pre-existing fractures and bone mass predict vertebral fracture incidence in women. Ann Intern Med 1991; 114:919–923.

49. Christiansen C. Prediction of future fracture risk. Presented at the 4th International Symposium on Osteoporosis. Abstract #50, 1993.

50. Cummings SR, Black DM, Nevitt MC, et al. Bone density and hip fractures in older women: a prospective study. Lancet 1993;341:72–75.

51. Lindsay R, Hart DM, Aitken JM, MacDonald EB, Anderson JB, Clarke AC. Long-term prevention of postmenopausal osteoporosis by oestrogen. Lancet 1976; 1:1038–1041.

52. Ettinger B, Genant HK, Cann CE. Long term estrogen therapy prevents fractures and preserves bone mass. Ann Intern Med 1985;102:319–324.

53. Christiansen C, Christiansen MS, McNair PL, Hagen C, Stocklund KE, Transbol I. Prevention of early postmenopausal bone loss: controlled 2-year study in

315 normal females. Eur J Clin Invest 1980;10:273–279.

54. Weiss NS, Ure CL, Ballard JH, Williams AR, Daling JR. Decreased risk of fractures of the hip and lower forearm with postmenopausal use of estrogen. N Engl J Med 1980;303:1195–1198.

55. Nachtigall LE, Nachtigall RH, Nachtigall RD, Beckman EM. Estrogen replacement therapy II: a prospective study in the relationship to carcinoma and cardiovascular and metabolic problems. Obstet Gynecol 1979;54:74–79.

56. Bergkvist L, Adami HO, Persson I, et al. The risk of breast cancer after estrogen and estrogen-progestin replacement. N Engl J Med 1989;321:293–297.

57. Barrett-Connor E, Bush TL. Estrogen and coronary heart disease in women. JAMA 1991;265:1861–1867.

58. Storm T, Thamsborg G, Steiniche T, Genant HK, Sorenson OH. Effect of intermittent cyclical etidronate therapy on bone mass and fracture rate in postmenopausal osteoporosis. N Engl J Med 1990:322: 1265–1271.

59. Overgaard K, Hansen MA, Jensen SB, Christiansen C. Effect of salcatonin given intranasally on bone mass and fracture rates in established osteoporosis: a dose-response study. Br Med J 1992;305: 556–561.

60. Riggs BL, Hodgson SF, O'Fallon WM, et al. Effect of fluoride treatment on fracture rate in postmenopausal women with osteoporosis. N Engl J Med 1990;322: 802–809.

61. Kleerekoper M, Peterson EL, Nelson DA, et al. A randomized trial of sodium fluoride as a treatment for postmenopausal osteoporosis. Osteoporosis Int 1990;1: 155–161.

62. Jacobson SJ, Goldberg J, Miles TP, Brody JA, Stiers W, Rimm AE. Regional variation in the incidence of hip fracture. JAMA 1990;264:500–502.

63. Danielson C, Lyon JL, Egger M, Goodenough GK. Hip fractures and fluoridation in Utah's elderly population. JAMA 1992;268:746–748.

64. Sowers MR, Clark MK, Jannasch ML, Wallace RB. A prospective study of bone mineral content and fracture in communities with differential fluoride exposure. Am J Epidemiol 1991;133:649–660.

65. Johnston CC, Miller JZ, Slemenda CW, et al. Calcium supplementation and increases in bone mineral density in children. N Engl J Med 1992;327:82–87.

66. Riis B, Thomsen K, Christiansen C. Does calcium supplementation prevent postmenopausal bone loss? A double-blind controlled clinical trial. N Engl J Med 1987;316:173–177.

67. Dawson-Hughes B, Dallal GE, Krall EA, Sadowski L, Sahyoun N, Tannenbaum S. A controlled trial of the effect of calcium supplementation on bone density in postmenopausal women. N Engl J Med 1990; 323:878–883.

68. Nordin BEC, Heaney RP. Calcium supplementation of the diet: justified by the present evidence. Br Med J 1990; 300:1056–1060.

69. Chapuy MC, Arlot ME. Duboeuf F, et al. Vitamin D_3 and calcium prevent hip fractures in elderly women. N Engl J Med 1992;327:1637–1642.

124 ◀

6 ▸ Ethnicity and Skeletal Health

▶ ▶ ▶ Marie Luz Villa

Diversity adds richness and color to the tapestry of human experience. In modern parlance, diversity is frequently defined by ethnic group or race. However, these two terms have very different meanings. *Race* refers to three major categories of human beings: Asian, black, and Caucasian. For purposes of serious investigation, dichotomy by race is highly problematic; it fails to account for the considerable variation within a single group or mixtures of groups. *Ethnicity* reflects a group's diversity and confers more specificity than race. It would distinguish Puerto Rican from Swede from Jew. Ethnicity may influence the incidence of some diseases; hypertension, diabetes, renal failure, neurologic and cardiovascular diseases, depression, and cancer are but a few of the maladies whose prevalence and severity vary among people of differing backgrounds (1–8). Ethnicity (often called ethnic group or ethnic background) refers to the distinction of a group by identifiable differences but makes no statement as to whether these differences are due to genetic or environmental causes (9). It refers not only to the group's race but includes all the layers of cultural complexity that both delight and confuse the onlooker. This chapter reviews the relationship between ethnicity and skeletal health, although unfortunately, it will at times be necessary to cite race without reference to ethnic background.

Defining an ethnic group for the purpose of a study may *appear* straightforward; many use the terms Hispanic, black, Asian, and Caucasian. However, use of these labels could miscategorize subjects or render data uninterpretable. Americans do not pigeonhole well. How one defines ethnicity can and does profoundly influence the quality and general applicability of collected information. "Hispanics" is a term used for the purpose of classifying Spanish-speaking peoples and may include Mexicans, Mexican-Americans, Chicanos, Puerto Ricans, Cubans, Cuban-Americans, Latinos, Central Americans, or South Americans. Families living for many generations in the southwestern United States, which at one time was Mexican territory, do not necessarily identify with *any* of the above terms.

Often ethnic groups are difficult to categorize. Some Spanish-speaking people are Europeans from Spain, and therefore not the typical "Hispanic." It is challenging to decide whether African-Americans from Puerto Rico are "Hispanic" or "black," and the differentiation between individuals with West African versus South African forebears is usually not made. One may ask if it is really acceptable to lump Indian, Filipino, Tongan, Southeast Asian, Chinese, and Japanese peoples under the common label "Asian." And there is always the question of how to describe individuals who are born into one ethnicity, but have a different ethnic background from most others in that region; if a study subject were born of Japanese parents but raised Brazilian, how would ethnicity be assigned?

In any study of the impact of ethnicity on measured variables, it is of utmost importance to define the study population. Given the difficulty of applying preset category labels to individuals, it makes more sense to ask people what their ethnicity is, as well as to which racial group they belong. Occasionally the specificity of a given research question may dictate more narrow selection by the investigator. For example, it may be necessary to include people whose parents and grandparents are *all* of a given race and ethnicity. However, it should be understood that such individuals may constitute a small minority in a "melting pot" country such as the United States and that conclusions may not be broadly applicable.

Importance of Acculturation

Studies that include measures of ethnicity and acculturation (loss of traditional cultural values) demonstrate striking variation in disease prevalence and severity associated with degree of maintenance of cultural values and habits (10,11). Most measures of acculturation have been applied to Hispanic and Asian groups using language and preservation of culture as indices of degree of acculturation. But groups that have been in America for many generations may also retain traditional foods, herbal remedies, and customs not necessarily in concordance with linguistic preservation. In addition to the impact on disease prevalence, ethnicity and resultant life-style choices may indirectly modify health outcomes. Epidemiologic studies confirm the clinical sentiment that Mexican-American and black American women tend toward obesity (12,13) and point out that body image is, to a large degree, culturally defined. When investigating risk factors for various human diseases, it is therefore valuable to include an evaluation of the impact of ethnicity and associated life-style factors.

Osteoporosis

It is expected that ethnic minorities will comprise an increasingly greater proportion of the population of aged persons in the United States. Data from the 1990 US Census indicated that there were approximately 2.5 million blacks, 1.25 million Hispanics, and 500,000 Asians over the age of 65 years (14). It is projected that in the next half century, the minority population aged 65 and older will *double* (15). Provision of health care to this kaleidoscopic population must consider the unique effects of cultural values.

Ethnic Aspects of Osteoporosis

▶ 127

Although osteoporosis looms centrally in the estimation of expected morbidity for aging Caucasians (16), much evidence points to a greatly differing experience for other ethnic groups. An early cross-national review found that osteoporosis, using radiographic estimates of metacarpal bone mass and fracture prevalence, was very rare in African countries and Jamaica (17). Japanese men and women, by contrast, frequently had fractures of the spine but less often fractures of the hip or wrist. Osteoporosis was relatively common in Europe and India, although osteomalacia contributed greatly to the fracture prevalence in India. Maggi and colleagues, in an excellent recent review of the international literature (18), illustrate that hip fracture incidence varies widely by geographic location, sex, and race [Table 6-1].

Observations within the United States, with its heterogeneous population, reflect international experience. It is estimated that costs stemming from osteoporotic fracture will consume an increasing proportion of health care dollars, especially as the population ages. Hip fractures comprise a large part of costs attributed to osteoporosis. Morbidity from other types of broken bones, especially of the spine, is expected to rise and exact its toll on the quality of life of elders. An understanding of the causes of ethnic variance in fracture incidence might therefore assist in developing preventive strategies for those most at risk for developing osteoporosis.

Ethnic Differences in Fracture Incidence

Many investigators have noted striking differences in the occurrence of osteoporotic fracture when comparing black Americans and Caucasians. Regional and national analysis of hospital discharge data have demonstrated dramatic gender and ethnic variation in hip fracture incidence. National incidence rates appear to be the highest for Caucasian women and are about 2 to 2.4 times rates for Caucasian men and blacks (19). Some regional studies find a lower rate of hip

TABLE 6-1   Age- and Sex-Specific Incidence Rates (per 100,000) of Hip Fracture

Geographic Area, Years of Survey	Women, Age (y)				Men, Age (y)			
	50–59	60–69	70–79	80+	50–59	60–69	70–79	80+
White populations								
Kuopio, Finland 1968	27	85	331	1130	24	54	154	559
Yorkshire, UK 1973–77	34	104	371	1200	20	51	140	548
New Zealand 1973–76	34	122	494	1988	27	51	186	862
Rochester, USA 1965–74	62	250	674	2108	37	92	192	1281
Funen, Denmark 1973–79	90	217	935	2533	48	129	307	1119
Oslo, Norway 1978–79	130	289	1022	2736	54	226	523	1598
Central Norway 1983–84	213	513	1611	5689	67	346	867	3234
Stockholm, Sweden 1972–81	79	227	820	2770	78	182	478	1419
Texas, USA 1980	45	235	726	2263	31	104	192	1641
California, USA 1983–84	65	213	726	2502	37	90	334	1209
Black populations								
Johannesburg, South Africa 1950–64	10	20	30	80	20	30	40	170
Texas, USA 1980		123	240	910				
California, USA 1983–84	35	80	270	990	46	84	190	816
Asian populations								
Singapore 1955–62	10	50	100	270	20	70	210	350
Hong Kong 1965–67	23	57	173	716	17	71	224	321
California, USA 1983–84	17	90	320	1930	16	49	155	739
Hong Kong 1985	32	135	501	1521	28	54	339	1156
Hispanic populations								
Texas, USA 1980	10	25	340	1423	18	31	214	816
California, USA 1983–84	16	60	250	960	15	34	150	600

(Reprinted by permission from Maggi S, Kelsey JL, Litvak J, Heyse SP. Incidence of hip fractures in the elderly: a cross national analysis. Osteoporosis Int 1991;1:232–241.)

fracture in black American men as compared to women (20–23). South African men and women have distinct rates of hip fracture depending on race, with an exceedingly small occurrence in black South Africans (24).

Reflecting the early observations of Nordin, it appears that ethnicity plays a critical role in the rate of occurrence of hip fracture in other groups as well. A lower incidence of hip fracture has been documented in elderly Japanese and Japanese-Americans (25,26), and for Mexican-Americans living in California and Texas (23,27), than for Caucasians. When looking at rates of hip fracture among the major US ethnic groups that have been studied (Native Americans and most Hispanic groups have been excluded), it appears that Asian Americans have an incidence intermediate to that of Caucasians and blacks, and that Mexican-Americans have a rate similar to that of blacks (22,23).

▶ 129

The gender difference in hip fracture incidence observed in Caucasians is not necessarily mirrored in other ethnic groups. One study demonstrated a higher incidence of hip fracture in Asian men than women (28), and the Maori of New Zealand exhibit no gender differences in fracture incidence, although compared to the local Caucasian population, their rate of fracture is greatly decreased (29).

In addition to differences due to gender or race, geographic diversity may play a role in osteoporotic fracture incidence. Bacon and colleagues found contrasts in Caucasian fracture incidence from one US census region to another (30) that might reflect residua from enclaves of people descended from specific immigrant groups. Black South Africans have a much lower rate of fracture than do black Americans; in contrast to trends noted in North America, black South African women historically are less likely to fracture than men (31).

Vertebral and other osteoporotic fracture incidence rates are more difficult to document because they do not typically involve hospitalization, nor do the majority of vertebral fractures necessitate presentation to health care facilities for treatment. There may be no difference in vertebral osteoporotic fracture rates between Asians and Caucasians (17,32). Smith and Rizek found a much lower prevalence of vertebral fractures in blacks than in Caucasians living in Michigan; a similar number of vertebral fractures in Puerto Rican nationals and Caucasians were observed (33). The only other US study of ethnic variation in vertebral fracture suggested that Mexican-Americans might have a lower occurrence of vertebral deformities than Caucasians (34), but the methods by which subjects were identified for this study raise questions about its applicability.

Hip fracture incidence does not always correlate with mortality rates; it has been noted that although Caucasian women have a higher incidence of hip fracture than Caucasian men and blacks, age-specific mortality rates for those hospitalized are highest for Caucasian and black men, intermediate for black women, and lowest for Caucasian women (20,35,36). The in-hospital death rates of men are about twice those observed for Caucasian women at any age (20), so gender and race differences in terms of mortality are attenuated. As ethnic groups come to comprise a larger proportion of the aged, this will become a pressing issue because extended-care facilities are not yet prepared for the varied needs of a diverse population.

The Basis of Ethnic Diversity in Skeletal Health

Several potential risk factors are invoked in seeking to explain the observed differences in fracture incidence. These include gradations in physical activity or dietary calcium; differences in vitamin D sufficiency related to latitude, skin pigment, or seasonal sunlight exposure; different patterns of obesity or muscle mass; and, perhaps most important, differences in the propensity to fall. It is thought that about 32% of Caucasian community-dwelling individuals aged 75 or above will fall at least once a year, with about 6% of those falls resulting in a fracture (37). Only a few ethnic studies of falls have been reported. Grisso and colleagues found that in an inner-city population of blacks, 28% of those who presented to an emergency room for evaluation following a fall had a resultant fracture, and many suffered significant postfall morbidity (38).

The Role of Bone Mass

Bone mineral density (BMD) predicts risk for fracture (39–41). The medical literature abounds with documentation of ethnic differences in bone mass, and it is thought that hereditary factors make significant contributions to these differences (9). Most investigators have found significantly greater BMD in Africans and black Americans than in Caucasians. Among older postmenopausal women, blacks consistently demonstrate a higher bone mass, which appears to correspond to their lower rate of hip fracture. Cross-sectional studies of older US and African women find a persistent black/white difference in bone mass, even when controlling for body mass index, age, and smoking history (24,42–45). Although some indicate a slower age-related decline of bone mass in Blacks, cohort effects may have contributed to these results. However, in a longitudinal study, Luckey and colleagues found that black women in early menopause have a lower rate of change in BMD than Caucasian women, a trend that did not continue into late menopause (43).

It is thought that skeletal mass begins to decline with age shortly after peak BMD is attained (46,47). Black premenopausal women apparently have denser bones than Caucasians. Although cross-sectional data raise the possibility that premenopausal black women *gain* bone while Caucasians *lose* it (44,48), an abstract describing a recent longitudinal study suggested that both groups undergo significant loss of bone from the radius and spine at similar rates (49).

The obvious place to look for elaboration of differences in bone mass is during skeletal development. Infants and young children sometimes demonstrate black/white differences in bone acquisition, but this issue remains controversial (50–56). Perhaps the inability to reach agreement about the early existence of ethnic differences in bone mass relates to the great difficulty in adjusting bone mass measurements for variation in body size. Assessment of BMD or bone mineral content (BMC) in older black and Caucasian children reveals that Tanner stage correlates highly with attainment of bone mass. When racial differences are found, they tend to be in adolescents (57,58).

▶ 131

One could readily conclude from the above discussion that blacks fracture at a lower rate than Caucasians due to the greater bone mass they enjoy. It would follow that Asians would have increased skeletal mass since they fracture less frequently, and that Mexican-Americans might have bone mass values equal to that of blacks since their fracture rates are equivalent. This concept may be true for the Maori of New Zealand (29,59), but in fact, most Asian groups have lower BMD than Caucasians (60–66). In addition, Mazess described a population of centenarians in Vilcabamba, Ecuador who have a minuscule incidence of fracture despite a mean value of bone mineral 15% lower than that of Caucasians (67).

Hirota and coworkers discovered a higher radial bone content for young Japanese women when compared to normative Caucasian values, but these findings were not replicated in other studies (68). Most healthy women beyond the age of 60 years in Japan are below the "fracture threshold" suggested for Caucasian women despite an occurrence of hip fracture 30% to 50% lower (60). Although low BMD may not correlate well with hip fracture in Asian populations, Ross and colleagues have found that decreased BMC did correlate with risk for vertebral fracture in Japanese-Americans (32).

Bone mineral density of Mexican-Americans does not appear to differ dramatically from that of Caucasians, although data are scanty. Bauer found some differences at the hip in premenopausal but not postmenopausal women (69). Benson and colleagues found no differences in adult cortical bone mass (70), and McCormick detected no significant variation between Hispanic and Caucasian children (56).

Bone mineral density can predict risk of vertebral fracture fairly well, but the considerable overlap with normal controls in hip fracture incidence indicates that other factors affecting bone strength contribute to risk for osteoporotic fracture at nonvertebral sites (16). Bone breaks when its structural integrity is threatened due to weakening or increased stress. When Beck and colleagues analyzed gender differences in cross-sectional hip strength, they found that women had significant age-related increases in stresses within the femoral neck, at three times the rate of men (71). Age-related loss of bone mass in men was offset by a compensatory increase in bone girth, thereby helping to maintain bone strength. This was not seen in women (71,72).

Recent analysis of data collected in the Study of Osteoporotic Fracture, suggests that geometric measurements of femoral size are related to fracture risk (73). Analysis of Eskimo BMC show it to be lower than that of Caucasians, but their low rate of fracture is thought to be due to relatively larger bone size (74). A cross-sectional study evaluating apparent ethnic variation in bone mass found that controlling for body habitus and medical history obliterated racial differences (75). Difference in body size appears as a persistent confounding variable in many studies; use of a mathematical correction for differences in bone size (76) from one population to another might therefore shed some light on the seeming discrepancies between bone mass and fracture risk.

Conventional bone mineral data are reported as BMD (in g/cm^2), that is, BMC divided by the projected area within the region of interest. This measure is more correctly called an *areal* density and is two dimensional. Bones of larger width and height are also thicker, and this third dimension of bone thickness is not factored into estimates of BMD. Therefore, reliance on BMD will overestimate the true *volumetric* (three dimensional) bone density of tall people and underestimate that of short people. Carter and coworkers (77) have proposed a way to express bone mineral data in a form that is less sensitive to differences in skeletal size. They defined another parameter, called the bone mineral apparent density (BMAD), that equals the BMC divided by estimates of bone volume based on the projected area measurements. These approximations have been applied to the data in a large multiethnic study of bone mineral status of postmenopausal women. In this study, black and Hispanic women were found to have higher BMD than Caucasian or Asian women, even when results were adjusted for age and body mass index. However, most ethnic differences in bone mineral lost significance when the data were corrected for approximate differences in bone size by calculating the BMAD, suggesting that ethnic variation in BMD status may reflect bone *size* rather than volumetric mineral density (Robert Marcus, personal communication). This was particularly interesting with respect to the observation that femoral neck BMD was significantly lower in Asian women than in all other groups, but that femoral neck BMAD was actually highest in Asians. As noted previously, hip fracture incidence is relatively low in Asian women despite an apparently low femoral BMD. The BMAD results from this study suggest that the reduction in bone mass may simply reflect a smaller bone size.

Bone mineral content within similar ethnic groups may vary, thereby suggesting that more than genetics is at play in determining skeletal mass (78). In a study of Japan-born and US-born persons of Japanese descent, Nomura and colleagues found significantly higher bone mass in the latter (65). It was thought that the differences between the two groups could be accounted for by environmental factors such as diet and medication use. This conclusion was supported by another study that found Japanese-American men and women to be consistently taller, heavier, and with greater BMC than Japanese nationals (79). Further evidence for environmental influence on bone mass comes from an elegant study of bone density and diet in four regions of rural China. Despite great genetic similarity, dramatic differences in BMD were detected among the four groups from different regions in which nutrient intakes varied widely (80). Bone mass correlated highly with dietary calcium intake, especially when dairy foods provided a substantial portion of ingested calcium. Conversely, it may be that for Caucasians living in the United States and Australia, life-styles have much in common because no significant differences in bone mass exist between the two populations (81).

The Role of Body Composition

Obesity, typically determined by body mass index (BMI), appears to protect against hip fracture (82). In a study of elderly women, underweight blacks had a significantly greater risk of hip fracture than their peers who were at or above ideal body weight (83). The mechanisms for this protection may be related to increased bone mass (due to greater weight bearing or to peripheral aromatization of androgens) or to buffering of the mechanical stress of falls (18,84). But even when comparing individuals defined as obese, ethnic differences in skeletal mass persist. Although obese women have significantly greater axial bone mass than the nonobese, black women's BMD is always higher than a comparable group of Caucasians even when differences in body size are considered (42,85–87).

The body mass index may be used to evaluate relative body size in a population. Depending on the investigator, a body mass index of about 28 kg/m² defines obesity in Caucasians. Most assume that an index value greater than 28 kg/m² reflects increased adiposity. Using this reference, a higher percentage of black and Mexican-American adults are defined as obese in comparison to Caucasians (12,13). Categorization of obesity in various ethnic groups using Caucasians as a standard is not necessarily appropriate, however, because body composition may differ from one group to another. It is likely that the standard body mass index is not a robust marker across ethnic groups.

Prevalence estimates for obesity, using a cutoff of 27.3 kg/m², are based on data gathered from the Second National Health and Nutrition Examination Survey (NHANES II), which used weights and heights of healthy Caucasian 20 to 29 year olds. The Hispanic Health and Nutrition Examination Survey (HHANES, 1982–1984) measured skinfolds, weight, and height in a cross-section of healthy Mexican-Americans, Cuban-Americans, and Puerto Ricans. Using the cutoff for obesity as being the 85th percentile of the 20- to 29-year-old women in HHANES, Lopez and Masse determined that the cutoffs for body mass index were 29.6 kg/m² for Mexican-American, 26.8 kg/m² for Cuban-American, and 29.2 kg/m² for Puerto Rican women (88). Using these group-specific standards, 14% fewer Mexican-American women were classified as overweight, with this pattern occurring in every age group.

Actual measurement of body composition, as opposed to use of an indirect gauge such as BMI, yields intriguing insights into racial contrasts. Using total body neutron activation analysis, Cohn and colleagues found that black men and women had higher absolute lean and skeletal body mass than Caucasians, but that the mean percent body fat did not differ between the two groups (86). Dual photon absorptiometry whole body scans of healthy women have demonstrated that in addition to higher total body calcium, blacks have significantly greater muscle mass than Caucasians (45).

Because muscle and skeletal mass are highly correlated (89), it could be that the increased BMD in blacks is due in part to the observed higher muscle mass. Furthermore, if muscle mass is conserved with aging, it may attenuate the acceleration of bone loss that occurs with menopause because muscle plays an important role in aromatization of androgens (90). Circulating androgens are independent predictors of peak bone mass in women as well as men (91), and some evidence suggests a decreased rate of hip fracture in women with higher circulating levels of serum testosterone and estradiol (92).

The Role of Dietary Calcium

One might posit that since a majority of the world's population develops lactose intolerance at an early age, calcium intake and hence conservation of bone mass would be significantly better in those areas where dairy food intake continues through adulthood. This hypothesis is not supported by examination of differences in dairy food intake between lactose absorbers and malabsorbers. It appears that alactasia plays no role in an individual's decision as to whether or not to drink milk (93,94), nor does lactase deficiency exert a detrimental effect on intestinal calcium absorption or bone mass in adults (95). Heaney pointedly remarks in his review of the role of calcium nutriture in osteoporosis that

> The alactasia argument . . . smacks of temporal provincialism. Dairy products are, indeed, the principal source of calcium in the contemporary diet of industrialized nations, but that does not mean that the primitive human was dependent upon dairy sources. . . . Over the long evolutionary history of humanity, it would appear that a low calcium intake is the exception, not the rule, and that we evolved, both as a species and as civilizations, in an environment which provided far more calcium than most of us get from our civilized diets (96).

▶ 135

Indeed, when analyses are made of dietary intake of calcium, it may be that the ability to accurately estimate calcium intake suffers from exclusion of appropriate foods on commonly used dietary intake questionnaires. In an analysis of nutrient intakes of Mexican-Americans, blacks, and Caucasians in Texas, it was found that Caucasians consumed a greater percentage of all nutrients from dairy sources than the other groups (97). This may be merely a reflection of culturally influenced preferences for food groups that have no real bearing on total intake of calcium.

Ethnicity and acculturation may be important predictors of food frequency consumption (98). In an analysis of the HHANES and NHANES II data, it was found that calcium intake in Hispanic diets were similar to those of non-Hispanic Caucasians, and somewhat higher than those of blacks (Anne Looker, personal communication). Examination of the diets of the three main Hispanic groups in the United States revealed striking differences in the dietary sources of calcium, although total calcium intakes did not vary significantly. Milk was the single greatest contributor in all three groups, but corn tortillas were the second in importance for Mexican-Americans alone. A listing of the top ten contributors to dietary calcium for Mexican-Americans also included flour tortillas and pinto beans, whereas for Cuban-Americans and Puerto Ricans, pizza and rice were major sources. The bioavailability of calcium in these diverse foods may vary highly. For some foods, such as pinto beans, calcium absorbability is less than that of milk (99), but the total intake of calcium from all sources may be sufficient to exceed gastrointestinal and renal losses.

Calcium intake does relate to bone mass, but it is difficult to assess given the vicissitude of responses to dietary intake questionnaires. Some have found that lifetime calcium intake, as determined by dietary recall, is a positive predictor of current bone mass (100,101). There is also evidence that Caucasian children with daily calcium intake of 1000 mg or more have higher BMDs than those ingesting less (102). In a study of ethnic variation in calcium absorption, Bell and colleagues found no racial differences in calcium absorption between black and Caucasian children, but the former had greater bone mass and lower urinary calcium excretion (103). Despite low dietary calcium intake, adult blacks have lower urinary calcium excretion than Caucasians as well as greater bone mass and fewer fractures (44,104–106). Others have found that greater calcium intakes do not predict higher BMD (107), and in fact, hip fractures are more prevalent in countries with high dairy calcium intake (18).

Adequacy of calcium intake may differ from one group to another depending on how well people adapt to variations in nutrient intake (96). Some populations may have sufficiently low dietary calcium intake that changes in food ingested will affect bone mass. Asians and Asian-Americans apparently have very low dietary calcium intake. In a study of elderly Japanese-Americans, it was found that average daily calcium intake was less than 500 mg. A weak but significant association of BMC with dietary calcium intake was demonstrated, even after adjusting for major confounders (108). Three-day diet reports by premenopausal Japanese women indicated that the significant dietary factors contributing to differences in bone mass were current intakes of calcium, protein, and energy, and that differences in BMD were intensified by whether or not the subjects drank milk in their childhood (68).

Overall calcium intake is relatively low in China. Hu and colleagues conducted a remarkably detailed analysis of diet in four rural Chinese regions that showed considerable variation in dietary calcium. The average calcium intake in one region with access to dairy products was almost twice that of other nonpastoral areas, and forearm bone mass was significantly higher in that region for all age groups (80). Rates of bone loss did not differ from one area to another despite dietary intake, and it was concluded that the differences in skeletal mass resulted from the effects of calcium intake on attainment of peak bone mass. Wide variation of dietary calcium and BMD notwithstanding, fracture rates were very low for all regions.

Another culturally mediated dietary factor that may affect calcium homeostasis is protein intake. Values for dietary protein in the United States and Europe are higher than for Asia and Africa. BMD of childhood and young adult Eskimos is similar to Caucasians, but they have a rate of bone loss 2% to 3% per decade greater (74,109). This has been attributed to the effects of increased metabolic acid production by the high protein diet of Eskimos (109). Abelow and associates demonstrated a striking cross-cultural relationship between animal protein intake and fractures in postmenopausal women, invoking the theory that animal protein leads to greater urinary acid excretion, promoting calciuresis (110). In addition, rural regions of China with greater animal protein intake have significantly greater urinary titratable acid and calcium excretion (111).

Cultural Values and Health Habits

Tobacco and alcohol use count among the putative risk factors for osteoporosis. Smoking has been postulated to reduce calcium absorption (112), and heavy smokers appear to have lower BMD than light or nonsmokers (113). Mexican-Americans smoke fewer cigarettes than Caucasians (3–5), but the relationship between smoking and bone mass of Mexican-Americans has not been studied. Elderly Japanese-American men demonstrate no relationship between alcohol intake and rate of bone loss, but have significantly faster loss rates associated with smoking (114). The association between alcohol consumption and osteoporosis could result from a direct toxic effect of ethanol on bone or may be related to other diseases associated with alcoholism (16). Caucasians have a much higher prevalence of drinking than blacks or Mexican-Americans, with men imbibing more than women (3–5,115), although greater acculturation leads to more alcohol consumption by Mexican-American women (116).

▶ 137

Some data suggest that non–insulin-dependent diabetes mellitus is positively associated with BMD in women (117). Mexican-Americans and blacks experience a proportionately greater amount of diabetes than do Caucasians (1,118), which may contribute to the observed differences in BMD. Prevalence of diabetes in Mexican-Americans is related to admixture with Native American genes (2), obesity (119), and acculturation (12). Hence, many factors may lead to differences in bone mass.

Calcium, Parathyroid Hormone, and Vitamin D

Differences in bone metabolism may contribute to the variation in fractures and bone mass observed between ethnic groups. Circulating concentrations of 25-hydroxyvitamin D, (25-(OH)D) are significantly lower in nonobese adult blacks than in Caucasians (104,106,120). It has been hypothesized that the lower levels are due to decreased dermal synthesis with increased skin pigmentation (121–123), but it appears that while melanin may constrain previtamin D formation when sun exposure is limited, maximal production may be independent of skin color (124). Circulating 25-(OH) D in black South Africans declines significantly when they visit the more northern latitude of Belgium, with a negative relationship between serum levels and length of stay (105). This effect is independent of dietary vitamin D intake.

In addition to lower 25-(OH)D and osteocalcin levels, data from Bell and coworkers show that black adults have significantly higher 1,25-dihydroxyvitamin D (calcitriol) and parathyroid hormone (PTH) concentrations, lower urinary excretion of calcium, but no difference in serum calcium or phosphate concentrations when compared to Caucasians (104). However, it may be that this secondary hyperparathyroidism resulted from a combination of marginal vitamin D levels and low dietary calcium intake, as this study's "typical" diet provided only 400 mg calcium daily (125). In a more comprehensive study of racial differences in calciotropic hormone status, Meier found that *both* black and Caucasian women with 25-(OH)D levels less than 10 ng/mL demonstrated an inverse relationship between dietary calcium and PTH. Irrespective of ethnic group, low dietary intake of calcium coupled with low circulating 25-(OH)D resulted in secondary hyperparathyroidism (106). There were no ethnic differences in PTH or calcitriol, although black women had statistically lower 25-(OH)D levels. Interestingly, no relationships between axial or appendicular BMD and calcitriol, PTH, or 25-(OH)D were found. Urinary calcium excretion, which was significantly lower in blacks, was inversely associated with forearm bone mass.

The finding of low plasma osteocalcin concentrations despite secondary hyperparathyroidism in blacks suggests a low rate of bone turnover. Weinstein and Bell found that rates of bone formation were significantly lower in blacks than in Caucasians when bone histomorphometric parameters were compared (126). In addition, the mineralization lag time and formation period were significantly prolonged, suggesting that diminished bone remodeling in blacks may protect skeletal mass. A black/white cross-sectional study of bone turnover in pre- and postmenopausal women also provided biochemical evidence for lower bone turnover in black women (44).

No studies have directly compared bone turnover between Asian and Caucasian groups, but it appears that the reported normal values for osteocalcin in Japanese women are lower than those of Caucasian women (66,104). In other ethnic comparisons of biochemical indices of bone turnover, Polynesians have similar levels of osteocalcin, PTH, and urinary excretion of hydroxyproline to Caucasians despite significantly higher BMD values (127). Reasner and colleagues found that young Mexican-American adults had significantly lower levels of 25-(OH)D than Caucasians, with evidence of secondary hyperparathyroidism (123). However, the typical dietary intake of calcium was only 400 mg/d, suggesting that the high PTH was a response to low vitamin D in conjunction with inadequate dietary calcium. Osteocalcin levels did not differ significantly between the two groups.

Summary

Fracture risk varies dramatically from one ethnic group to another and often within a given regional population. Although it is tempting to attribute responsibility for fracture protection to differences in bone mass, other factors may contribute equally. Some groups with high skeletal mass have few fractures, but others, such as the centenarians of Vilcabamba, have relatively low BMD but protection against fracture. Within some ethnicities, fractures at one site occur less frequently than at another. Perhaps there are differences in the shape of bones that confer protection against fracture, but data exploring this hypothesis are scanty. Further investigation addressing the etiology of differential fracture risk among human populations must include evaluation of bone size and shape, distribution of mechanical stresses, and other factors such as fall risk. The number of minority aged within the US population will double in the next 50 years. It follows that the biology and epidemiology of osteoporosis in ethnic groups must be explored. Additionally, in future studies consideration must be given to culturally determined factors, such as diet and life-style choices, all of which influence bone health.

▶ 139

Acknowledgments

The author gratefully acknowledges Ji-Fan Hu of Cornell University, Anne Looker of the National Center for Health Statistics, and Robert Marcus of Stanford University for graciously sharing in-press data.

References

1. Hanis CL, Ferrell RE, Barton SA, et al. Diabetes among Mexican Americans in Starr County, Texas. Am J Epidemiol 1983;118:659–672.

2. Gardner LI, Stern MP, Haffner SM, et al. Prevalence of diabetes in Mexican Americans: relationship to percent of gene pool derived from Native American sources. Diabetes 1984;33:86–92.

3. Friis R, Nanjundappa G, Prendergast TJ, Welsh MJ. Coronary heart disease, mortality and risk among Hispanics and non-Hispanics in Orange County, California. Public Health Rep 1981;96:418–422.

4. Mitchell BD, Stern MP, Haffner SM, Hazuda HP, Patterson JK. Risk factors for cardiovascular mortality in Mexican Americans and non-Hispanic Whites. Am J Epidemiol 1990;131:423–433.

5. Haffner SM, Stern MP, Hazuda HP,

Rosenthal M, Knapp JA. The role of behavioral variables and fat patterning in explaining ethnic differences in serum lipids and lipoproteins. Am J Epidemiol 1986;123:830–839.

6. Linn MW, Hunter KI, Linn BS. Self-assessed health, impairment and disability in Anglo, black and Cuban elderly. Med Care 1980;18:282–288.

7. VanDerZwagg R, Runyan JW, Davidson JK, Delcher HK, Mainzer I, Baggett HW. A cohort study of mortality in two clinic populations of patients with diabetes mellitus. Diabetes Care 1983;6:341–346.

8. Reed DM, Brody JA. Amyotrophic làteral sclerosis and Parkinson's dementia in Guam, 1945–1972. Am J Epidemiol 1975;101:287–301.

9. Pollitzer WS, Anderson JJ. Ethnic and genetic differences in bone mass: a review with a hereditary vs environmental perspective [published erratum appears in Am J Clin Nutr 1990;52:181]. Am J Clin Nutr 1989;50:1244–1259.

10. Espino DV, Maldonado D. Hypertension and acculturation in elderly Mexican Americans: results from 1982–84 Hispanic HANES. J Gerontol 1990;45:M209–213.

11. Lubben JE, Weiler PG, Chi I. Gender and ethnic differences in the health practices of the elderly poor. J Clin Epidemiol 1989;42:725–736.

12. Stern MP, Rosenthal M, Haffner SM, Hazuda HP, Franco LJ. Sex differences in the effect of sociocultural status on diabetes and cardiovascular risk factors in Mexican Americans: the San Antonio heart study. Am J Epidemiol 1984;120:834–851.

13. Kumanyika S. Obesity in black women. Epidemiol Rev 1987;9:31–51.

14. Barresi CM, Stull DE, eds. Ethnic elderly and long-term care. New York: Springer, 1993.

15. Fowles DG, ed. Aged America: trends and projections; US Department of Health and Human Services, DHHS Publication No. (FCoA) 91-28001, 1991.

16. Cummings SR, Kelsey JL, Nevitt MC, O'Dowd KJ. Epidemiology of osteoporosis and osteoporotic fractures. Epidemiol Rev 1985;7:178–207.

17. Nordin BEC. International patterns of osteoporosis. Clin Orthop 1966;45: 17–30.

18. Maggi S, Kelsey JL, Litvak J, Heyse SP. Incidence of hip fractures in the elderly: a cross-national analysis. Osteoporos Int 1991;1:232–241.

19. Farmer ME, White LR, Brody JA, Bailey KR. Race and sex differences in hip fracture incidence. Am J Public Health 1984;74:1374–1380.

20. Kellie SE, Brody JA. Sex-specific and race-specific hip fracture rates. Am J Public Health 1990;80:326–328.

21. Jacobsen SJ, Goldberg J, Miles TP, Brody JA, Stiers W, Rimm AA. Hip fracture incidence among the old and very old: a population-based study of 745,435 cases. Am J Public Health 1990;80:871–873.

22. Bauer RL. Ethnic differences in hip fracture: a reduced incidence in Mexican Americans. Am J Epidemiol 1988;127: 145–149.

23. Silverman SL, Madison RE. Decreased incidence of hip fracture in Hispanics, Asians, and blacks: California hospital discharge data. Am J Public Health 1988; 78:1482–1483.

24. Solomon L. Bone density in aging Caucasian and African populations. Lancet 1979;2:1326–1330.

25. Fujino H, Yamamoto K, Ieshima R, Kishimoto H, Kuranobu K, Nakamura T. The incidence of fractures of the proximal femur and the distal radius in Tottori prefecture, Japan. Arch Orthop Trauma Surg 1990;109:43–44.

26. Ross PD, Norimatsu H, Davis JW, et al. A comparison of hip fracture incidence among native Japanese, Japanese Americans, and American Caucasians. Am J Epidemiol 1991;133:801–809.

27. Bauer RL, Diehl AK, Barton SA, Brender J, Deyo RA. Risk of postmenopausal hip fracture in Mexican American women. Am J Public Health 1986;76: 1020–1021.

28. Wong PCN. Fracture epidemiology in a mixed Southeastern Asian community (Singapore). Clin Orthop 1966; 45:55–61.

29. Stott S, Gray DH, Stevenson W. The incidence of femoral neck fractures in New Zealand. N Z Med J 1980;91:6–9.

30. Bacon WE, Smith GS, Baker SP. Geographic variation in the occurrence of hip fractures among the elderly white US population. Am J Public Health 1989;79: 1556–1558.

31. Solomon L. Osteoporosis and fracture of the femoral neck in the South African Bantu. J Bone Joint Surg (Br) 1968; 50:2–13.

32. Ross PD, Wasnich RD, Vogel JM. Detection of prefacture spinal osteoporosis using bone mineral absorptiometry. J Bone Miner Res 1988;3:1–11.

33. Smith RW, Rizek J. Epidemiologic studies of osteoporosis in women of Puerto Rico and southeastern Michigan with special reference to age, race, national origin, and to other related or associated findings. Clin Orthop 1966;45:31–48.

34. Bauer RL, Deyo RA. Low risk of vertebral fracture in Mexican American women. Arch Intern Med 1987;147:1437–1439.

35. Jacobsen SJ, Goldberg J, Miles TP, Brody JA, Stiers W, Rimm AA. Race and sex differences in mortality following fracture of the hip. Am J Public Health 1992;82:1147–1150.

36. Myers AH, Robinson EG, Van NM, Michelson JD, Collins K, Baker SP. Hip fractures among the elderly: factors associated with in-hospital mortality. Am J Epidemiol 1991;134:1128–1137.

37. Tinetti ME, Speechley M, Ginter SF. Risk factors for falls among elderly persons living in the community. N Engl J Med 1988;319:1701–1707.

38. Grisso JA, Schwartz DF, Wolfson V, Polansky M, LaPann K. The impact of falls in an inner-city elderly African-American population. J Am Geriatr Soc 1992;40:673–678.

39. Hui SL, Slemenda CW, Johnston CC Jr. Age and bone mass as predictors of fracture in a prospective study. J Clin Invest 1988;81:1804–1809.

40. Cummings SR, Black DM, Nevitt MC, et al. Appendicular bone density and age predict hip fracture in women. The study of osteoporotic fractures research group. JAMA 1990;263:665–668.

41. Ross PD, Davis JW, Vogel JM, Wasnich RD. A critical review of bone mass and the risk of fractures in osteoporosis. Calcif Tissue Int 1990;46:149–161.

42. DeSimone DP, Stevens J, Edwards J, Shary J, Gordon L, Bell NH. Influence of body habitus and race on bone mineral density of the midradius, hip, and spine in aging women. J Bone Miner Res 1989;4: 827–830.

43. Luckey M, Meier D, Wallenstein S, Lapinski R. Racial differences in early postmenopausal bone loss. J Bone Miner Res 1992;7(suppl):S140. Abstract.

44. Meier DE, Luckey MM, Wallenstein S, Lapinski RH, Catherwood B. Racial differences in pre- and postmenopausal bone homeostasis: association with bone density. J Bone Miner Res 1992;7:1181–1189.

45. Ortiz O, Russell M, Daley TL, et al. Differences in skeletal muscle and bone mineral mass between black and white females and their relevance to estimates of body composition. Am J Clin Nutr 1992;55:8–13.

46. Meier DE, Orwoll ES, Jones JM. Marked disparity between trabecular and cortical bone loss with age in healthy men. Ann Intern Med 1984;101:605–612.

47. Riggs BL, Wahner HW, Melton LJ III, Richelson LS, Judd HL, Offord KP. Rates of bone loss in the appendicular and axial skeletons of women: evidence of substantial vertebral bone loss before menopause. J Clin Invest 1986;77:1487–1491.

48. Luckey MM, Meier DE, Mandeli JP, DaCosta MC, Hubbard ML, Goldsmith SJ. Radial and vertebral bone density in white and black women: evidence for racial differences in premenopausal bone homeostasis. J Clin Endocrinol Metab 1989;69: 762–770.

49. Meier D, Luckey M, Wallenstein S, Papinski R. Significant premenopausal bone loss in white and black women: a longitudinal study. J Bone Miner Res 1992; 7(suppl):S135. Abstract.

50. Laraque D, Arena L, Karp J, Gruskay

D. Bone mineral content in black preschoolers: normative data using single photon absorptiometry. Pediatr Radiol 1990; 20:461–463.

51. Patel DN, Pettifor JM, Becker PJ, Grieve C, Leschner K. The effect of ethnic group on appendicular bone mass in children. J Bone Miner Res 1992;7:263–272.

52. Prentice A, Laskey MA, Shaw J, Cole TJ, Fraser DR. Bone mineral content of Gambian and British children aged 0–36 months. Bone Miner 1990;10:211–224.

53. Garn SM, Sandusky ST, Nagy JM, McCann MB. Advanced skeleton development in low-income and Negro children. J Pediatr 1972;80:965–969.

54. Li JY, Specker BL, Ho ML, Tsang RC. Bone mineral content in black and white children 1 to 6 years of age. Early appearance of race and sex differences. Am J Dis Child 1989;143:1346–1349.

55. Garn SM, Lifelong black-white differences in bone size and cortical area. Am J Dis Child 1990;144:750–751.

56. McCormick DP, Ponder SW, Fawcett HD, Palmer JL. Spinal bone mineral density in 335 normal and obese children and adolescents: evidence for ethnic and sex differences. Bone Miner Res 1991;6: 507–513.

57 Southard RN, Morris JD, Mahan JD, et al. Bone mass in healthy children: measurement with quantitative DXA. Radiology 1991;179:735–738.

58. Gilsanz V, Roe TF, Mora S, Costin G, Goodman WG. Changes in vertebral bone density in black and white girls during childhood and puberty. N Engl J Med 1991;325:1597–1600.

59. Reid IR, Mackie M, Ibbertson HK. Bone mineral content in Polynesian and white New Zealand women. BMJ 1986; 292:1547–1548.

60. Norimatsu H, Mori S, Uesato T, Yoshikawa T, Katsuyama N. Bone mineral density of the spine and proximal femur in normal and osteoporotic subjects in Japan. Bone Miner 1989;5:213–222.

61. Russell-Aulet M, Wang J, Thornton J, Colt EW, Pierson RJ. Bone mineral density and mass by total-body dual-photon absorptiometry in normal white and Asian men. J Bone Miner Res 1991;6:1109–1113.

62. Kin K, Kushida K, Yamazaki K, Okamoto S, Inoue T. Bone mineral density of the spine in normal Japanese subjects using dual-energy x-ray absorptiometry: effect of obesity and menopausal status. Calcif Tissue Int 1991;49:101–106.

63. Yano K, Wasnich RD, Vogel JM, Heilbrun LK. Bone mineral measurements among middle-aged and elderly Japanese residents in Hawaii. Am J Epidemiol 1984;119:751–764.

64. Sugimoto T, Tsutsumi M, Fujii Y, et al. Comparison of bone mineral content among Japanese, Koreans, and Taiwanese assessed by dual-photon absorptiometry. J Bone Miner Res 1992;7:153–159.

65. Nomura A, Wasnich RD, Heilbrun LK, Ross PD, Davis JW. Comparison of bone mineral content between Japan-born and US-born Japanese subjects in Hawaii. Bone Miner 1989;6:213–223.

66. Hagino H, Yamamoto K, Teshima R, Kishimoto H, Kagawa T. Radial bone mineral changes in pre- and postmenopausal healthy Japanese women: cross-sectional and longitudinal studies. J Bone Miner Res 1992;7:147–152.

67. Mazess RB. Bone mineral in Vilcabamba, Ecuador. Am J Roentgenol 1978; 130:671–674.

68. Hirota T, Nara M, Ohguri M, Manago E, Hirota K. Effect of diet and lifestyle on bone mass in Asian young women. Am J Clin Nutr 1992;55:1168–1173.

69. Bauer RL, Haffner SM. Axial skeletal bone density in Mexican American and non-hispanic white women. J Bone Miner Res 1992;7:(suppl):S195. Abstract.

70. Benson BW, Prihoda TJ, Glass BJ. Variations in adult cortical bone mass as measured by a panoramic mandibular index. Oral Surg Oral Med Oral Pathol 1991;71:349–356.

71. Beck TJ, Ruff CB, Scott WJ, Plato CC, Tobin JD, Quan CA. Sex differences in geometry of the femoral neck with aging: a structural analysis of bone mineral data. Calcif Tissue Int 1992;50:24–29.

142

72. Martin RB, Atkinson PJ. Age and sex-related changes in the structure and strength of the human femoral shaft. J Biomech 1977;10:223–231.

73. Faulkner KG, Cummings SR, Black D, Palermo L, Glüer C-C, Genant HK. Simple measurement of femoral geometry predicts hip fracture: the study of osteoporotic fractures. J Bone Miner Res 1993;8:1211–1217.

74. Harper AB, Laughlin WS, Mazess RB. Bone mineral content in St Lawrence Island Eskimos. Hum Biol 1984;56:63–78.

75. Russell-Aulet M, Wang J, Thornton JC, Colt EWD, Pierson RN. Bone mineral density and mass in a cross-sectional study of white and Asian women. J Bone Miner Res 1993;8:575–582.

76. Katzman DK, Bachrach LK, Carter DR, Marcus R. Clinical and anthropometric correlates of bone mineral acquisition in healthy adolescent girls. J Clin Endocrinol Metab 1991;73:1332–1339.

77. Carter DR, Bouxsein ML, Marcus R. New approaches for interpreting projected bone densitometry data. J Bone Miner Res 1992;7:137–145.

78. Krall EA, Dawson-Hughes B. Heritable and life-style determinants of bone mineral density. J Bone Miner Res 1993;8:1–9.

79. Ross PD, Orimo H, Wasnich RD, et al. Methodological issues in comparing genetic and environmental influences on bone mass. Bone Miner 1989;7:67–77.

80. Hu J-F, Schwartz R, Zhao X-H, Parpia B, Campbell TC. Dietary calcium and bone density among middle aged and elderly women in China. Am J Clin Nutr 1993;58:219–227.

81. Pocock NA, Eisman JA, Mazess RB, Sambrook PN, Yeates MG, Freund J. Bone mineral density in Australia compared with the United States. J Bone Miner Res 1988;3:601–604.

82. Farmer ME, Harris T, Madans JH, Wallace RB, Cornoni-Huntley J, White LR. Anthropometric indicators and hip fracture: the NHANES I epidemiologic follow-up study. J Am Geriatr Soc 1989;37:9–16.

83. Pruzansky ME, Turano M, Luckey M, Senie R. Low body weight as a risk factor for hip fracture in both black and white women. J Orthop Res 1989;7:192–197.

84. Harris S, Dallal GE, Dawson-Hughes B. Influence of body weight on rates of change in bone density of the spine, hip, and radius in postmenopausal women. Calcif Tissue Int 1992;50:19–23.

85. Liel Y, Edwards J, Shary J, Spicer KM, Gordon L, Bell NH. The effects of race and body habitus on bone mineral density of the radius, hip, and spine in premenopausal women. J Clin Endocrinol Metab 1988;66:1247–1250.

86. Cohn SH, Abesamis C, Zanzi I, Aloia JF, Yasumura S, Ellis KJ. Body elemental composition: comparison between black and white adults. Am J Physiol 1977;232:E419–422.

87. Nelson DA, Kleerekoper M, Parfitt AM. Bone mass, skin color and body size among black and white women. Bone Miner 1988;4:257–264.

88. Lopez LM, Masse B. Comparison of body mass indexes and cutoff points for estimating the prevalence of overweight in Hispanic women. J Am Diet Assoc 1992;92:1343–1347.

89. Ellis KJ, Cohn SH. Correlation between skeletal calcium mass and muscle mass in man. J Appl Physiol 1975;38:455–460.

90. Matsumine H, Hirato K, Yanaihara T, Tamada T, Yoshida M. Aromatization by skeletal muscle. J Clin Endocrinol Metab 1986;63:717–720.

91. Buchanan JR, Myers CA, Lloyd T, Leuenberger P, Demers LM. Determinants of peak trabecular bone density in women: the role of androgens, estrogen, and exercise. J Bone Miner Res 1988;3:673–680.

92. Davidson BJ, Ross RK, Paganini-Hill A, Hammond GD, Siiteri PK, Judd HL. Total and free estrogens and androgens in postmenopausal women with hip fractures. J Clin Endocrinol Metab 1982;54:115–120.

93. Woteki CE, Weser E, Young EA. Lactose malabsorption in Mexican American adults. Am J Clin Nutr 1977;30:470–475.

94. Rorick MH, Scrimshaw NS. Comparative tolerance of elderly from differing ethnic backgrounds to lactose-containing and lactose-free dairy drinks: a double-blind study. J Gerontol 1979;34:191–196.

95. Slemenda CW, Christian JC, Hui S Fitzgerald J, Johnston CC. No evidence for an effect of lactase deficiency on bone mass in pre- or postmenopausal women. J Bone Miner Res 1991;6:1367–1371.

96. Heaney RP. Calcium, bone health and osteoporosis. In: Peck WA, ed. Bone and mineral research. Amsterdam-New York-Oxford: Elsevier, 1986:255–301.

97. Borrud LG, Pillow PC, Allen PK, McPherson RS, Nichaman MZ, Newell GR. Food group contributions to nutrient intake in whites, blacks, and Mexican Americans in Texas. J Am Diet Assoc 1989;89:1061–1069.

98. Bartholomew AM, Young EA, Martin HW, Hazuda HP. Food frequency intakes and sociodemographic factors of elderly Mexican Americans and non-Hispanic whites. J Am Diet Assoc 1990;90:1693–1696.

99. Heaney RP, Weaver CM. Plant constituents and good calcium absorbability. J Bone Miner Res 1992;7(suppl):S136. Abstract.

100. Halioua L, Anderson JJ. Lifetime calcium intake and physical activity habits; independent and combined effects on the radial bone of healthy premenopausal caucasian women. Am J Clin Nutr 1989; 49:534–541.

101. Sandler RB, Slemenda CW, LaPorte RE, et al. Postmenopausal bone density and milk consumption in childhood and adolescence. Am J Clin Nutr 1985;42:270–274.

102. Chan GM. Dietary calcium and bone mineral status of children and adolescents. Am J Dis Child 1991;145:631–634.

103. Bell NH, Yergey AL, Vieira N, Shary JR. Calcium absorption is the same and urinary calcium is lower in black than white children: mechanism for calcium retention and greater bone mass in blacks. J Bone Miner Res 1991;7(suppl):S150. Abstract.

104. Bell NH, Greene A, Epstein S, Oexman MJ, Shaw S, Shary J. Evidence for alteration of the vitamin D-endocrine system in blacks. J Clin Invest 1985; 76:470–473.

105. M'Buyamba-Kabangu JR, Fagard R, Lijnen R, Bouillon R, Lissens W, Amery A. Calcium, vitamin D-endocrine system, and parathyroid hormone in black and white males. Calcif Tissue Int 1987;41:70–74.

106. Meier DE, Luckey MM, Wallenstein S, Clemens TL, Orwoll ES, Waslien CI. Calcium, vitamin D, and parathyroid hormone status in young white and black women: association with racial differences in bone mass. J Clin Endocrinol Metab 1991;72:703–710.

107. Lacey JM, Anderson JJ, Fujita T, et al. Correlates of cortical bone mass among premenopausal and postmenopausal Japanese women. J Bone Miner Res 1991;6: 651–659.

108. Yano K, Heilbrun LK, Wasnich RD, Hankin JH, Vogel JM. The relationship between diet and bone mineral content of multiple skeletal sites in elderly Japanese-American men and women living in Hawaii. Am J Clin Nutr 1985;42:877–888.

109. Mazess RB, Mather W. Bone mineral content of North Alaskan Eskimos. Am J Clin Nutr 1974;27:916–925.

110. Abelow DJ, Holford TR, Insogna KL. Cross-cultural association between dietary animal protein and hip fracture: a hypothesis. Calcif Tissue Int 1992;50:14–18.

111. Hu J-F, Zhao X-H, Parpia B, Campbell TC. Dietary intakes and urinary excretion of calcium and acids: a cross-sectional study in China. Am J Clin Nutr 1993;58:398–406.

112. Krall EA, Dawson-Hughes B. Smoking and bone loss among postmenopausal women. J Bone Miner Res 1991; 6:331–338.

113. Slemenda CW, Hui SL, Longcope C, Johnston CJ. Cigarette smoking, obesity, and bone mass. J Bone Miner Res 1989;4:737–741.

114. Davis JW, Ross PD, Vogel JM, Wasnich RD. Effects of smoking and alcohol on the rates of bone loss among elderly

144 ◀

Japanese-American men. J Bone Miner Res 1992;7(suppl):S138. Abstract.

115. Molgaard CA, Nakamura CM, Stanford EP, Peddecord KM, Morton DJ. Prevalence of alcohol consumption among older persons. J Community Health 1990; 15:239–251.

116. Marks G. García M, Solis JM. Health risk behaviors of Hispanics in the United States: findings from HHANES 1982–84. Am J Public Health 1990;80 (suppl):20–26.

117. Barrett-Conner E, Holbrook TL. Sex differences in osteoporosis in older adults with non-insulin dependent diabetes mellitus. JAMA 1992;268:3333–3337.

118. Lieberman LS, ed. Diabetes and obesity in elderly black americans. In: Jackson JS, ed. The black american elderly. New York: Springer, 1988:150–189.

119. Stern MP, Gaskill SP, Hazuda HP, Gardner LI, Haffner SM. Does obesity explain excess prevalence of diabetes among Mexican Americans? Results of the San Antonio heart study. Diabetologia 1983; 24:272–277.

120. Epstein S, Bell NH, Shary J, Shaw S, Breene A, Oexmann MJ. Evidence that obesity does not influence the vitamin D-endocrine system in blacks. J Bone Miner Res 1986;1:181–184.

121. Loomis WF. Skin-pigment regulation of vitamin-D biosynthesis in man. Science 1967;157:501–506.

122. Clemens TL, Henderson SL, Adams JS, Holick MF. Increased skin pigment reduces the capacity of skin to synthesize vitamin D_3. Lancet 1982;1:74–76.

123. Reasner C, Dunn JF, Fetchick DA, et al. Alteration of vitamin D metabolism in Mexican-Americans. J Bone Miner Res 1990;5:13–17.

124. Brazerol WF, McPhee AJ, Mimouni F, Specker BL, Tsang RC. Serial ultraviolet B exposure and serum 25-hydroxyvitamin D response in young adult American blacks and whites: no racial differences. J Am Coll Nutr 1988;7:111–118.

125. Fuleihan GE, Gundberg C, Gleason R, Porrino N, Bacon EM. Parathyroid hormone dynamics in black subjects. J Bone Miner Res 1992;7(suppl):S237. Abstract.

126. Weinstein RS, Bell NH. Diminished rates of bone formation in normal black adults. N Engl J Med 1988;319:1698–1701.

127. Reid IR, Cullen S, Schooler BA, Livingston NE, Evans MC. Calcitropic hormone levels in polynesians: evidence against their role in interracial differences in bone mass. J Clin Endocrinol Metab 1990;70:1452–1456.

▶ 145

7 ▸ Osteoporosis in Men

▸ ▸ ▸ Eric S. Orwoll

Robert F. Klein

Ever since its initial description in the postmenopausal period by Albright and colleagues in 1941 (1), osteoporosis has been considered a disease of women. Nevertheless, in the earliest reports of the epidemiology of fractures associated with osteoporosis it was clear that the classical age-related increase in fractures seen in women is apparent in men as well. Only in the last few years has it been recognized that the problem of osteoporosis in men represents an important public health issue and that it also presents a unique array of scientific challenges and opportunities. In this chapter, the issue of osteoporosis in men is examined by attempting to compare its pathophysiology and clinical presentation with parallel processes in women.

The Male Skeleton

Growth and Development

The development of the male skeleton during childhood is similar to that in girls in that there is a nearly linear increase in bone mass until adolescence, when a rapid increase leads to adult (peak) proportions. The determinants of peak bone mass are incompletely understood, but in both boys and girls nutritional factors (calcium, protein, etc), physical activity, genetic potential, and other influences are probably important. Sexual differences in the magnitude, character, and timing of this process may influence the subsequent risk of osteoporosis, and in part may help to explain the differences in osteoporosis incidence between men and women (see Chapter 4).

The development of bone mass depends on changes in both density and size, and sexual differences are primarily related to differences in size. Bone mineral density (BMD) has received considerable attention recently, and varying interpretations of experimental results have generated some controversy.

Bonjour and colleagues and others demonstrated that women exhibit a dramatic increase in bone mass that begins during adolescence and is essentially complete when puberty ends. In men, a similar relationship of bone mass accretion to adolescence holds, and since the chronological onset of puberty is later in boys than girls, the achievement of peak bone mass is also later. The magnitude of increase in bone density appears to be essentially the same in men and women in axial, primarily trabecular, compartments. Vertebral mineral density determined by quantitative computed tomography (QCT, a true volumetric assessment) is very similar in men and women (2). Kelly (3) showed that when the effects of size on BMD measures were considered, proximal femoral density in men was the same as in women, and vertebral density was even slightly lower! ► 147 Likewise, histomorphometric studies of vertebral bone volume and trabecular connectivity reveal no differences between young adult men and women (4). Whereas vertebral density by areal measures (dual energy x-ray absorptiometry [DXA]) appears to reach slightly higher levels in men, the male advantage disappears (or is even slightly reversed) once those values are corrected for differences in vertebral dimensions. Similarly, in the proximal femur, absolute measures of mineral density reach nearly identical levels in men and women, and when differences in body size are considered, female levels may slightly exceed those in men (3,5). On the other hand, in appendicular, primarily cortical bone areas, men have been noted to have greater density even at very early ages. Measures of metacarpal cortical thickness, radial bone density, and total body bone density are consistently higher in men throughout adolescence and early adulthood. However, Ruff and Hayes and others have pointed out that these measures of density all depend on the assessment of bone area as an assumed surrogate for bone volume, an assumption that is frequently not valid (3,6). When density is examined as a function of true measures of volume, the sexual differences in "density" at the femoral mid-shaft disappear. Hence, the apparent male advantage in density may be illusory, and the sexual dichotomy in peak appendicular bone mass relates simply to differences in cortical thickness and diameter. Nevertheless, these differences in size may have profound implications for the determination of fracture risk. For instance, resistance to vertebral compressive fracture is related to both density *and* size, and the tensile resistance of a long bone to fracture is *exponentially* related to its diameter. Thus, the larger size of male bones adds greatly to strength. These sex differences in peak bone mass and size underlie in part the differences in fracture patterns that emerge later in life.

The acquisition of peak bone mass in men, as in women, is influenced by genetic factors. Krall and Dawson-Hughes estimated heritability to be 40% to 83% at several measurement sites in men (5). The subsequent loss of bone with aging, however, is apparently not influenced by genotype (7), as discussed by Slemenda (see Chapter 5) in this volume.

Aging

In addition to differences in peak bone mass, sexual differences in the pattern of age-related bone loss affect eventual fracture risk. Adult men experience a fairly linear decrease in cortical bone mass as age increases (8–12), but there may be an acceleration in the rate of bone loss in the most elderly men (8,11). The reduction may not be as rapid as in women, thereby accentuating the sexual differences in cortical mass present in early adulthood. For instance, cross-sectional measures of radial (13) and total body (9) bone mass suggest a lesser decline with age in men. On the other hand, some reports indicate similar rates of change (10). The loss of appendicular bone mass in men as reported from longitudinal studies is considerably more rapid (5% to 10%/decade) (8,12,14) than previously estimated from cross-sectional studies (1% to 3%/decade) (10,11,13). The differences noted in longitudinal versus cross-sectional studies may reflect the difficulty in adequately estimating time-dependent processes by cross-sectional methods, but also suggest that there is an increasingly greater rate of bone loss in men (8). The decline in mass is to some extent compensated by changes in cortical *dimensions*. In both sexes, there is an age-related increase in cortical width, and since fracture resistance is so dependent on geometry, this change is beneficial. In a two-decade study Garn and colleagues found that the rate of metacarpal cortical loss in men was similar to that in women, but periosteal apposition was also somewhat greater, yielding a lesser loss of thickness and overall mass (15). The sex-related differences in the rate of density change with age are in accord with the fracture patterns observed in the elderly, when appendicular fractures are distinctly less common in men than women.

The decline in axial bone density was initially also considered to be relatively slow in men, primarily as a result of cross-sectional studies of spinal bone mass using techniques that assess total spinal bone mass (dual photon absorptiometry [DPA]). Vertebral bone density as measured by QCT, however, suggested a much more rapid rate of bone loss with aging in normal men (16; Figure 7-1). Subsequently, the results derived from DXA were shown to be influenced by artifacts in measurement introduced by extravertebral calcifications, and that if men with such calcifications were excluded, the relationship of spinal bone density with age is similar in men and women (17). Longitudinal studies verify a rapid rate of vertebral bone loss with aging in normal men (8). The rate and magnitude of decline in density with age at proximal femoral sites is similar (slightly less) in men compared to women (a menopausal acceleration of loss obviously does not occur in men) (13,18). Similarly, bone volume in the iliac crest declines at very similar rates in men and women (Figure 7-2). Thus, little sexual dimorphism exists in axial bone density in the elderly. Nevertheless, the microstructural nature of axial (trabecular) bone loss may be different in men

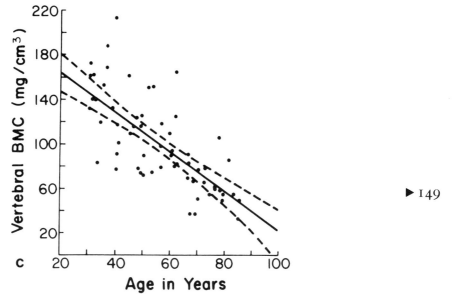

▶ 149

FIGURE 7-1 Regression of vertebral bone mineral content (BMC) with age in healthy men. BMC was measured with quantitative computed tomography. *(Reproduced by permission from Meier DE, Orwoll ES, Jones JM. Marked disparity between trabecular and cortical bone loss with age in healthy men: measurement by vertebral computed tomography and radial photon absorptiometry. Ann Intern Med 1984;101:605–612.)*

and women. Using histomorphometric methods to analyze vertebral bone, Moskilde found that whereas density is not particularly different between older men and women, the microarchitectural pattern of trabecular loss is distinct. Women tend to experience both trabecular thinning and trabecular loss (particularly horizontal elements), whereas men experience trabecular thinning without quite as much trabecular loss (19). Similar results have been described in iliac crest biopsy specimens (4,20,21), although Parfitt and Matthews reported that the major cause of the reduction in iliac crest bone volume with age in both men and women is loss of trabeculae rather than thinning (22).

Fracture Epidemiology

Incidence of Fractures

The incidence of all fractures is actually higher in men than women early in life, probably as a result of trauma (23,24). At about age 40 to 50 years, this trend reverses with fractures in general, but in particular fractures of the pelvis, hu-

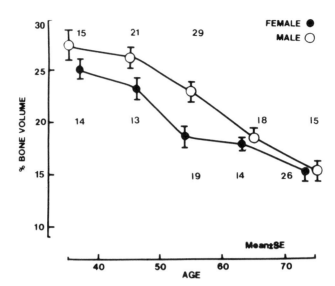

FIGURE 7-2 The decrease in trabecular bone volume in the iliac crest with age in men and women. The number of subjects in each decade is shown. (*Reproduced by permission from Aaron JE, Makins NB, Sagreiya K. The microanatomy of trabecular bone loss in normal aging men and women. Clin Orthop Rel Res 1987;215: 260–271.*)

merus, forearm, and femur become much more common in women. Fractures due to minimal or moderate trauma are uncommon in men in youth and early adulthood, but the incidence of selected fractures (particularly hip and spine) increases rapidly thereafter (Figure 7-3), and reflects an increasing prevalence of skeletal fragility.

HIP

Hip fracture is the most important site of osteoporotic fracture and about which the most complete data are available. It is clear that the incidence of hip fracture increases exponentially in men with aging, as it does in women (Figure 7-4). However, the age at which the incidence begins to increase dramatically is slightly older (~5 years) in men (25). In US men older than 65 years, the incidence of hip fracture is 4 to 5/1000 (26,27) compared with 8 to 10/1000 in like-aged US women. A similar 2:1 female to male ratio has been reported in Northern Europe, although in other geographic areas the ratio has been noted to be much lower (28). In Southern European areas, the incidence of hip fracture is relatively lower in both sexes, and men have as many hip fractures as do women (29). Since there are fewer older men than women, the absolute number of hip fractures tends to be proportionately less in men (165,000/yr in men versus 580,000/yr in women in the United States in 1984 to 1987, or 22% of the total

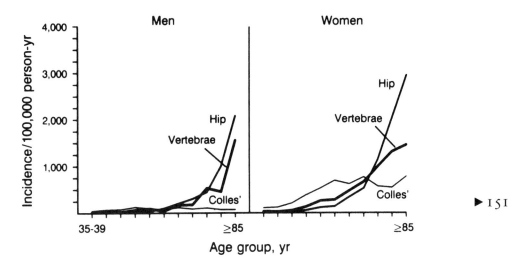

FIGURE 7-3 Age-specific rates of fracture in Rochester Minnesota, men and women. (*Reproduced by permission from Cooper C, Atkinson EJ, O'Fallon WM, Melton LJ. Incidence of clinically diagnosed vertebral fractures: a population-based study in Rochester, Minnesota, 1985–1989. J Bone Miner Res 1992;7:221–227.*)

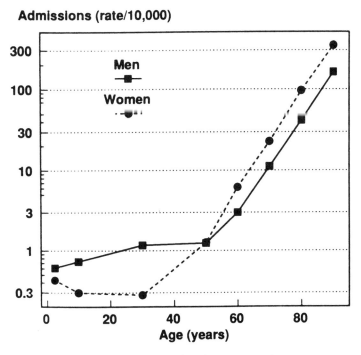

FIGURE 7-4 Annual admission rates for hip fractures in the Trent region of England, 1989 to 1990. (*Reproduced by permission from Kanis JA. The incidence of hip fracture in Europe. Osteoporosis Int 1993;3:S10–S15.*)

in men) (27). It has been estimated that approximately 30% of hip fractures worldwide occur in men (30). Currently, the lifetime risk of a hip fracture in the United States (Rochester, Minnesota) has been calculated to be 6% in men and 17.5% in women from age 50 onward (31), and 2.4% in men and 9% in women in Canada (Saskatchewan and Manitoba) (32). This risk increases (with fewer years left to live) to 4% in men and 11.7% in women at age 70 (32). Perhaps as a result of a higher prevalence of concomitant disease, the mortality associated with a hip fracture in the elderly (aged 75 and older) is considerably higher in men than in women (30% versus 9%) (33). Whereas in Europe the incidence of fracture is at least twice as great in women, the death rates for femoral neck fractures are approximately equal, again suggesting a greater risk of mortality in men (34).

Unfortunately, the number of hip fractures is projected to increase dramatically as the elderly population expands (35). Compounding matters, the incidence of hip fractures has also been noted to be increasing. The increase in incidence in some populations is more pronounced in men (24,36,37), but in general there appears to be similar trends in both sexes (29,38,40). In Canada, there was an increase of 42.2% in the age-adjusted incidence rate of proximal femur fracture in men (59.7% in women) between 1972 and 1984 (32). Increases of similar magnitude were noted in several European regions (29).

There are also clear racial differences in the incidence of hip fracture. For instance, African-American men experience hip fractures at a rate only half that of Caucasians (27). There is no extensive comparative data concerning other races, but evidence clearly suggests a lower rate of hip fracture in Japanese men compared to Caucasian men from the United States (39).

VERTEBRAE

Vertebral fracture is also an important sequel of osteoporosis. Since the diagnostic criteria for a vertebral fracture are unsettled, and vertebral fracture infrequently results in hospitalization, consistent epidemiologic information is somewhat limited. Although previously considered uncommon in men, recent information suggests the incidence and prevalence of osteoporotic vertebral fractures in US men is about half that in women—similar to hip fractures (40,41). In other geographic areas the prevalence of thoracic vertebral fractures is nearly as high in men as in women (41,42). In younger adults, the prevalence of vertebral fracture is actually higher in men than women, but in later life women experience a greater rate of increase in fracture prevalence (41,42). Vertebral and femoral BMD is reduced in men with vertebral fractures compared with non-fractured controls (43), indicating that vertebral fracture in men is not merely the result of a higher rate of trauma, but is related to the presence of osteopenia (Figure 7-5). There is only one study of bone density in men with vertebral fracture (43), but it suggests that the average bone density in fractured men ($\sim$1.0 g/cm^2) is somewhat higher than that previously reported in similar studies in women ($\sim$0.8 g/cm^2), perhaps reflecting an artifact induced by size. Fractures are primarily in low thoracic vertebrae in men, but are found at all levels. Most fractures are anterior compression in type (43) with vertebral crush fractures occurring less frequently than is reported in women. Vertebral epiphysitis

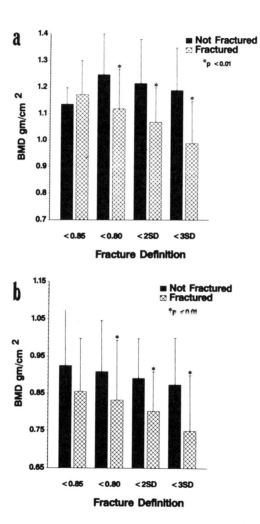

FIGURE 7-5 Lumbar spine (a) and femoral neck (b) bone mineral density in men with and without vertebral deformity. (*Reproduced by permission from Mann T, Oviatt SK, Wilson D, Orwoll ES. Vertebral deformity in men. J Bone Miner Res 1992; 7:1259–1265.*)

(Scheuermann's disease) is an uncommon cause of significant vertebral deformity in men (43).

OTHER FRACTURES

Other fractures (radius/ulna, humerus, pelvis, femoral shaft) share a similar epidemiologic pattern. Men experience more of these fractures in youth, but with unusual exceptions (eg, humerus) the incidence remains relatively stable with aging, while rising markedly in women (38,44,45). Why men are relatively resistant to these fractures with aging, while experiencing increases in hip and vertebral fractures, is not totally clear but probably relates to the relatively higher peak appendicular bone mass in men and the slower rate of subsequent loss from this compartment. Importantly, the occurrence of a limb fracture in an older man indicates a considerably increased risk of other fractures (46), presumably as a result of diffuse osteopenia or an increased risk of falling, or both.

Determinants of Fracture

BONE DENSITY

In women, BMD is clearly shown to be related to fracture risk in both retrospective case-controlled studies and prospective trials. Less data are available in men, but those available are consistent with a similar relationship of osteopenia to fracture. For instance, in men with spinal fractures assessments of femoral cortical area and Singh grade (47), proximal femoral DPA (43), vertebral QCT (2), vertebral DPA (8,48), and total body bone density as determined by DXA (49) have all revealed reduced mean values compared to control men. Whereas in women it is suggested that levels of spinal bone density greater than 2 standard deviations below the mean of young normal subjects can be considered abnormal (31) (more than 90% of patients with vertebral fractures have vertebral densities below this level), there is not enough experience to determine if this is a reasonable approach in men as well. As in women, there is a clear overlap in bone density in men with fractures and control subjects, indicating that bone density is not the sole determinant of fracture risk. There are few specific data concerning the measurement of bone mass in men with hip fracture, although Chevalley and colleagues and Karlsson and coworkers recently showed that hip and spine BMD were clearly reduced in a series of men with hip fracture when compared with age-matched controls (50,51). In a prospective study, Gardsell and coworkers showed that forearm bone density measures at both proximal and distal sites were lower in men who had sustained osteoporotic fractures (vertebrae, hip, proximal humerus, forearm, pelvis, and tibial condyle) in the subsequent 10-year study (52).

Osteoporosis

As discussed above, there are microscopic changes in bone architecture with aging that in all likelihood influence fracture risk. The decline in vertebral trabecular number and thickness with age is associated with a reduction in compressive strength (53), and men with vertebral and femoral fractures have a lower trabecular plate density (22). In men and women there is a generalized loss of trabeculae, but loss of horizontal elements (number and thickness) is particularly marked, in turn resulting in less support to vertical, load-bearing trabeculae (19; Figure 7-6). Similar changes in trabecular structure in other locations (proximal femur) probably also contribute to fracture risk. In fact, the quantitation of proximal femoral trabecular patterns reveals a definite loss of trabeculation with age in men and that men with osteoporotic fractures have less trabeculation than control men (54). In addition to trabecular loss, the appearance of microfractures increases with age and may also contribute to fracture risk (55). In cortical bone, men experience an increase in porosity at a rate similar to that seen in women (56). This results in a reduction in density, probably in mechanical strength, and presumably increases fracture risk.

▶ 155

FALLS

In addition to bone mass, the risk of falling has been identified as a major determinant of fracture in women. In men, there are no prospective data that directly relate fall propensity to subsequent fractures, but a variety of factors indirectly related to risk of falling have been related to fracture. For instance, Nguyen found that men who had experienced a nontraumatic fracture had more body sway and lower grip strength (as well as lower bone density) than nonfracture controls (57). Similarly, in a study of men with hip fractures (58) a number of factors associated with falls were found to be more prevalent than in controls. These included neurologic disease, confusion, "ambulatory problems," and alcohol use. As in women, the use of several classes of psychotropic drugs has been associated with hip fracture risk in men (59,60). Finally, men with hip fracture appear to be of lower weight, to have lower fat and lean body mass, and more commonly to live alone than control subjects (51). These differences suggest a body habitus and life-style more conducive to falls and injury, as well as the possibility of other interacting risk factors (nutritional).

Why are Fractures Less Common in Men than in Women?

The cause of the greater fracture rate in women is complex. First, accumulation of skeletal mass during growth, particularly in puberty, is greater in men than

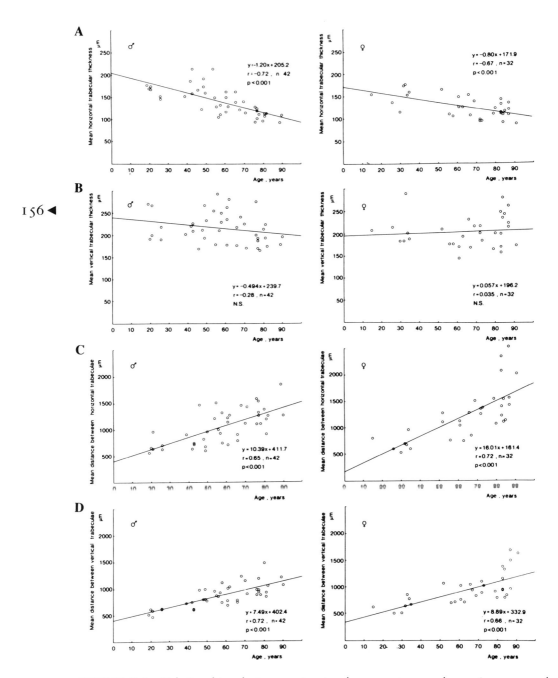

FIGURE 7-6 Relationships between structural parameters and age in men and women. (A) Horizontal trabecular thickness. (B) Vertical trabecular thickness. (C) Distance between horizontal trabeculae. (D) Distance between vertical trabeculae. (*Reproduced by permission from Mosekilde L. Sex differences in age-related loss of vertebral trabecular bone mass and structure—biomechanical consequences. Bone 1989;10:425–432.*)

Osteoporosis

in women, resulting in larger bones. This is especially true in tubular bones, where there is a greater total width (20% in the second metacarpal) (61) and greater cortical width in early adulthood. This difference persists throughout life. Because resistance to fracture in tubular bones is related both to total diameter and cortical thickness, it follows that long bone fractures should be more common in women. Secondly, women lose more bone mineral with aging than do men, a phenomenon also most apparent in long bones. Both sexes increase the periosteal diameter while losing at the endosteal surface, a process found to be present even in paleopathologic studies of ancient populations. However, women lose more at the endosteal surface than do men, increasing their relative risk of fracture. At some long bone sites (the femoral diaphysis) women gain less periosteally than do men, and thus gain less biomechanical benefit (6,62). Interestingly, femoral neck girth increases with age in men but may not in women (63,64; Figure 7-7). This difference at the proximal femur may help explain the lower hip fracture rate in men, particularly because there is little sexual difference in peak hip mineral density or in the rate of age-related decline in hip density. Thirdly, a sexual difference in the character of age-related changes in trabecular bone structure probably contributes to a greater fracture risk in women. Whereas in men the age-related fall in BMD at trabecular sites (which is almost as impressive as in women) is the result of generalized trabecular thinning as well as loss of trabeculae (19,20,65), in women there is a more marked loss of trabecular elements.

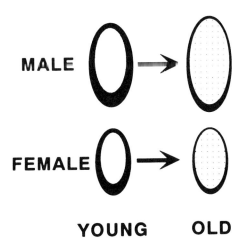

FIGURE 7-7   Depiction of the typical pattern of age-related change observed in cross-sections of the femoral neck in men and women. Both sexes show cortical thinning, but men show compensatory increases in section breadth. (*Reproduced by permission from Beck TJ, Ruff CB, Scott WWJ, Plato CC, Tobin JD, Quan CA. Sex differences in geometry of the femoral neck with aging: a structural analysis of bone mineral data. Calcif Tissue Int 1992;50:24–29.*)

Osteoporosis in Men

Osteoporosis in men is a heterogeneous condition, encompassing a wide variety of etiologies and clinical presentations. In practice, it is common to encounter several potential explanations for bone loss and fractures in a single patient. For the sake of clarity, we have chosen to discuss those individual causes of bone disease commonly encountered in men, recognizing that each will be rarely encountered in its pure form in clinical situations.

Senile Osteoporosis

Bone loss that occurs with aging is an important feature of osteoporosis in men and women. In some men, age-related bone loss may alone suffice to cause non-traumatic fractures, but age-related bone loss is frequently accentuated by other conditions that adversely affect fracture risk. Presumably those men who achieve relatively low levels of peak bone mass, and lose at more rapid rates thereafter, are at greater risk for eventual fracture. Even when other causes of bone loss are present (hypogonadism, alcoholism, etc), the universal loss of bone that accompanies aging certainly contributes to the eventual propensity for fractures.

As discussed above (see also Chapter 5), aging in normal men is associated with detectable appendicular and substantial axial bone loss. The cause of this loss is unknown, but has been speculated to be related to a number of factors similar to those thought to be influential in aging women. In both sexes there appears to be a reduction in bone formation (mean wall thickness) (4,66–69,70) that probably contributes to the decline in bone mass with aging. This reduction is considered a function of aging, but it is of unknown etiology. It appears to occur to a similar extent in men and women (70). An additional age-related increase in bone resorption in men appears less likely (66,71). In addition to these putative intrinsic remodeling abnormalities, several other factors have been suggested to contribute to the process of senile bone loss. These include nutritional deficiencies, inactivity, and loss of gonadal function.

CALCIUM NUTRITION AND BONE LOSS

The average level of dietary calcium necessary to maintain mineral balance is relatively low in young men (mean 400 to 500 mg/d) but the range is large and data suggest a higher requirement in older men (72,73). Although men achieve a mean dietary calcium intake considerably greater than that of women (~800 versus ~500 mg/d in the 1978 Health and Nutritional Examination Survey), these data still indicate that about one half of men ingest less than the recommended daily allowance (800 mg), and many ingest much less. In addition, aging in men has been associated with increased parathyroid hormone (PTH) levels (74,75), reduced 25-hydroxyvitamin D (25-(OH)D) levels (76), and (in some studies) subnormal 1,25-dihydroxyvitamin D (1, 25(OH)$_2$ D) levels (77). Further validation of the importance of changes in mineral metabolism in aging men comes from a report from the Baltimore Longitudinal Study of Aging (78), in which lower radial bone density was related to higher PTH levels and lower 25-(OH)D concentrations. Osteocalcin levels and urinary pyridinoline excretion (79) gradually increase with age in men, raising the possibility that increased bone turnover, possibly associated with these changes in mineral homeostasis, plays a role in age-related bone loss (80). The potential for negative calcium balance therefore exists as a determinant of age-related bone loss in men as well as in women.

▶ 159

Several reports have linked dietary calcium intake to levels of bone density or fracture rates in men. Kelly and Pocock (81) found that 24% and 42% of the variation of lumbar spine and femoral neck bone density in men, respectively, could be explained by calcium intake. Other (82), but not all (83), studies yield similar findings. The relationship between fracture incidence and calcium intake also suggests a beneficial effect of calcium in men. Holbrook and colleagues (84) found that the relative risk of hip fracture in male residents in a southern California retirement community in the upper tertile of dietary calcium intake was 0.3 compared to those in the lower tertiles. In another study, a higher calcium intake was associated with lower hip fracture rates in Chinese men (85). In the only prospective trial of calcium supplementation of men, 1200 mg calcium carbonate daily was ineffective in altering the rate of bone loss at radial or vertebral sites over 3 years. This study was limited in that the mean daily dietary calcium intake in the men studied was relatively high (1100 mg) and thus the effectiveness of calcium supplementation in men with lower intakes could not be assessed. Albeit incomplete, the data are consistent with a role for dietary calcium insufficiency in the determination of the rate of bone loss and fractures in men.

OTHER NUTRIENTS

By virtue of dietary excess or insufficiency, a number of nutrients are speculated to be responsible for accelerating age-related bone loss. Particularly in men, the experimental evidence for these putative relationships is meager. Increased dietary protein intake has been theoretically linked to reduced calcium balance and bone mass, and in men a variety of studies have demonstrated the dependence of urinary calcium excretion and calcium balance on dietary protein intake (86).

The magnitude of the effect of dietary protein when ingested as part of a mixed meal is probably modest, but a high protein intake (particularly of animal protein) has the potential to induce negative calcium balance and contribute to bone loss. Inadequate protein intake is suggested to affect bone adversely (86), and aging is associated with evidence of protein undernutrition in some individuals (increased protein requirements without adequate intake) (73). In fact, Albright initially considered senile osteoporosis to be a consequence of protein insufficiency (resulting in a failure to produce bone matrix) (1). Garn reported osteopenia in a group of malnourished male prisoners of war and suggested that protein malnutrition may have contributed (87), but obviously other factors were perhaps important. A fall in serum albumin concentrations with age has been linked to bone mass in men, but apparently not because of a deficiency in dietary protein intake, and dietary protein intake was not related to the rate of bone loss in a longitudinal study in men (8). An excess of dietary phosphorous, as part of a modern, highly processed diet, may be associated with secondary hyperparathyroidism in women (88), but balance experiments in normal young men suggest that high levels of dietary phosphate (as part of mixed meals) do not significantly influence calcium metabolism even at low dietary calcium intakes (89,90). Other elements surmised to affect bone and mineral metabolism (boron, copper, zinc, selenium, etc) have not been specifically studied in men.

WEIGHT AND PHYSICAL ACTIVITY

Mechanical force has major effects on bone mass, and it may be one of the fundamental variables responsible for the sexual dimorphism in bone mass and structure. In cross-sectional studies, bone mass is greater in physically active men (91–96), an effect that can be demonstrated at the regional (the particular anatomic region affected) and systemic level. Longitudinal studies tend to corroborate the effect of mechanical force on skeletal character in men (97) but are very few in number. Muscle strength and lean body mass in men also correlate with bone density both regionally and systemically (91). Furthermore, muscle strength is related to bone bending stiffness in men, an index of strength measured independent of mass, suggesting that mechanical force has effects not only on bone mass but also quality (98). As in women, body weight itself is highly correlated with bone density in men (16), an effect that could be related to the mechanical effect exerted by mass alone or to a particular aspect of body composition (lean versus fat mass, adipose distribution, etc). Reid and colleagues (99) suggested that there are sexual differences in the relative effects of body composition on skeletal morphology. In their studies bone mass was associated with fat mass in women, but not in men (lean mass was not associated with bone mass in either sex). They speculated that androgens may contribute to the lack of fat/bone correlation in men because androgen action is associated with an increase in bone mass but a fall in adiposity. The data strongly suggest a powerful effect of weight and mechanical force on the male skeleton. In view of the clear decline in physical activity and muscle strength with aging (100–102), senile osteopenia in men may in part relate to a diminution of the trophic effects of mechanical force on skeletal tissues. In fact, the character of senile bone loss closely mimics that of chronic disuse (103).

GONADAL DYSFUNCTION

Aging in men is associated with changes in the hypothalamic-pituitary-gonadal axis that result in notable declines in total and free testosterone levels (104,105). These changes have given rise to considerable speculation as to whether several of the concomitants of aging are the result, at least in part, of the decline in testosterone levels. For instance, the well-documented declines in muscle strength and bone mass with aging have been suggested to be potential sequelae (106). Several lines of evidence firmly link androgen action to skeletal mass in men (see below), and there have been several attempts to link bone mass to testosterone levels. Kelly and Pocock (81) found that free testosterone levels correlated with ultradistal bone density (but not with a variety of other densitometric measurement sites) in a group of men aged 21 to 79 even after the effects of age were considered. Similarly, in a study of randomly selected older men in England, androgen levels were found to correlate (albeit weakly) with proximal femoral BMD (107). However, these findings have not been corroborated by other investigators (108,109). In an attempt to test the hypothesis that relative androgen deficiency had a skeletal impact in older men, Tenover reported in a small study (13 men) that parenteral testosterone supplementation reduced urinary hydroxyproline excretion (110). In a much larger trial of transdermal testosterone supplementation in older normal men, more sensitive and specific indices of bone metabolism (serum osteocalcin and procollagen, urinary N-telopeptide) were unchanged (111). Hence, the issue of the importance of gonadal insufficiency in the genesis of senile osteopenia in men remains unresolved.

Osteoporosis Secondary to Other Disorders

The pathophysiologic character of osteoporosis in men is minimally explored, but several series have examined the risk factors present for bone disease in small patient populations. In the available series (47,112,113) 30% to 60% of men evaluated for vertebral fractures had "secondary" causes (underlying illness) contributing to the presence of bone disease. It must be recognized that these studies are of selected subjects—men presenting for health care in the United

States or Great Britain because of vertebral fracture. Hence, the findings may not accurately represent the spectrum of disease in other community settings. A major deficit is that there have been no similar studies of the character of the bone disease present in men sustaining femoral or other fractures. The principal conditions found in men with osteopenia are shown in Table 7-1. Prominent are glucocorticoid excess, hypogonadism, alcoholism, gastrectomy and other gastrointestinal disorders, and hypercalciuria. Similar attempts to examine the contributing factors in osteoporotic women suggest that the spectrum of disorders is somewhat different (38,114,115), but glucocorticoid excess, premature hypogonadism, and gastrointestinal disorders are prominent in women as well. It has been suggested that the number of men with "secondary" osteoporosis is higher than in women (115), but in other more objective evaluations (114) the proportion of women with major illnesses contributing to the development of bone disease is actually similar to findings in male osteoporotics.

GLUCOCORTICOID EXCESS

In the largest series of men evaluated for spinal osteoporosis, glucocorticoid excess (particularly exogenous) is the most prominent of the secondary causes identified, accounting for 16% to 18% of the men evaluated (47,112). Glucocorticoids are commonly prescribed to men for disorders such as collagen vascular diseases, chronic obstructive pulmonary disease, among others. The pathophysiology of glucocorticoid–induced osteoporosis is discussed in Chapter 8, and presumably the events that lead to bone loss in men and women are in many ways similar. In men, impotence and loss of libido frequently occur in the clin

TABLE 7-1 Osteoporosis in Men

I.	Primary
II.	Secondary
	Hypogonadism
	Glucocorticoid excess
	Alcoholism
	Gastrointestinal disorders
	Hypercalciuria
	Smoking
	Anticonvulsants
	Thyrotoxicosis
	Immobilization
	Osteogenesis imperfecta
	Homocystinuria
	Systemic mastocytosis
	Neoplastic diseases
	Rheumatoid arthritis

ical settings in which glucocorticoids are administered and are attributed to the effects of the chronic illness. However, these symptoms may actually be due to glucocorticoid-induced hypogonadism, which in turn may contribute substantially to the mechanism resulting in osteopenia. Exogenous glucocorticoids markedly reduce testosterone levels in men (116–118; Figure 7-8) by mechanisms that have not been fully defined, but may include central inhibition of gonadotropin-releasing hormone (GnRH) release, suppression of pituitary sensitivity to GnRH, and direct antagonism of testicular steroidogenesis (117–120). Clinicians who care for men with osteoporosis should be aware of this phenomenon and recognize it as an important cause of a low serum testosterone level. Furthermore, because administration of testosterone to hypogonadal men improves bone mass, such therapy in glucocorticoid-treated men may be useful to prevent and treat glucocorticoid-induced osteoporosis.

▶ 163

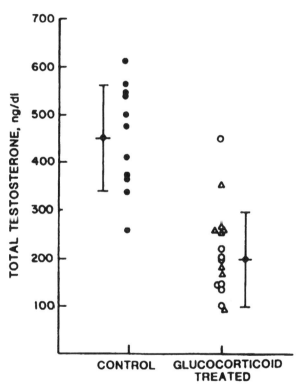

FIGURE 7-8 Chronic glucocorticoid therapy reduces circulating testosterone levels. Total testosterone levels in 11 control male patients with chronic obstructive pulmonary disease (*closed circles*) and 16 age- and disease-matched patients receiving glucocorticoid therapy either daily (*open circles*) or on alternating days (*open triangles*) are shown. The horizontal lines indicate mean ± SD. (*Reproduced by permission from MacAdams MR, White RH, Chipps BE. Reduction of serum testosterone levels during chronic glucocorticoid therapy. Ann Intern Med 1986;104:648–651.*)

Sex steroids have major influences on the regulation of bone metabolism. The obvious importance of menopause to osteoporosis drew early attention to the role of estrogen, but more recently both clinical and basic observations have also highlighted the importance of androgens in bone physiology in both sexes. Several lines of evidence firmly link androgen action to skeletal mass in men. First, there is an expanding understanding of the cellular effects of androgens on bone remodeling. Androgen receptors are present in physiologically relevant concentrations in osteoblastic cells (116,121), and androgens affect a variety of osteoblastic functions, including proliferation, growth factor and cytokine production, and bone matrix protein production (collagen, osteocalcin, osteopontin) (122–126). Hence, there is an excellent foundation in basic research for the precept that androgens are active in bone.

Prepubertal Hypogonadism: With adolescence, bone mass increases dramatically in both sexes that is closely related to gonadal maturation (127). Increases are seen in both cancellous and cortical bone (128). Strongly supporting the importance of androgen action in the achievement of peak bone mass in men is the fact that genetic males with complete androgen insensitivity (testicular feminization) experience increased pubertal growth but achieve a bone mass typical of genetic women (J. Wilson, personal communication). Probably as a result of androgen action, boys experience a particularly vigorous increase in cortical bone and attain greater peak bone densities at cortical sites than girls (81; Figure 7-9). Osteopenia is found in men who experience an abnormal puberty (Klinefelter's and Kallman's syndromes) (129–131), and the bone deficit is more marked in cortical compartments than is the osteopenia of adult-onset hypogonadism (129). The apparent emphasis on cortical bone mass in boys suggests that androgen action is especially important in the modeling drifts that add periosteal new bone during growth. It is proposed that the failure to acquire peak bone mass with puberty is the primary abnormality in these forms of early onset hypogonadism (129). In fact, even constitutionally delayed puberty is associated with permanent reductions in bone density (132). A reasonable hypothesis is that androgens increase trabecular bone formation at epiphyseal areas and strongly promote the addition of cortical thickness through periosteal and endosteal growth—processes that then are impaired in the presence of hypogonadism.

A single animal study examines indirectly the effects of prepubertal hypogonadism. Hock and Gera (133) examined trabecular and cortical bone mass in rats castrated (or sham operated) just before sexual maturation (4 weeks). In both compartments, bone mass in the hypogonadal rats continued to increase but at a rate considerably slower than in the controls. This unique experiment is

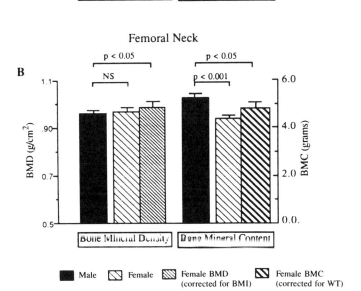

FIGURE 7-9 Comparison of BMD and BMC values in the lumbar spine (A) and femoral neck (B) with and without correction for sex differences in body mass index (BMI) and weight (Wt) in twins of differing sex. (*Reproduced by permission from Kelly PJ, Twomey L, Sambrook PN, Eisman JA. Sex differences in peak adult bone mineral density. J Bone Miner Res 1990;5:1169–1175.*)

consistent with the hypothesis that hypogonadism impairs the pubertal stimulus to bone mass accumulation. It provides no histomorphometric or structural information. Another study of rats during adolescence reports histomorphometric analyses of cortical bone (including fluorescent labeling) and suggests that periosteal bone formation and cortical thickness decreased in adolescent males following castration (134). This indicates that a reduction in bone formation contributes to osteopenia in hypogonadal adolescent animals. Certainly the fact that male rats have markedly greater cortical mass than do females, and that the differences are eliminated by castration (134), strongly supports a prominent role for androgens in the phase of cortical bone accumulation.

Postpubertal Hypogonadism: Androgens also appear essential for the maintenance of bone mass in adult men because the development of hypogonadism in mature men is associated with osteopenia. Hypogonadism is present in 5% to 33% of men evaluated in vertebral fractures and osteoporosis (47,112,135), and hip fractures in elderly men apparently occur more commonly in the setting of hypogonadism (136). Reduced bone mass and fractures are associated with many forms of hypogonadism, including castration, hyperprolactinemia, anorexia, and hemachromatosis (137–140). Vertebral and appendicular bone mass are both reduced, but in adult-onset hypogonadism vertebral loss is relatively more pronounced. In addition to the link between primary testicular dysfunction and osteopenia, reduction in gonadal function secondary to several other conditions is now postulated to contribute to the development of bone loss. For instance, hypogonadism is suspected to contribute to the osteopenia associated with glucocorticoid excess, renal insufficiency, and other conditions (141,142).

The Character of Hypogonadal Bone Disease in Men: The histologic pattern of hypogonadal bone loss in men is poorly described. In fact, there are no reported studies characterizing the bone deficit in hypogonadism of preadolescent onset. There is some limited information on adult-onset hypogonadism. A single report examines skeletal metabolism in the period shortly after gonadal failure. Stepan and Lachman (140) studied a small group of men in the years immediately following castration. The subjects were osteopenic and had clear biochemical indications of increased bone remodeling (increased serum osteocalcin levels and urinary hydroxyproline excretion). Unfortunately, no direct histomorphometric analyses were reported. Several reports have described the histomorphometric character of hypogonadal, osteopenic men, but they are uncontrolled, and are from subjects in whom hypogonadism was of varied causation (both early and late onset) and of long duration. For instance, in a study of 13 men with long-standing hypogonadism, Francis and Peacock found that bone remodeling and formation were reduced, and $1,25(OH)_2D$ levels were low in those with fractures (143). With testosterone therapy, $1,25(OH)_2D$ levels increased and there was some indication of an increase in "formation" parameters. Similarly, Delmas and Meunier reported decreased rates of formation in a small group of hypogonadal men (144), and formation rates were low in a single case reported by Baran and colleagues (vitamin D metabolite levels were not available in these reports [145]). These data raise the issue of whether androgens provide an important stimulus to bone formation. In contrast, Jackson and colleagues (146) reported histomorphometric analyses of a small group of osteoporotic, chronically hypogonadal men with normal vitamin D levels. In these patients no apparent defect in mineralization was observed, and the authors speculated that nutritional vitamin D deficiency may be a factor in the European studies of Francis and Delmas. They found a slight increase in mean remodeling rate and concluded that androgen deficiency induces a remodeling defect similar to that of estrogen deficiency in the postmenopausal period. In both the series from Jackson and Francis, trabecular number was reduced in the hypogonadal men, indicating that trabecular loss is a feature of androgen deficiency as it is in estrogen deficiency (22). There are no reports of cortical remodeling dynamics. Actually, the remodeling character of all these study ▶ 167 populations was heterogeneous, and in view of the variability in the small groups, the presence of other confounding clinical conditions, and the lack of adequate controls, no firm conclusions can be drawn concerning the remodeling defect induced by hypogonadism in men.

The data from Stepan and Lachman in the early stages of hypogonadism (140) are most consistent with a model of adult-onset hypogonadism with an early stage of increased bone turnover and bone loss. An early increase in remodelling is also consistent with recent reports of the biochemical and cellular events associated with androgen action—a suppression of cytokine production and osteoclast formation (147). The histomorphometric data (primarily from patients with long-standing hypogonadism) and the better documented sequence of events that follows gonadal hypofunction in menopause suggest that this period of increased remodeling is followed by a subsequent phase of reduced turnover, possibly accompanied by a decline in bone formation.

Animal studies provide limited additional information. The cellular events in cortical bone following castration in animals are unclear. Studies have been reported in male rates (postpubertal but during rapid adolescent growth) castrated at both 2 months (134,148–150) and 12 to 13 months at maximum adult skeletal mass (149,151), but the resulting model of skeletal events remains incomplete. As a reflection of cortical bone metabolism, change in femoral ash weight is similar to that seen after oophorectomy (12% to 15% less than control 4 to 6 months after castration), apparently in part as a result of increased porosity and considerable endosteal resorption (151).

Cancellous bone volume appears to be lost following castration in mature male rats. Histomorphometric measurements of cancellous bone after orchiectomy in mature rats so far include only static parameters. These studies are from one group, but are somewhat inconsistent. In an early description in postpubertal growing animals (134), trabecular bone area was similarly reduced in males and females (~50%) following castration, but changes in metaphyseal remodeling were minimal in males, suggesting that a reduction in trabecular formation contributed to the osteopenia. Later, in similar experiments, it was reported (148) that static indices of both formation and resorption were increased following orchiectomy, and accompanied the previously observed reductions in trabecular bone volume. Indirect evidence of increased resorption was reported in older rats (151). Other studies examining calcium dynamics similarly indicate an increase in remodeling rates following castration (149). Although an increase in remodeling is suggested in animal as well as human studies, the cellular events following hypogonadism remain unresolved.

Therapy: The effectiveness of androgen replacement therapy in hypogonadal men is unclear. There have been several reports of small increases in BMD with androgen replacement in hypogonadal adult men (138,152,153), but the influence of such variables as time since onset of gonadal disease and age are not controlled. One experience with a small number of hypogonadal adolescents suggested an improvement in bone mass, which was lacking in untreated subjects (131). Finally, reversal of hyperprolactinemia and the subsequent achievement of eugonadism in men with pituitary adenomas led to an improvement in vertebral bone mass (139). In general, the response of BMD to androgen replacement has been modest (Figure 7-10). The histomorphometric response to

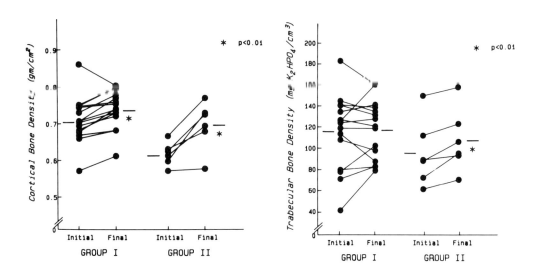

FIGURE 7-10 Cortical and trabecular (vertebral) bone density before and after treatment of men with isolated GnRH deficiency; patients who initially had fused epiphyses (group I) and those who initially had open epiphyses (group II). *(Reproduced by permission from Finkelstein JS, Klibanski A, Neer RM, et al. Increases in bone density during treatment of men with idiopathic hypogonadotropic hypogonadism. J Clin Endocrinol Metab 1989;69:776–783.)*

androgen replacement is unknown, but a single case report suggested that an impairment in bone formation was improved (145). All these reports suggest that at least in the short term, androgen replacement therapy may have beneficial effects on bone mass. However, it is not certain that all men respond, or whether other factors (age, duration of hypogonadism) influence the success of treatment.

The most appropriate route of androgen administration, and the minimally effective dose, have not been examined for this indication. Moreover, all studies that suggest beneficial effects of androgen therapy are of short duration (1 to 5 years) and whether there is a sustained increase in bone mass with therapy, or whether bone mass ever reaches eugonadal levels, is uncertain. In fact, in patients with Klinefelter's syndrome evidence suggests that bone mass does not recover after therapy is begun (154). Of great importance, the potential risks of androgen replacement therapy, particularly in the elderly, are uncertain in relation to the possible skeletal benefits to be gained. Nevertheless, the concern of bone loss and fractures should represent one of the indications for androgen therapy of gonadal failure.

There is essentially no experience with the therapy of hypogonadal bone disease in men with other agents. The character of hypogonadal bone loss in men suggests it is similar to that in women (an early phase of resorption followed by lower turnover) and so approaches that have been effective in the postmenopausal period (bisphosphonates, calcitonin) may be useful in men as well. In a study of the early hypogonadal period in men, Stepan and Lachman (140) found that calcitonin therapy reduced biochemical evidence of increased resorption, but measures of bone mass were not assessed.

ALCOHOLISM

It is well established that long-term alcohol consumption can result in a host of abnormal clinical, biochemical, and physiologic findings that stem from the toxic effects of ethanol on the liver, gonads, marrow, heart, and brain. The fact that prolonged abuse of alcohol is also detrimental to skeletal integrity in men has only recently been recognized.

Numerous studies over the past quarter century have demonstrated a reduction in bone mass in alcoholics, especially in the iliac crest, calcaneus, vertebral column, and hip (112,155–168)—all areas with a high proportion of metabolically active, trabecular bone. Saville first recognized a relationship between osteoporosis and alcohol abuse (155). Using postmortem material from 198 cadavers, he observed that fat-free bone mass was significantly reduced in alcoholics as compared to controls. More recent quantitative measures of bone mass have substantiated the presence of osteopenia in alcoholics. Laitinen and colleagues (169) observed that BMD at all axial sites decreased in parallel with duration of drinking in 27 noncirrhotic male alcoholics. Diamond and colleagues (166) found that 38% of ambulatory patients with alcoholic liver disease had reduced BMD of the spine, forearm, or both, and Bikle and coworkers (167) found the mean BMD of vertebral trabecular bone was 58% of normal in 8 men with long-standing histories of alcohol abuse, whereas appendicular cortical bone density was 90% of normal. It should be pointed out, however, that the studies cited above can be criticized for their small size and for being poorly controlled.

More extensive studies have attempted to estimate the prevalence of skeletal fracture in the alcoholic population. Spencer and colleagues (162) reviewed thoracolumbar spine x-rays of 96 ambulatory men with chronic alcoholism and noted osteopenia or fracture or both in 47%. One half of those affected were under the age of 50. Lindsell and coworkers (163) compared chest x-rays of 72 subjects with alcoholic cirrhosis to those of 149 controls. Rib fractures were four times more common in the alcoholic population (28% versus 7%). Similarly, Israel and colleagues (164) found 29% of 198 male alcoholics had rib or vertebral fractures on x-ray compared to 2% of nonalcoholic control males. Finally, Crilly and colleagues (165) evaluated 50 male alcoholics and found that 25 had at least two atraumatic spinal crush fractures. Thus, osteopenia is evident on routine x-rays in a significant percentage of individuals (25% to 50%) whose drinking habits have prompted them to seek medical help. The degree to which bone disease is present in the entire population of alcoholics remains uncertain, and determination of the true incidence of alcohol-induced osteopenia in men must await a survey of a large number of cases. But the habitual consumption of alcoholic beverages is clearly recognized as a significant negative determinant of bone mass in epidemiological surveys of men (14,112,168,170) and has been shown in longitudinal studies to be associated with increased rates of bone loss (14; Figure 7-11). Thus, the link between alcohol abuse and bone disease is well established.

Mechanism of Ethanol-Induced Bone Disease: Although a definite relationship exists between alcohol abuse and bone disease, the mechanisms by which alcohol induces bone disease remain unclear. An association between alcoholism and accidental injury is well recognized. Acute intoxication, impaired judgment, withdrawal seizures, and hypoglycemic episodes, as well as unstable locomotion and poor motor control due to neuropathy, myopathy and cerebellar degeneration, all conspire to increase the likelihood of trauma and resultant skeletal fracture in alcoholic men. However, emerging evidence now suggests that in addition to the increased incidence of trauma, the high incidence of fracture in this population may also stem from a generalized skeletal fragility. The in vivo rate of skeletal protein synthesis of young male rats is reduced by 25% to 30%

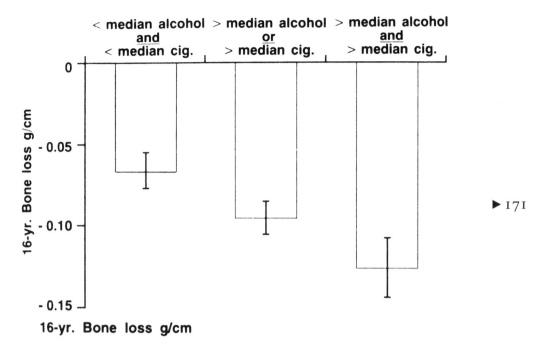

▶ 171

FIGURE 7-11 Effects on bone loss by cigarette smoking and alcohol use in men. *(Reproduced by permission from Slemenda CW, Christian JC, Reed T, Reister TK, Williams CJ, Johnston CC Jr. Long-term bone loss in men: effects of genetic and environmental factors. Ann Intern Med 1992;117:286–291.)*

in response to acute ethanol exposure (171). Furthermore, the chronic administration of ethanol to rats produces ultrastructural changes in the bone microarchitecture that compromise mechanical strength (172,173). Bone histomorphometric studies have provided further insight into the specific nature of the skeletal disorder induced by ethanol. Iliac crest biopsy usually reveals significant reductions in trabecular bone volume, osteoid matrix, number of osteoblasts, mineral apposition, and overall rate of bone formation (165–167,174). Marrow fibrosis is uncommon and there is generally no evidence of osteomalacia, except in patients who have previously undergone gastric surgery (175). Parameters reflecting osteoclast activity (eg, eroded surface, resorption depth, and resorption period) are, for the most part, spared (165–167,174). Since the osteoblast is the cell responsible for bone formation, the histomorphometric findings in alcoholic patients with bone disease suggest that the osteoblast may be specifically targeted by alcohol.

Nutritional deficiencies are common in alcoholics. However, poor nutrition alone does not induce osteoporosis in experimental animals (176), and none of the histomorphometric studies cited above demonstrated any evidence for nutritional deficiency. Mild hypocalcemia, hypophosphatemia, and hypomagnesemia are frequently present in ambulatory alcoholic men because of poor dietary intake, malabsorption, and increased renal excretion (122,123,125, 167, 169, 177). Hypocalcemia, if severe enough, could result in osteopenia by inducing a state of secondary hyperparathyroidism. However, evidence for hyperparathyroidism with accelerated bone remodeling is not seen on bone biopsies of affected patients (165–167,174). Recently, acute alcohol intoxication has been reported to reduce intact PTH levels (178). The relevance of this finding is unclear because the reduction in PTH levels lasts only a few hours, and osteopenia is not observed in hypoparathyroid patients. Early studies found circulating levels of the vitamin D metabolites to be low (158,159,179), but subsequent investigation has excluded vitamin D deficiency as a major cause of alcohol-induced bone disease by demonstrating normal vitamin D absorption (180) and conversion to 25-(OH)D (181) in alcoholic individuals and, more directly, by the measurement of normal free concentrations of 25-(OH)D and 1,25(OH)$_2$D in patients with alcoholic cirrhosis and alcoholic bone disease (167,182,183). These findings do not exclude the possibility of an alcohol-induced vitamin D–resistant state, but again the lack of histomorphometric evidence of osteomalacia in vitamin D–replete osteopenic alcoholic subjects (166,167) argues strongly against such a possibility.

Hypogonadism is clearly a risk factor for osteoporosis in men (see above). Chronic alcoholic men suffer from impotence, sterility, and testicular atrophy (184). Most studies of alcoholic men with bone disease, however, report normal androgen levels (167,169). But, reduced serum free testosterone concentrations in alcoholic subjects with osteoporosis were reported by Diamond and colleagues (166). The testosterone levels were on average lower than those of the male control subjects but still fell within the normal range for the general male population overall. Male hypogonadism is usually associated with accelerated bone resorption (146), but the effects of modest reductions in gonadal steroid levels on bone physiology are currently unknown.

Recent studies suggest that ethanol exerts its toxic effects directly at the cellular level in bone. Ethanol induces a dose-dependent reduction in cellular protein and DNA synthesis in human osteoblasts in vitro (185). Further evidence implicating a direct effect of ethanol on osteoblast activity comes from studies examining circulating bone Gla protein (BGP, osteocalcin) levels in alcoholic subjects. BGP is a small peptide synthesized by active osteoblasts, a portion of which is released into the circulation. BGP levels are positively correlated with histomorphometric parameters of bone formation in normal individuals (186) and in patients with metabolic bone disease (187). Chronic alcoholic patients exhibit significantly lower BGP levels than age-matched controls (188). Moreover, alcohol has a dose-dependent suppressive effect on circulating BGP levels (178,189,190; Figure 7-12). The consumption of 50 g ethanol (equivalent to four "shots" of scotch whiskey) over 45 minutes results in a

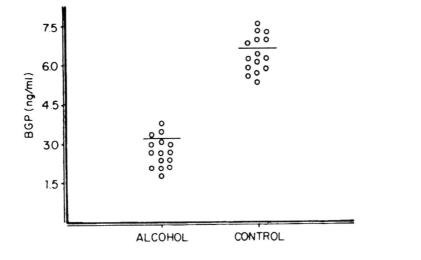

▶ 173

FIGURE 7-12 Alcohol impairs synthesis of osteocalcin. Shown are circulating osteocalcin values in 15 patients with acute alcohol intoxication and in 15 control subjects. The horizontal lines indicate mean values for each group. (*Reproduced by permission from Rico H, Cabranes JA, Cabello J, Gomez-Castresana F, Hernandez ER. Low serum osteocalcin in acute alcohol intoxication: a direct effect of alcohol on osteoblasts. Bone Miner 1987;2:221–225.*)

30% decrease in serum BGP concentration that is detectable 2 hours later (190). Beyond these fragmentary attempts at characterization, however, little is known about phenotypic regulation by ethanol in the osteoblast.

To summarize, the habitual consumption of ethanol is clearly linked with osteopenia, yet no alteration in the hormonal regulation of calcium homeostasis is evident in alcoholics with bone disease. Biochemical and histomorphometric evaluation of alcoholic subjects reveal a marked impairment in osteoblastic activity (reduced BGP levels and collagen synthesis; reduced osteoblast number and bone formation rate) with normal osteoclastic activity. Laboratory studies on isolated osteoblasts demonstrate a potent inhibitory effect of ethanol on the proliferation of isolated osteoblasts in vitro. Acute ethanol exposure depresses in vivo skeletal protein synthesis in rats and BGP levels in human beings. Taken together this body of evidence argues strongly that a primary target of ethanol's adverse effects on the skeleton is the osteoblast. Because bone remodeling and mineralization are dependent on osteoblasts, it follows that the deleterious effect of alcohol on these cells will lead to slowed bone formation, ultimately resulting in osteopenia and fracture.

Therapy: The prevention and treatment of osteoporosis in alcoholic men is similar to that recommended for idiopathic osteoporosis. Nevertheless, several points deserve emphasis. Osteoporosis should be suspected in every chronic alcohol abuser and patients with "idiopathic" osteoporosis should be routinely and thoroughly questioned about drinking habits. Alcoholism is a subtle disease in most patients and the diagnosis may be missed unless the patient is specifically questioned. A history of sporadic alcohol ingestion should arouse suspicion. Symptoms such as low back pain, which can indicate the presence of osteoporosis, may be minimized or overlooked in these patients because of the more obvious acute and chronic complications of alcoholism. Once the diagnosis of alcohol-induced bone disease has been established, a number of measures are recommended. Aggressive medical and psychiatric treatment should be pursued in the hopes of interrupting the cycle of chronic alcohol ingestion and thereby diminish the risk of further skeletal deterioration. Unfortunately, the personality disturbances and low compliance of most alcohol abusers reduces the long-term success of such therapeutic interventions (191), especially in patients without adequate social and economic support. A careful dietary history should be followed by an adequate well-balanced diet rich in milk and calcium-containing products. Evidence that calcium supplementation will improve the bone disease of alcoholics has not been reported, but it is reasonable to minimize other potential risk factors for bone loss if possible. Adequate vitamin D nutrition and physical exercise should be encouraged. Tobacco use and excessive consumption of phosphate-binding antacids should be discouraged.

Presumably, the cessation of alcohol intake will stop further progression of osteopenia, but data are scant. Moreover, no evidence has been reported that bone, once lost, will be restored when alcohol abuse is discontinued. Studies on alcohol abstainers have demonstrated a rapid recovery of osteoblast function (as assessed histomorphometrically and by biochemical parameters of bone remodeling) within as little as a week after cessation of drinking, but no significant differences in bone mineral content were observed between abstainers and actively drinking men (160,166,169). The relatively short period of abstinence, however, makes these results inconclusive.

The challenge in alcohol-induced bone disease is to stimulate bone formation. Most of the drugs currently used to treat other forms of osteoporosis work primarily by inhibiting osteoclastic bone resorption. Agents such as fluoride, PTH, or growth hormone may stimulate bone formation, but such regimens remain investigational and no therapeutic trials in alcoholic men have been reported. The toxic effects of alcohol and fluoride on the gastrointestinal tract may likely preclude its use in the individual who continues to drink.

GASTROINTESTINAL DISORDERS

In both sexes, disorders of gastrointestinal function have been associated with skeletal disease, frequently as a result of malabsorption of calcium, vitamin D, or other nutrients. In men, a particularly striking relationship has been observed between gastrectomy and vertebral osteoporosis (47,112), although some data actually support the precept that the female skeleton is more severely affected by gastrectomy (192). Nevertheless, men are overrepresented in most studies of postgastrectomy bone disease. This may reflect the increased frequency of peptic ulcer disease, and hence gastrectomy, in men. Estimates of prevalence of osteopenia range from less than 10% to greater than 40% (193,194), depending on the population studied and the methods used for diagnosis. Similarly, bone disease commonly results from a variety of small bowel disorders (195,196), but there is little evidence that men are more affected than are women. Large bowel disorders are rarely associated with osteopenia (197). ▶ 175

Mechanisms of Gastrointestinal Bone Disease: The etiology of gastrointestinal bone disease remains unclear. Proposed causes include malabsorption of vitamin D (198–200) or calcium (201–203), a decreased intake of vitamin D (204,205) or calcium (206,207), inadequate contact between nutrients and their absorptive sites, either because of altered anatomy or rapid transit (3,208–210), and reduced exposure to sunlight (208). A single functional lesion that results in bone disease in the majority of patients has not been convincingly demonstrated, although classic vitamin D deficiency and osteomalacia appear most commonly associated with frank malabsorption.

Unfortunately, most investigations of postgastrectomy bone disease have dealt with heterogeneous populations, sometimes including both sexes, widely varying ages, and a number of surgical procedures. In some cases no attempt has been made to identify other factors that might predispose to bone disease, such as endocrinopathy, small bowel or liver disease, or chronic use of corticosteroids. Furthermore, techniques to characterize the bone and mineral abnormalities have often been inadequate, casting doubt on the validity of the conclusions. For instance, rarely has comprehensive bone histomorphometry been done. Finally, some studies have been restricted to patients with classical findings, thereby ignoring those who have significant bone disease without symptoms or biochemical or radiologic changes (194,211,212).

Despite the lack of comprehensive studies, it is clear that the osteopenia seen in men with gastrointestinal disorders is heterogeneous in nature. Osteomalacia is commonly reported, but osteoporosis and less well-characterized forms of osteopenia have been described (193,194,197,204,206,213–216). In fact, frank osteomalacia may represent a small portion of the affected population. Several studies have clearly demonstrated significant osteopenia in gastrectomized patients in the absence of vitamin D deficiency, even after more conservative surgical procedures (Bilroth I)(192,197,217,218). The histomorphometric character of "gastrectomy" bone disease is unusual in that there is evidence of a mineralization abnormality in the absence of obvious defects in mineral homeostasis (vitamin D deficiency, hyperparathyroidism, hypophosphatemia, etc.) (217,218). Parfitt has characterized these forms of osteomalacia as focal (increased osteoid thickness without a proportionate increase in osteoid surface) or atypical (increased osteoid surface without increased osteoid thickness) (219). In both cases the mineralization rate is depressed. These forms of osteomalacic bone disease are similar to those described in small bowel disease (196,220–222). Their pathophysiologies are unknown, suggesting there are yet unidentified mechanisms for skeletal abnormalities in the presence of gastrointestinal malfunction. Finally, a common form of osteopenia in men with bowel disease is low-turnover osteoporosis (196). Its causation is also unknown.

Therapy: The therapeutic approach to osteopenia in men with gastrectomy or small bowel disease should be based on an understanding of gastrointestinal function and mineral metabolism. Vitamin D insufficiency should be treated with replacement doses sufficient to restore adequate serum 25-(OH)D levels. Dietary calcium intake should be supplemented when necessary, but the amounts needed to achieve adequate calcium balance vary greatly. PTH levels and rates of urinary calcium excretion may help to gauge the severity of dietary calcium deficiency and the adequacy of replacement doses. With this therapy for classic hypovitaminosis D, improvement in bone mass should be expected, but the bone deficit existing before therapy is, to a large extent, irreversible (65). In patients with osteopenia who show either histomorphometric evidence of a mineralization defect or low-turnover osteoporosis in the absence of vitamin D insufficiency, there is no therapy yet shown to be effective in restoring bone mass. Many patients with osteopenia and mineralization defects with normal vitamin D levels fail to improve with calcium–vitamin D replacement therapy (223).

HYPERCALCIURIA

Several reports have linked hypercalciuria or nephrolithiasis in men to a reduction in BMD (111,224–227). It is not clear whether this apparent increase in bone disease in men is a result of a greater impact of hypercalciuria in men or merely reflects the fact that hypercalciuria is more than twice as common in men than women (228). In fact, hypercalciuria has also been linked to osteoporosis in women (229).

Mechanisms of Hypercalciuric Bone Disease: The etiology of the osteopenia is unclear but has been postulated to involve an alteration in mineral metabolism, including an increase in 1,25-(OH)$_2$D levels in absorptive hypercalciurics

(230,231) and a negative calcium balance with secondary hyperparathyroidism in renal hypercalciurics (230,232,233). This is supported by the finding that lower dietary calcium intakes in men with hypercalciuria are associated with a further reduction in bone mass (234). On the other hand, in some patients hypercalciuria may be only part of a more diffuse metabolic abnormality that may affect bone metabolism in other ways. For instance, renal tubular acidosis may be present with hypercalciuria and osteopenia in the presence of complex abnormalities of mineral and bone metabolism (235), hypercalciuria has been linked to phosphate wasting disorders causing osteopenia (236), and medullary sponge kidney is not uncommonly associated with increased urinary calcium excretion and disordered parathyroid function (237–239).

▶ 177

In most subjects with idiopathic hypercalciuria, the depression in bone mass is quite modest, and of itself is unlikely to result in clinically significant bone disease. On the other hand, renal lithiasis has been associated with osteopenia and fractures in men (112). In a small series of relatively young men (5 subjects, aged 27 to 57 years) Perry and colleagues (240) found osteoporosis in association with moderate hypercalciuria in the absence of other risk factors for bone loss. In all patients hyperabsorption appeared to be a contributor to the hypercalciuria. Histomorphometric analysis revealed an increased rate of bone remodeling in the face of no apparent alteration in mineral metabolism. In a somewhat different experience, Zerwekh and coworkers (231) reported that of 16 men (mean 50 ± 11) referred for evaluations of osteoporosis, 9 were hypercalciuric without any other obvious cause of bone disease. Further examination showed that all of the hypercalciuric group had evidence of an element of absorptive hypercalciuria, and 4 actually had increased gastrointestinal calcium absorption and 1,25-(OH)$_2$D levels. In the hypercalciuric subgroup, bone formation rates were depressed (reduced bone formation rate, increased mineralization lag time) in comparison to normals or normocalciuric osteoporotics, with no differences in indices of bone resorption (Figure 7-13). Similar findings have been reported in men with idiopathic hypercalciuria (241). In other groups of men with unexplained osteoporosis, some have been reported to be hypercalciuric (158,242). Thus, suggestive but still preliminary data link hypercalciuria to bone loss and osteoporosis in men. The specific pathophysiology involved and the clinical spectrum of bone disease produced remain somewhat unclear.

Therapy: Attempts to treat osteopenia associated with idiopathic hypercalciuria are not yet reported. Because the most likely cause of defects in bone remodeling are related to the mineral abnormalities induced by the renal calcium disturbance, it seems prudent to prevent hypercalciuria. In those with either renal or absorptive hypercalciuria, thiazide diuretics would be appropriate (and their use is associated with positive effects on bone density in other settings).

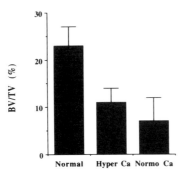
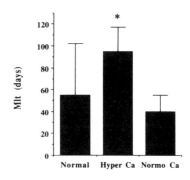

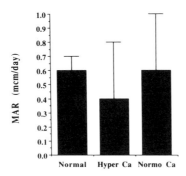
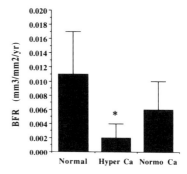

FIGURE 7-13 Selected histomorphometric parameters in osteoporotic men with hypercalciuria and normocalciuria, and normal men. BFR, bone formation rates; BV/TV, bone volume; MAR, mean absorption rate; Mlt, mineralization lag time. (*Adapted and reproduced by permission from Zerwekh JE, Sakhaee K, Breslau NA, Gottschalk F, Pak CYC. Impaired bone function in male idiopathic osteoporosis: further reduction in the presence of concomitant hypercalciuria. Osteoporosis Int 1992;2:128–134.*)

TOBACCO USE

Tobacco use has been associated with lowered bone mass and fractures in women (243–246). Tobacco was also linked to an increased prevalence of vertebral fractures in men in the cohort studies of Seeman and coworkers (112), in which the relative risk of vertebral fracture in smokers was 2.3. This risk was independent of alcohol consumption, and in fact, the risk imparted by the two variables was multiplicative. In the case of both these risk factors, adverse effects were noted only in subjects over 60 years of age and the average duration of smoking was 36 years, suggesting that long-term exposure was needed for an effect on fracture to become apparent. In support of the adverse effects of smoking on bone health in men, Slemenda and coworkers (11) found that the rate of bone loss from the radius was significantly greater (140%) in subjects who smoked than in nonsmokers (see Figure 7-11). In fact, there was a correlation between the number of cigarettes smoked and the rapidity of bone loss, and identical twins who smoked lost more bone than did their nonsmoking siblings. In this study the adverse effects of smoking and alcohol use were independent.

Mechanism of Tobacco Use in Bone Disease: The mechanism by which smoking affects bone in men is unclear. In women, tobacco use has been associated with lower weight, calcium absorption, and estrogen levels, all of which are negatively associated with bone mass (243,244,247). Alternatively, smoking may impair respiratory function and hence bone metabolism, or a direct toxic effect of smoking on bone metabolism may exist. No data are available concerning the effects of tobacco use in other forms (chewing, snuff). Whether smoking adversely affects androgen levels or other potential effectors of bone remodeling in men is unknown.

▶ 179

Therapy: The ideal approach to osteoporosis associated with tobacco use is smoking cessation. Whether cessation leads to reduced rates of bone loss or to a gain in bone mass is unknown. In the studies by Slemenda and coworkers (14) there was apparently a protective effect of heavy physical activity on the bone loss induced by smoking. Other interventions (nutritional supplements, antiresorptive drugs) might potentially reduce the incidence of osteopenia in men who did not abstain, but this possibility is untested.

MISCELLANEOUS DISORDERS

A variety of other illnesses or medications have been associated with bone loss or fractures in men, including anticonvulsant use (47,112,248), thyrotoxicosis (249), immobilization (44), liver and renal disease (113), homocystinuria (47), and others. However, there is little evidence that the skeletal abnormalities induced by these conditions affect men any differently (qualitatively or quantitatively) than women.

Idiopathic (Primary) Osteoporosis in Men

Osteoporosis in men has been termed idiopathic if no known cause of bone disease can be identified on clinical and laboratory grounds. Although metabolic bone disease in men has been traditionally considered to be more commonly related to "secondary" causes (250), this impression is not well validated. In fact, the frequency with which osteoporosis in men has been found to be idiopathic is high. In the largest series of osteoporotic men, most patients (almost 60%) were considered to have bone disease of unknown etiology—70 of 105 subjects (112), 40 of 94 subjects (47), and 60 of 95 subjects (113). Idiopathic osteoporosis has been reported to be more commonly encountered in men than in women (251).

The age of men with primary, or idiopathic, osteoporosis varies widely (23 to 86 years), with an average age in the mid-60s. This age range overlaps that of "senile" osteoporosis, and differentiation of idiopathic and senile osteoporosis is somewhat arbitrary. Riggs and Melton (115) defined senile (or type II) osteoporosis as occurring in either sex after the age of 70, but this definition obviously does not exclude the potential for pathophysiologic overlap between older and younger patients. The universal decline in bone mass that happens as a concomitant of aging has the potential for eventually producing clinical osteoporosis in all individuals, and some idiopathic osteoporosis may represent this age-related process (also poorly understood) or its premature onset.

The character of idiopathic osteoporosis in men is relatively indistinct. After major contributors to bone loss have been eliminated, more detailed biochemical and histomorphometric analyses of men with idiopathic disease fail to reveal consistent features (47,113,158,252). Some patients have slightly increased serum alkaline phosphatase activity (47,113). Reduced intestinal calcium absorption has been reported in the presence of lowered $1,25-(OH)_2D$ levels (47), but calcium balance has not been systematically examined in male osteoporotics. Histomorphometrically, there is a suggestion that osteoblastic function is defective in osteoporotic men (158,252). Bordier and colleagues reported studies of a series of 11 patients with idiopathic osteoporosis, 10 of whom were men. In those subjects, histomorphometric parameters clearly suggested that defective bone formation contributed to bone loss (253). However, osteoblastic dysfunction is not a consistent finding in idiopathic male osteoporosis (47,231), and Nordin and coworkers have also suggested that resorption is a primary mediator (254). They compared the forming and resorbing surfaces in iliac crest samples from young and old normal men (autopsy specimens) and men with idiopathic osteoporosis. The extent of forming surface was similar in the osteoporotic and older men (both were lower than the young men) while the resorbing surface extent was greater in the osteoporotic men than in either the young or old normal men. Unfortunately, the osteoporotic men were not well characterized and remodeling was assessed with only static parameters. There are no data concerning the levels of contemporary biochemical indices of bone remodeling in osteoporotic men (serum osteocalcin or procollagen extension peptide, urinary pyridinoline excretion).

These apparently discrepant results may in part be explicable by findings reported by Aaron and colleagues (255) who noted that young men (aged 49 years or less) with idiopathic osteoporosis had reductions in bone forming parameters (osteoid surface, mean wall thickness), while older men had forming parameters similar to age-matched controls but with evidence of slightly increased resorption. Thus, the histomorphometric pathomechanisms of early on-set primary osteoporosis in men may be different when the disorder appears later in life. The late-onset form appears to be similar to the bone loss that occurs with normal aging, albeit at a more accelerated pace.

Finally, the microarchitectural features of idiopathic osteoporosis in men have not been defined. Francis and coworkers (47) and Aaron and colleagues (255) did report that men with primary osteoporosis had a reduction in iliac crest bone volume and surface primarily because of a reduced trabecular number rather than a decline in thickness. The issue of trabecular connectivity was not formally evaluated.

▶ 181

Therapy: Idiopathic osteoporosis in men is a perplexing and difficult disorder for the clinician. In addition to the lack of knowledge of the pathophysiology of the disorder, there have been essentially no attempts to define appropriate treat-ments. In the absence of contributory factors that can be addressed, the basic issues of nutritional adequacy (calcium and vitamin D) and physical activity (both for its trophic effects on the skeleton as well as the desire to maintain strength and coordination to prevent falls) should be addressed. Because os-teopenia must have its genesis in a remodeling imbalance, it may be appropriate to consider antiresorptive agents (biphosphonates, calcitonin). Unfortunately, the efficacy of those (or any other) drugs in the treatment of idiopathic or senile osteoporosis in men has not been examined.

The Evaluation of Osteoporotic Men

Guidelines for the most efficient, cost-effective approach for the evaluation of the patient with osteoporosis, or the patient suspected of having osteoporosis, are poorly validated for either sex. Recommendations are therefore based on ex-isting knowledge of disease epidemiology and clinical characteristics (256,257) rather than on models that have been carefully tested in prospective studies. Within these constraints, it is possible to formulate an approach to the male os-teoporotic. Of necessity it derives from the more mature knowledge base avail-able concerning osteoporosis in women but departs in several key areas.

THE DIAGNOSIS OF OSTEOPENIA IN MEN

In some men the diagnosis of an osteopenic metabolic bone disease can be made with basic clinical information. Most important is a clear history of low trauma fractures (multiple fractures, documented low trauma) in the absence of evidence of a focal pathologic process (malignancy, infection, Paget's disease, etc).

In several clinical situations the presence of osteoporosis cannot be confidently determined but should be considered likely. In these circumstances further diagnostic steps are appropriate. These situations include the presence of suspicious (low trauma) fractures, radiographic osteopenia, and conditions known to be associated with increased risk of bone loss.

Fractures: In women a wide variety of fractures (256,257) are associated with low bone mass, and thus can practically be termed osteoporotic (258). In men there are fewer data, but the publications that have examined the relationships between bone mass, bone structure, mechanical strength, and fracture in men support this contention (19,52). The presence of a low trauma fracture should raise the probability of metabolic bone disease and prompt further evaluation (densitometry, etc). Certainly the occurrence of classic osteoporotic fractures (vertebral, proximal, femoral) in the absence of focal pathology should raise immediate concern.

The incidental finding of vertebral deformity in men warrants comment because the prevalence of these deformities is relatively high (259). It was the previous contention that many of these deformities are the result of excessive trauma, or developmental deformity (Scheurmann's disease), and hence should not be considered the consequence of osteopenia. However, recent studies show that men with even relatively small degrees of vertebral deformity (vertebral height reduction of 2 standard deviations or more) have mean BMD values significantly below subjects without deformities (259). This information suggests the finding of vertebral abnormality (eg, on chest radiography) should raise the concern that an osteopenic disorder is present, and further evaluation should be considered.

It is of course important to consider the other possible causes of vertebral deformity in addition to metabolic bone disease. The most important focal pathologic causes to be recognized are infection and neoplasia (260–262). These causes are sometimes difficult to differentiate from osteoporosis, but usually are heralded by clinical and radiographic signs not associated with metabolic bone disorders.

Radiographic Osteopenia: Osteopenia detected radiographically, even in the absence of a fracture, is of concern because the loss of bone must be well advanced before it is detectable with routine x-ray procedures. If, in fact, diffuse osteopenia is noted radiographically it indicates the presence of clinically significant osteopenia and should prompt a diagnostic evaluation. Although useful to observe when present, radiographic estimates of osteopenia are qualitative, and the actual quantitation of bone density provides a more definitive estimate of disease severity and a baseline from which to gauge subsequent change.

Clinical Conditions Associated with Osteopenia: On the basis of limited epidemiologic information (47,112), it is apparent that there are a number of causes of increased risk for osteoporosis, including glucocorticoid excess, alcoholism, hypogonadism, etc (discussed above). The presence of one, or particularly several, of these conditions should prompt concern, and the consideration for further characterization of the skeletal status.

Bone Mineral Density Measurements: In men presenting with findings that suggest the presence of metabolic bone disease (low trauma fractures, radiographic osteopenia, or conditions associated with bone loss), the measurement of BMD should be strongly considered.

▶ 183

For the reasons that have been previously elaborated (263) BMD measures provide valuable data that cannot be deduced from other clinical information and can cement the diagnosis of osteopenia. The validity of this contention is derived from studies in women, but the basic tenets should be applicable in men as well. Specifically, (1) low bone mass is related to fracture, (2) bone mass measures predict fracture risk, (3) bone mass can be accurately measured, (4) an understanding of bone mass may influence the therapeutic approach, and (5) treatment of osteoporosis affects fracture risk. Although not as well founded as in women, some of these assumptions (namely, 1 to 3) can be adequately supported in men as well. Tenets 4 and 5 are virtually unexplored in men. Nevertheless, there are no conceptual reasons to deny their applicability in devising a diagnostic strategy in men.

DIFFERENTIAL DIAGNOSIS

The intent at this stage of the evaluation should be to determine with reasonable certainty the histologic cause of the osteopenic disorder and to identify the etiologic factors contributing to it.

Osteomalacia: In women, the vast majority of patients with osteopenic fractures have histologic osteoporosis, but a small proportion are found to be osteomalacic (264–266). Similarly, a fraction of men with fracture have osteomalacia (264–266). Whereas it can be confidently stated that osteomalacia is less common than osteoporosis in both sexes, the specific magnitude of the problem of osteomalacia is unclear. Some have suggested that women with femoral fractures are more frequently osteomalacic than men (264,265), but others report a similar proportion (266). Reports suggest osteomalacia to be present in from under 4% to 47% of men with femoral fractures, with most reports being 20% or less (264–268). Most studies find that increasing age is associated with an increasing prevalence of osteomalacia (266). Thus far, the only patients who have been carefully surveyed are those with femoral fractures, and it is not known whether populations with other fractures (vertebral) would include similar proportions of osteoporotic and osteomalacic individuals.

Although the exact magnitude of the problem presented by osteomalacia in men is uncertain, it is clear that the process of the differential diagnosis of osteopenia and fractures in men must consider the possibility. This becomes particularly imperative because the treatment for osteomalacia differs considerably from that of osteoporosis (269).

History, Physical, Routine Biochemical Measures: The history, physical, and routine biochemical profile can be helpful in directing a focused evaluation of an osteopenic man. The intent of this stage of the evaluation should be to determine the specific diagnosis (whether the cause of the osteopenia is osteoporosis or osteomalacia) and to identify contributing factors in the genesis of the disorder. Of particular importance in the history and physical, therefore, are clinical signs of genetic, nutritional/environment, social (alcohol, tobacco), medical, or pharmacologic factors that may be present to aid in these goals. A variety of approaches for the differential diagnosis of osteopenia have been suggested using standard clinical and biochemical information (114,269,270). Certainly, if there is evidence for medical conditions associated with bone loss (malignancy, Cushing's syndrome, thyrotoxicosis, malabsorption, etc), a definitive diagnosis should be pursued with appropriate testing.

Comprehensive Evaluation: It has been considered appropriate to be diagnostically aggressive in osteopenic men in whom no clear pathophysiology is identified by routine methods, primarily because the potential occult "secondary" causes of osteoporosis may be higher in men. However, the incidence of occult causes of osteoporosis in men, and whether it is greater than it is for women, is poorly studied, and the yield of extensive biochemical studies in the man with apparently "idiopathic" osteoporosis is unknown. Without this information, a reasonable evaluation (based on the major risk factors associated with osteoporosis in men and the practicality of testing) should include:

- 24-hour urine calcium and creatinine
- 24-hour urine cortisol
- serum 25-(OH)D level
- serum testosterone and luteinizing hormone levels
- serum thyroid stimulating hormone level
- serum protein electrophoresis (in those over 50 years old)

Histomorphometric Characterization: Transiliac bone biopsy is a safe and effective means of assessing skeletal histology and remodeling characteristics

(271). Some have suggested a transiliac bone biopsy is indicated in those men in whom a thorough biochemical evaluation has failed to reveal an etiology for osteoporosis (135). The rationale for this approach is based on the need to accomplish several objectives: (1) to ensure that occult osteomalacia is not present; (2) to identify unusual causes of osteoporosis that may be revealed only by histologic analysis, such as mastocytosis (272,273); and (3) to yield information concerning the remodeling rate, which in turn may further direct the differential diagnosis (for instance unappreciated thyrotoxicosis or secondary hyperparathyroidism may be suggested by the presence of increased turnover) or may be helpful in designing the most appropriate therapeutic approach. Considerable histologic heterogeneity exists among men with osteoporosis. Whether distinct histologic patterns represent different stages of a single disease entity, separate subtypes of the disease, or simply an arbitrary subdivision of a normal distribution of remodeling rates is unknown.

▶ 185

Vigorous attempts have been made to substitute sensitive and specific biochemical markers of skeletal metabolism for histomorphometric estimates of bone turnover. Serum levels of osteocalcin and procollagen peptides and urinary pyridinoline excretion correlate well with remodeling rates (79). For aiding in the diagnosis of high turnover states and for guiding therapeutic choice (274), these or other biochemical parameters may supplant the histomorphometric analysis of biopsy specimens. The practical feasibility of this promise is not yet clear. Measurement of serum osteocalcin may also be helpful in the evaluation of osteomalacia in men (275), but it appears to offer no more sensitivity than more conventional biochemical tests (alkaline phosphatase, 25-(OH)D).

With this information, a reasonable approach to the evaluation of men with apparent idiopathic osteoporosis is to combine the advantages of the biochemical markers of bone turnover with those of bone biopsy. An initial biochemical assessment of bone turnover should provide an understanding of remodeling rate. In the presence of an increase in biochemical indices of remodeling (osteocalcin, pyridinoline), a bone biopsy may be appropriate to identify unusual causes of osteopenia (eg, osteomalacia, mastocytosis). Bone biopsy may be particularly helpful if there is any clinical concern for occult osteomalacia. If osteocalcin levels or pyridinoline excretions are reduced, the probability of osteomalacia or an unexpected disorder associated with increased bone resorption is probably low. Nevertheless, even in this situation, a bone biopsy can reveal unanticipated osteomalacia, particularly in older men (266).

Therapy of Osteoporosis in Men

Therapy of osteoporotic disorders in men is virtually unexplored. As discussed above, some information suggests that treatment of underlying conditions associated with osteopenia is effective in stabilizing or improving bone mass in osteoporotic men, but the data are scarce. The effects of these therapies on fracture risk is unknown. In primary osteoporosis in men, similarly little data are available. Few trials of specific osteoporosis therapies have been performed in male populations, although some men with osteoporosis have been included in mixed populations treated with a variety of agents. In general, it is difficult to independently assess the specific success of these approaches in the male subjects.

PREVENTION OF AGE-RELATED BONE LOSS

186 ◄

Although it has recently become apparent that bone loss and fractures with aging in men is an important public health issue, there is very little information available concerning its prevention. Reasonable guidelines can be developed on the basis of current pathophysiologic models, and on experience in women, but these approaches lack validation.

1. In men (as in women) an important component of bone loss is that contributed by associated medical illnesses (gastrointestinal disturbance, renal disease, hypogonadism, etc) or drugs/toxins (glucocorticoids, ethanol, tobacco). It is straightforward to recommend the treatment or avoidance of these risk factors whenever possible.

2. Although an exercise prescription is difficult to generate with currently available information, activity is probably beneficial in several ways. Reductions in strength and coordination probably contribute to fracture via an increased risk of falling (276). In addition, inactivity is associated with bone loss, and exercise may increase or maintain bone mass. Specific exercise prescriptions to accomplish these goals have not been well validated, although it is clear that strength can be dramatically increased, and risk of falls reduced, in the elderly with achievable levels of exercise (276).

Calcium nutrition is probably of benefit in the preservation of bone mass in men (above). The level of calcium intake that should be recommended is unclear. Only one prospective study has addressed the issue and found no benefit of calcium supplements in an already well-nourished population, in which dietary calcium intake was greater than 800 mg/d (86). In the absence of definitive data, a reasonable approach is to suggest a calcium intake of at least 800 to 1000 mg/d. The major concern regarding dietary calcium supplementation has been the possible precipitation of calcium stone disease in susceptible individuals. However, recent data suggest dietary calcium intake is actually negatively correlated with the risk of nephrolithiasis in men (277), potentially by increasing gastrointestinal oxalate binding.

CALCITONIN

There has been one trial of calcitonin therapy in a small group of men with idiopathic osteoporosis (278) in which total body calcium tended to increase during a 24-month treatment interval (100 IU/d with a calcium and vitamin D supplement). However, the change was not significantly different than the control groups (receiving calcium plus vitamin D supplements or vitamin D alone), and there were no changes in radial bone mass. Men have been included in several other trials of calcitonin therapy, but the effects in men are not separable from those in the women (275,279,280).

Stepan and Lachman (141) treated castrated men with calcitonin and ▶ 187 showed biochemical evidence of a reduction in bone turnover, but there are few if any studies of men with other forms of secondary bone disease treated with calcitonin. Men have comprised the majority of subjects in some series of patients receiving glucocorticoids who responded to calcitonin (281).

Although there are few data in men, calcitonin should be effective in reducing osteoclastic activity in at least some patients with osteoporosis or the risk of bone loss.

BISPHOSPHONATES

There have been no trials of any bisphosphonate performed exclusively in men. Male patients with osteoporosis have been included in mixed patient populations and have seemed to experience beneficial effects on calcium balance and lumbar spine bone density during treatment with pamidronate (282). Similarly, men have been included (in fact the majority of subjects were men) in a trial of pamidronate for glucocorticoid induced bone loss, in which therapy had a beneficial effect on metacarpal cortical area and vertebral bone density (283). Although specific data are lacking, there is no theoretical reason bisphosphonates would not be effective in reducing osteoclastic work in men as in women (284).

PARATHYROID HORMONE

Parathyroid hormone administration to osteoporotic subjects has been shown to increase trabecular bone formation and bone volume in concert with an increase in calcium balance (266,285–287). Slovik and coworkers reported that in a small group of men with idiopathic osteoporosis combined administration of PTH and $1,25(OH)_2D$ increased trabecular (spinal) bone mass and improved intestinal calcium absorption (288). Although the role of PTH, alone or in concert with other agents (287), in the treatment of osteoporosis remains unclear, the potential appears similar in men and women.

Growth hormone may have anabolic actions on the skeleton in the elderly (289) and in subjects with osteoporosis, but the available data are inconclusive (290). Low levels of insulin-like growth factor I (IGF-I) have been reported to be present in men with idiopathic osteoporosis (291), and in a study of healthy men over 60 years of age with low IGF-I levels, Rudman and colleagues (292) found that in addition to positive effects on lean mass, fat mass, and skin thickness, vertebral BMD was increased slightly (1.6%) by the administration of growth hormone for 6 months. Radial and proximal femoral density was unaffected. In either sex, growth hormone therapy may be of potential, but as of yet unproved, usefulness.

188 ◄

References

1. Albright F, Smith PH, Richardson AM. Postmenopausal osteoporosis. JAMA 1941;116:2465–2474.

2. Genant HK, Gordon GS, Hoffman PGJ. Osteoporosis part I. Advanced radiologic assessment using quantitative computed tomography—Medical Staff Conference, University of California, San Francisco. West J Med 1983;139:75–84.

3. Kelly TL. Bone mineral density reference databases for American men and women. J Bone Miner Res 1990;1:549. Abstract.

4. Aaron JE, Makins NB, Sagreiya K. The microanatomy of trabecular bone loss in normal aging men and women. Clin Orthop Rel Res 1987;215:260–271.

5. Krall EA, Dawson-Hughes B. Heritable and life-style determinants of bone mineral density. J Bone Miner Res 1993;8:1–9.

6. Ruff CB, Hayes WC. Sex differences in age-related remodeling of the femur and tibia. J Orthop Res 1988;6:886–896.

7. Christian JC, Yu P-L, Slemenda CW, Johnston CCJ. Heritability of bone mass: a longitudinal study in aging male twins. Am J Hum Genet 1989;44:429–433.

8. Orwoll ES, Oviatt SK. The rate of bone mineral loss in normal men and the effects of calcium and cholecalciferol supplementation. Ann Intern Med 1990;112:29–34.

9. Gotfredsen A, Hadberg A, Nilas L, Christiansen C. Total body bone mineral in healthy adults. J Lab Clin Med 1987; 110:362–368.

10. Hannan MT, Felson DT, Anderson JJ. Bone mineral density in elderly men and women: results from the Framingham osteoporosis study. J Bone Miner Res 1992; 7:547–553.

11. Mazess RB, Barden HS, Drinka PJ, Bauwens SF, Orwoll ES, Bell NH. Influence of age and body weight on spine and femur bond mineral density in US white men. J Bone Miner Res 1990;5:645–652.

12. Davis JW, Ross PD, Vogel JM, Wasnich RD. Age-related changes in bone mass among Japanese-American men. Bone Miner 1991;15:227–236.

13. Riggs BL, Wahner HW, Dunn WL, Mazess RB, Offord KP, Melton LJI. Differential changes in bone mineral density of the appendicular and axial skeleton with aging. J Clin Invest 1981;67:328–335.

14. Slemenda CW, Christian JC, Reed T, Reister TK, Williams CJ, Johnston CC Jr. Long-term bone loss in men: effects of genetic and environmental factors. Ann Intern Med 1992;117:286–291.

15. Garn SM, Sullivan TV, Decker SA, Larkin FA, Hawthorne VM. Continuing bone expansion and increasing bone loss over a two-decade period in men and

women from a total community sample. Am J Human Biol 1992;4:57–67.

16. Meier DE, Orwoll ES, Jones JM. Marked disparity between trabecular and cortical bone loss with age in healthy men: measurement by vertebral computed tomography and radial photon absorptiometry. Ann Intern Med 1984;101:605–612.

17. Orwoll ES, Oviatt SK, Mann T. The impact of osteophytic and vascular calcifications on vertebral mineral density measurements in men. J Clin Endocrinol Metab 1990;70:1202–1207.

18. Elliott JR, Gilchrist NL, Wells JE, et al. Effects of age and sex on bone density at the hip and spine in a normal Caucasian New Zealand population. N Z Med J 1990; 103:33–37.

19. Mosekilde L. Sex differences in age-related loss of vertebral trabecular bone mass and structure—biomechanical consequences. Bone 1989;10:425–432.

20. Compston JE, Mellish RWE, Garrahan NJ. Age-related changes in iliac crest trabecular microanatomic bone structure in man. Bone 1987;8:289–292.

21. Compston JE, Mellish RWE, Croucher P, Newcombe R, Garrahan NJ. Structural mechanism of trabecular bone loss in men. Bone 1989;8:339–350.

22. Parfitt A, Mathews HE. Relationships between surface, volume, and thickness of iliac trabecular bone in aging and in osteoporosis. J Clin Invest 1983;72:1396–1409.

23. Arneson TJ, Melton LJI, Lewallen DG, O'Fallon WM. Epidemiology of diaphyseal and distal femoral fractures in Rochester, Minnesota, 1965–1984. Clin Orthop Rel Res 1988;234:188–194.

24. Melton LJI, O'Fallon WM, Riggs BL. Clinical investigations: secular trends in the incidence of hip fractures. Calcif Tiss Int 1987;41:57–64.

25. Farmer ME, White LR, Brody JA, Bailey KR. Race and sex differences in hip fracture incidence. Am J Public Health 1984;74:1374–1380.

26. Bacon WE, Smith GS, Baker SP. Geographic variation in the occurrence of hip fractures among the elderly white US population. Am J Public Health 1989; 79:1556–1558.

27. Jacobsen SJ, Goldberg J, Miles TP, Brody JA, Stiers W, Rimm AA. Hip fracture incidence among the old and very old: a population-based study of 745,435 cases. Am J Public Health 1990;80:871–873.

28. Gallagher JD, Melton LJ, Riggs BL. Epidemiology of fracture of the proximal femur in Rochester, MN. Clin Orthop Rel Res 1980;150:163–171.

29. Kanis JA. The incidence of hip fracture in Europe. Osteoporosis Int 1993; 3:S10–S15.

30. Cooper C, Campion G. Hip fractures in the elderly: a world-wide projection. Osteoporosis Int 1992;2:285–289.

31. Melton LJ III, Chrischilles EA. Perspective: how many women have osteoporosis? J Bone Miner Res 1992;7:1005–1010.

32. Martin AD, Silverthorn KG, Houston CS, Bernhardson S, Wajda A, Roos LL. The incidence of fracture of the proximal femur in two million Canadians from 1972 to 1984. Clin Orthop Rel Res 1991; 266:111–118.

33. Melton LJI, Riggs BL. Epidemiology of age-related fractures. In: Avioli LV, ed. The osteoporotic syndrome. New York: Grune & Stratton, 1983:45.

34. Heyse SP. Epidemiology of hip fracture in the elderly: a cross-national analysis of mortality rates for femoral neck fractures. Osteoporosis Int 1993;1:S16–S19.

35. Schneider EL, Guralnik JM. The aging of America: impact on health care costs. JAMA 1990;263:2335–2340.

36. Obrant KJ, Bengner U, Johnell O, Nilsson BE, Sernbo I. Increasing age-adjusted risk of fragility fractures: a sign of increasing osteoporosis in successive generations? Calcif Tiss Int 1989;44:157–167. Editorial.

37. Simonen O. Incidence of femoral neck fractures: senile osteoporosis in Finland in the years 1970–1985. Calcif Tiss Int 1991;49:S8–S10.

38. Melton LJI, Cummings SR. Heterogeneity of age-related fractures: implications for epidemiology. Bone Miner 1987; 2:321–331.

39. Ross PD, Norimatsu H, Davis JW, et al. A comparison of hip fracture incidence among native Japanese, Japanese Americans, and American Caucasians. Am J Epidemiol 1991;133:801–809.

40. Cooper C, Atkinson EJ, O'Fallon WM, Melton LJ. Incidence of clinically diagnosed vertebral fractures: a population-based study in Rochester, Minnesota, 1985–1989. J Bone Miner Res 1992;7:221–227.

41. Kanis JA, McCloskey EV. Epidemiology of vertebral osteoporosis. Bone 1992; 13:S1–S10.

42. Santavirta S, Konttinen YT, Heliovaara M, Knekt P, Luthje P, Aramaa A. Determinants of osteoporotic thoracic vertebral fracture. Acta Orthop Scand 1992; 63:198–202.

43. Orwoll ES, Oviatt SK, Biddle JA. Precision of dual energy x-ray absorptiometry: the development of quality control rules and their application in longitudinal studies. J Bone Miner Res 1993;8:693–699.

44. Donaldson CL, Hulley SB, Vogel JM. Effect of prolonged bed rest on bone mineral. Metabolism 1970;19:1071–1084.

45. Buhr AJ, Cooke AM. Fracture patterns. Lancet 1959; March 14:531–536.

46. Mallmin H, Ljunghall S, Persson I, Naessen T, Jrusemo U-B, Bergstrom R. Fracture of the distal forearm as a forecaster of subsequent hip fracture: a population-based cohort study with 24 years of follow-up. Calcif Tissue Int 1993;52:269–272.

47. Francis RM, Peacock M, Marshall DH, Horsman A, Aaron JE. Spinal osteoporosis in men. Bone Miner 1989; 5:347–357.

48. Riggs BL, Wahner HW, Seeman E, et al. Changes in bone mineral density of the proximal femur and spine with aging. J Clin Invest 1982;70:716–723.

49. Hamdy RC, Moore S, Cancellaro V, et al. Osteoporosis in men—prevalence and biochemical parameters. Program and Abstracts of the 14th Annual Meeting American Society for Bone and Mineral Research Program and Abstracts, Minneapolis, Minn, 1992.

50. Chevalley T, Rizzoili R, Nydegger V, et al. Preferential low bone mineral density of the femoral neck in patients with a recent fracture of the proximal femur. Osteoporosis Int 1991;1:147–154.

51. Karlsson MK, Johnell O, Nilsson BE, Sernbo I, Obrant KJ. Bone mineral mass in hip fracture patients. Bone 1993; 14:161–165.

52. Gardsell P, Johnell O, Nilsson BE. The predictive value of forearm bone mineral content measurements in men. Bone 1990;11:229–232.

53. Mosekilde L, Viidik A, Mosekilde L. Correlation between the compressive strength of iliac and vertebral trabecular bone in normal individuals. Bone 1985; 6:291–295.

54. Singh M, Riggs BL, Beabout JW, Jowsey JD. Femoral trabecular-pattern index for evaluation of spinal osteoporosis. Ann Intern Med 1972;77:63–67.

55. Frost HM. Suggested fundamental concepts in skeletal physiology. Calcif Tissue Int 1993;52:1–4.

56. Laval-Jeantet A-M, Bergot C, Carroll R, Garcia-Schaefer F. Cortical bone senescence and mineral bone density of the humerus. Calcif Tissue Int 1983;35:268–272.

57. Nguyen TV, Sambrook PN, Kelly PJ, Lord S, Freund J, Elsman JA. Body sway and bone mineral density are predictors of fracture prevalence: the DUBBO osteoporosis epidemiology study. J Bone Miner Res 1992;7(1):S112.

58. Grisso JA, Chiu GY, Maislin G, Steinmann WC, Portale J. Risk factors for hip fractures in men: a preliminary study. J Bone Miner Res 1991;6:865–868.

59. Ray WA, Griffin MR, Schaffner W, Baugh DK, Melton LJ III. Psychotropic drug use and the risk of hip fracture. N Engl J Med 1987;316:363–370.

60. Ray WA, Griffin MR, Downey W. Benzodiazepines of long and short elimination half-life and the risk of hip fracture. JAMA 1989;262:3303–3307.

61. Garn SM. The earlier gain and the later loss of cortical bone in nutritional perspective. Springfield, Ill: Charles C Thomas, 1970:44–59.

62. Martin RB, Atkinson PJ. Age and sex-related changes in the structure and

strength of the human femoral shaft. J Biomech 1977;10:223–231.

63. Smith RWJ, Walker RR. Femoral expansion in aging women: implications for osteoporosis and fractures. Science 1964; 145:156–157.

64. Beck TJ, Ruff CB, Scott WWJ, Plato CC, Tobin JD, Quan CA. Sex differences in geometry of the femoral neck with aging: a structural analysis of bone mineral data. Calcif Tissue Int 1992;50:24–29.

65. Parfitt AM, Rao DS, Stanciu J, Villanueva AR, Kleerekoper M, Frame B. Irreversible bone loss in osteomalacia—comparison of radial photon absorptiometry with iliac bone histomorphometry during treatment. J Clin Invest 1985; 76:2403–2412.

66. Eriksen EF. Normal and pathological remodeling of human trabecular bone: three dimensional reconstruction of the remodeling sequence in normals and in metabolic bone disease. Endocr Rev 1986; 7:379–408.

67. Eriksen EF, Mosekilde L, Melsen F. Trabecular bone resorption depth decreases with age: differences between normal males and females. Bone 1985;6:141–146.

68. Croucher PI, Mellish RWE, Vedi S, Garrahan NJ, Compston JE. The relationship between resorption depth and mean interstitial bone thickness: age-related changes in man. Calcif Tissue Int 1989; 45:15–19.

69. Melsen F, Melsen B, Mosekilde L, Bergmann S. Histomorphometric analysis of normal bone from the iliac crest. Acta Path Microbiol Scand 1986;86:70–81.

70. Kragstrup J, Melsen F, Mosekilde L. Thickness of bone formed at remodeling sites in normal human iliac trabecular bone: variations with age and sex. Metab Bone Dis Rel Res 1983;5:17–21.

71. Melsen F, Melsen B, Mosekilde L, Bergmann S. Histomorphometric analysis of normal bone from the iliac crest. Acta Path Microbiol Scand 1978;86:70–81.

72. Irwin MI, Kienholz EW. A conspectus of research on calcium requirements of man. J Nutr 1973;103:1019–1095.

73. Morley JE. Nutritional status of the elderly. Am J Med 1986;81:679–695.

74. Young G, Marcus R, Minkoff JR, Kim LY, Segre GV. Age-related rise in parathyroid hormone in man: the use of intact and midmolecule antisera to distinguish hormone secretion from retention. J Bone Miner Res 1987;2:367–374.

75. Endres DB, Morgan CH, Garry PJ, Omdahl JL. Age-related changes in serum immunoreactive parathyroid hormone and its biological action in healthy men and women. J Clin Endocrinol Metab 1987; 65:724–731.

76. Orwoll ES, Meier DE. Alterations in calcium, vitamin D, and parathyroid hormone physiology in normal men with aging: relationship to the development of senile osteopenia. J Clin Endocrinol Metab 1986;63:1262–1269.

77. Slovik DM, Adams JS, Neer RM, Holick MF, Potts JR. Deficient production of 1,25-dihydroxyvitamin D in elderly osteoporotic patients. N Engl J Med 1981; 305:372.

78. Sherman SS, Tobin JD, Hollis BW, Gundberg CM, Roy TA, Plato CC. Biochemical parameters associated with low bone density in healthy men and women. J Bone Miner Res 1992;7:1123–1130.

79. Delmas PD. Clinical use of biochemical markers of bone remodeling in osteoporosis. Bone 1992;13:S17–S21.

80. Orwoll ES, Deftos LJ. Serum osteocalcin levels in normal men: a longitudinal evaluation reveals an age-associated increase. J Bone Miner Res 1990;5:259–262.

81. Kelly PJ, Pocock NA. Dietary calcium, sex hormones, and bone mineral density in men. Br M J 1990;300:1361–1363.

82. Kroger H, Laitinen K. Bone mineral density measured by dual-energy x-ray absorptiometry in normal men. Eur J Clin Invest 1992;22:454–460.

83. Wickham CAC, Walsh K, Cooper C, et al. Dietary calcium, physical activity, and risk of hip fracture: a prospective study. BMJ 1989;299:889–892.

84. Holbrook TL, Barrett-Connor E, Wingard DL. Dietary calcium and risk of hip fracture: 14-year prospective population study. Lancet 1988;ii:1046–1049.

▶ 191

85. Lau E, Donnan S, Barker DJP, Cooper C. Physical activity and calcium intake in fracture of the proximal femur in Hong Kong. BMJ 1988;297:1441–1443.

86. Orwoll ES. The effects of dietary protein insufficiency and excess on skeletal health. Bone 1992;13:343–350.

87. Garn SM, Kangas J. Protein intake, bone mass, and bone loss. In: DeLuca HF, Frost HM, Lee WSS, Johnston CC, Parfitt AM, eds. Osteoporosis: recent advances in pathogenesis and treatment. Baltimore: University Park Press, 1981:257.

88. Calvo MS, Kumar R, Heath HI. Persistently elevated parathyroid hormone secretion and action in young women after four weeks of ingesting high phosphorus, low calcium diets. J Clin Endocrinol Metab 1990;70:1334–1340.

89. Spencer H, Kramer L, Osis D. Do protein and phosphorus cause calcium loss? J Nutr 1988;118:657–660.

90. Parfitt AM. Dietary risk factors for age-related bone loss and fractures. Lancet 1983;2:1181–1185.

91. Snow-Harter C, Whalen R, Myburgh K, Arnaud S. Marcus R. Bone mineral density, muscle strength, and recreational exercise in men. J Bone Miner Res 1992;7:1291–1296.

92. Colletti LA, Edwards J, Bordon L, Shary J, Bell NH. The effects of muscle-building exercise on bone mineral density of the radius, spine and hip in young men. Calcif Tissue Int 1989;45:12–14.

93. Block JE, Genant HK, Black D. Greater vertebral bone mineral mass in exercising young men. West J Med 1986; 145:39–42.

94. Block JE, Friedlander AL, Brooks GA, Steiger P, Stubbs HA, Genant HK. Determinants of bone density among athletes engaged in weight-bearing and non-weight-bearing activity. J Appl Physiol 1989;67:1100–1105.

95. Jones HH, Priest JD, Hayes WC, Tichenor CC, Nagel DA. Humeral hypertrophy in response to exercise. J Bone Joint Surg 1977;59A:204–208.

96. Orwoll ES, Ferar J, Oviatt SK, McClung MR, Huntington K. The relationship of swimming exercise to bone mass in men and women. Arch Intern Med 1989; 149:2197–2200.

97. Williams JA, Wagner J, Wasnich R, Heilbrun L. The effect of long-distance running upon appendicular bone mineral content. Med Sci Sports Exerc 1984; 16:223–227.

98. Myburgh KH, Zhou L-J, Steele CR, Arnaud S, Marcus R. In vivo assessment of forearm bone mass and ulnar bending stiffness in healthy men. J Bone Miner Res 1992;7:1345–1350.

99. Reid IR, Plank LD, Evans MC. Fat mass is an important determinant of whole body bone density in premenopausal women but not in men. J Clin Endocrinol Metab 1992;75:779–782.

100. Nevitt MC, Cummings SR, Kidd S, Black D. Risk factors for recurrent nonsyncopal falls. JAMA 1989;261:2663–2668.

101. Larsson L, Sjodin B, Karlsson J. Histochemical and biochemical changes in human skeletal muscle with age in sedentary males, age 22–65 years. Acta Physiol Scand 1978;103:31–39.

102. Aniansson A, Gustaffson E. Physical training in elderly men with special reference to quadriceps muscle strength and morphology. Clin Physiol 1981;1: 89–98.

103. Frost HM. The role of changes in mechanical usage set points in the pathogenesis of osteoporosis. J Bone Miner Res 1992;7:253–261.

104. Vermeulen A. Clinical review 24: androgens in the aging male. J Clin Endocrinol Metab 1991;73:221–223.

105. Vermeulen A, Kaufman JM. Role of the hypothalamopituitary function in the hypoandrogenism of healthy aging. J Clin Endocrinol Metab 1992;75:704–706. Editorial.

106. Bardin CW, Swerdloff RS, Santen RJ. Androgens: risk and benefits. J Clin Endocrinol Metab 1991;73:4–17.

107. Murphy S, Khaw K-T, Cassidy A, Compston JE. Sex hormones and bone mineral density in elderly men. Bone Miner 1992;20:133–140.

108. Drinka PJ, Olson J, Bauwens S, Voeks S, Carlson I, Wilson M. Lack of association between free testosterone and bone density separate from age in elderly males. Calcif Tissue Int 1993;52:67-69.

109. Meier DE, Orwoll ES, Keenan EJ, Fagerstrom RM. Marked decline in trabecular bone mineral content in healthy men with age: lack of association with sex steroid levels. J Am Geriatr Soc 1987;35:189-197.

110. Tenover JS. Effects of testosterone supplementation in the aging male. J Clin Endocrinol Metab 1992;75:1092-1098.

111. Orwoll ES, Oviatt S, Biddle J, Janowsky J. Transdermal testosterone supplementation in normal older men. Endocrine Society 7th Annual Meeting Programs and Abstracts (Abstract #1071), San Antonio, Tex;319.

112. Seeman E, Melton LJ, O'Fallon WM, Riggs BL. Risk factors for spinal osteoporosis in men. Am J Med 1983; 75:977-983.

113. Resch H, Pietschmann P, Woloszczuk W, Krexner E, Bernecker P, Willvonseder R. Bone mass and biochemical parameters of bone metabolism in men with spinal osteoporosis. Europ J Clin Invest 1992;22:542-545.

114. Johnson BE, Lucasey B, Robinson RG, Lukert BP. Contributing diagnoses in osteoporosis. Arch Intern Med 1989; 149.1069-1072.

115. Riggs BL, Melton LJ. Medical progress: involutional osteoporosis. New Engl J Med 1986;314:1676-1686.

116. Doerr P, Pirke KM. Cortisol-induced suppression of plasma testosterone in normal adult males. J Clin Endocrinol Metab 1976;43:622-629.

117. MacAdams MR, White RH, Chipps BE. Reduction of serum testosterone levels during chronic glucocorticoid therapy. Ann Intern Med 1986;104:648-651.

118. Veldhuis JD, Lizarralde G, Iranmanesh A. Divergent effects of short term glucocorticoid excess on the gonadotropic and somatotropic axes in normal men. J Clin Endocrinol Metab 1992;74:96-102.

119. Sakakura M, Takebe K, Nakagawa S. Inhibition of luteinizing hormone secretion induced by synthetic LRH by long-term treatment with glucocorticoids in human subjects. J Clin Endocrinol Metab 1975;40:774-779.

120. Evain D, Morera AM, Saez JM. Glucocorticoid receptors in interstitial cells of the rat testis. J Steroid Biochem 1976; 7:1135-1139.

121. Tabor CW, Tabor H. Polyamines. Ann Rev Biochem 1984;53:749-790.

122. Kalbfleisch JM, Lindeman RD, Ginn HE, Smith WO. Effects of ethanol administration on urinary excretion of magnesium and other electrolytes in alcoholic and normal subjects. J Clin Invest 1963;42:1472-1475.

123. Avery DH, Overall JE, Calil HM, Hollister LE. Plasma calcium and phosphate during alcohol intoxication. J Stud Alcohol 1983;44:205-214.

124. Pegg AE, McCann PP. Polyamine metabolism and function in mammalian cells and protozoans. ISI Atlas Sci Biochem 1988;11-18.

125. Anderson R, Cohen M, Haller R, Elms J, Carter NW, Knochel JA. Skeletal muscle phosphorus and magnesium deficiency in alcoholic myopathy. Miner Elect Metab 1980;4:106-112.

126. Pegg AE. Recent advances in the biochemistry of polyamines in eukaryotes. Biochem J 1986;234:249-262.

127. Krabbe S, Hummer L, Christiansen C. Longitudinal study of calcium metabolism in male puberty. Acta Poediatr Scand 1984;73:750-755.

128. Bonjour J-P, Theintz G, Buchs B, Slosman D, Rizzoli R. Critical years and stages of puberty for spinal and femoral bone mass accumulation during adolescence. J Clin Endocrinol Metab 1991; 73:555-563.

129. Finkelstein JS, Klibanski A, Neer RM, Greenspan SL, Rosenthal DI, Crowley WFJ. Osteoporosis in men with idiopathic hypogonadotropic hypogonadism. Ann Intern Med 1987;106:354-361.

130. Smith DAS, Walker MS. Changes in plasma steroids and bone density in Kleinfelter's syndrome. Calcif Tissue Int 1977;22(suppl):225-228.

131. Arisaka O, Arisaka M. Effect of testosterone on radial bone mineral density in adolescent male hypogonadism. Acta Poediatr Scand 1991;80:378–380.

132. Finkelstein JS, Neer RM, Biller BMK, Crawford JD, Klibanski A. Osteopenia in men with a history of delayed puberty. N Engl J Med 1992;326:600–604.

133. Hock JM, Gera I. Human parathyroid hormone (1-34) increases bone mass in ovariectomized and orchidectomized rats. Endocrinology 1988;122:2899–2904.

134. Turner RT, Hammnon KS. Differential effects of gonadal function in bone histomorphometry in male and female rats. J Bone Miner Res 1989;4:557–563.

135. Jackson JA, Kleerekoper M. Osteoporosis in men: diagnosis, pathophysiology, and prevention. Medicine 1990; 69:137–152.

136. Stanley HL, Schmitt BP, Poses RM, Deiss WP. Does hypogonadism contribute to the occurrence of a minimal trauma hip fracture in elderly men? J Am Geriatr Soc 1991;39:766–771.

137. Greenspan SL, Neer RM, Ridgway EC, Klibanski A. Osteoporosis in men with hyperprolactinemic hypogonadism. Ann Intern Med 1986;104:777–782.

138. Diamond T, Stiel D, Posen S. Effects of testosterone and venesection on spinal and peripheral bone mineral in six hypogonadal men with hemochromatosis. J Bone Miner Res 1991;6:39–43.

139. Greenspan SL, Oppenheim DS, Klibanski A. Importance of gonadal steroids to bone mass in men with hyperprolactinemic hypogonadism. Ann Intern Med 1989; 110:526–531.

140. Stepan JJ, Lachman M. Castrated men with bone loss: effect of calcitonin treatment on biochemical indices of bone remodeling. J Clin Endocrinol Metab 1989; 69:523–527.

141. Laitiren K, Lamberg-Allardt C, Tunninen R, Harkonen M, Vlaimaki M. Bone mineral density and abstention-induced changes in bone and mineral metabolism in noncirrhotic male alcoholics. Am J Med 1992;93:642–650.

142. Lukert BP, Raisz LG. Glucocorticoid-induced osteoporosis: pathogenesis and management. Ann Intern Med 1990; 112:352–364.

143. Francis RM, Peacock M. Osteoporosis in hypogonadal men: role of decreased plasma 1,25-dihydroxyvitamin D, calcium malabsorption, and low bone formation. Bone 1986;7:261–268.

144. Delmas P, Meunier PJ. L'osteoporose au course du syndrome de Klinefelter. Donnees histologiques osseuses quantitative dans cinq cas. Relation avec la carence hormonale. Nour Presse Med 1981;10:687.

145. Baran DT, Bergfeld MA, Teitelbaum SL, Avioli LV. Effect of testosterone therapy on bone formation in an osteoporotic hypogonadal male. Calcif Tissue Res 1978;26:103–106.

146. Jackson JA, Kleerekoper M, Parfitt AM, et al. Bone histomorphometry in hypogonadal and eugonadal men with spinal osteoporosis. J Clin Endocrinol Metab 1987;65:53–58.

147. Girasole G, Passeri G. Upregulation of osteoclastogenic potential of the marrow is induced by orchidectomy and is reversed by testosterone replacement in the mouse. J Bone Miner Res 1992;7:S96.

148. Wakley GK, Schutte HDJ, Hannon KS, Turner RT. Androgen treatment prevents loss of cancellous bone in the orchidectomized rat. J Bone Miner Res 1991; 6:325–330.

149. Verhas M, Schoutens A. The effect of orchidectomy on bone metabolism in aging rats. Calcif Tissue Int 1986;39:74–77.

150. Turner RT, Wakley GK. Differential effects of androgens on cortical bone histomorphometry in gonadectomized male and female rats. J Orthopaed Res 1990;8:612–617.

151. Wink CS, Felts WJL. Effects of castration on the bone structure of male rats: a model of osteoporosis. Calcif Tissue Int 1980;32:77–82.

152. Finkelstein JS, Klibanski A, Neer RM, et al. Increases in bone density during treatment of men with idiopathic hypogonadotropic hypogonadism. J Clin Endocrinol Metab 1989;69:776–783.

153. Devogelaer JP, Cooman SE, de Deuxchaisnes CN. Low bone mass in hypogonadal males. Effect of testosterone

substitution therapy, a densitometric study. Maturitas 1992;15:17–23.

154. Wong FHW, Pun KK, Wang C. Loss of bone mass in patients with Klinefelter's syndrome despite sufficient testosterone replacement. Osteoporosis Int 1993;3:3–7.

155. Saville PD. Changes in bone mass with age and alcoholism. J Bone Joint Surg 1965;47A:492–499.

156. Dalen N, Lamke B. Bone mineral losses in alcoholics. Acta Orthop Scand 1976;47:469–471.

157. Nilsson BE. Conditions contributing to fracture of the femoral neck. Acta Chir Scand 1970;136:383–384.

158. DeVernejoul MC, Bielakoff J, Herve M, et al. Evidence for defective osteoblastic function. A role for alcohol and tobacco consumption in osteoporosis in middle-aged men. Clin Orthop 1983;179:107–115.

159. Lalor BC, France MW, Powell D, et al. Bone and mineral metabolism and chronic alcohol abuse. Q J Med 1986;59: 497–511.

160. Feitelberg S, Epstein S, Ismail F, et al. Deranged bone mineral metabolism in chronic alcoholism. Metabolism 1987; 36:322–326.

161. Crilly RG, Richardson-Delaquerriere L. Current bone mass and body weight changes in alcoholic males. Calcif Tiss Int 1990;46:169–172.

162. Spencer H, Rubio N, Rubio E, et al. Chronic alcoholism. Frequently overlooked cause of osteoporosis in men. Am J Med 1986;80:393–397.

163. Lindsell DR, Wilson AG, Maxwell JD. Fractures on the chest radiograph in detection of alcoholic liver disease. BMJ 1982;285:597–599.

164. Israel Y, Orrego H, Holt S, et al. Identification of alcohol abuse: thoracic fractures on routine chest x-rays as indicators of alcoholism. Alcoholism 1980; 4:420–422.

165. Crilly RG, Anderson C, Hogan D, et al. Bone histomorphometry, bone mass, and related parameters in alcoholic males. Calcif Tiss Int 1988;43:269–276.

166. Diamond T, Stiel D, Lunzer M, et al. Ethanol reduces bone formation and may cause osteoporosis. Am J Med 1989; 86:282–288.

167. Bikle DD, Genant HK, Cann CE, et al. Bone disease in alcohol abuse. Ann Intern Med 1985;103:42–48.

168. Hernandez-Avila M, Colditz GA, Stampfer MJ, Rosner B, Speizer FE, Willett WC. Caffeine, moderate alcohol intake, and risk of fractures of the hip and forearm in middle-aged women. Am J Clin Nutr 1991;54:157–163.

169. Laitinen K, Lamberg-Allardt C, Tunnninen R, Harkonen M, Valimaki M. Bone mineral density and abstention-induced changes in bone and mineral metabolism in noncirrhotic male alcoholics. Am J Med 1992;93:642–650.

170. Grisso JA, Chiu GY, Maislin G, Steinmann WC, Portale J. Risk factors for hip fractures in men: a preliminary study. J Bone Miner Res 1991;6:865–868.

171. Preedy VR, Marway JS, Salisbury JR, Peters TJ. Protein synthesis in bone and skin of the rat are inhibited by ethanol: implications for whole body metabolism. Alcohol Clin Exp Res 1990;14:165–168.

172. Peng T-C, Kusy RP, Hirsch PF, Hagaman JR. Ethanol-induced changes in the morphology and strength of femurs of rats. Alcohol Clin Exp Res 1988;12:655–659.

173. Pierce RO, Perry A. The effect of ethanol on bone mineral. J Natl Med Assoc 1991;83:505–508.

174. Lindholm J, Steiniche T, Rasmussen E, et al. Bone disorder in men with chronic alcoholism: a reversible disease? J Clin Endocrinol Metab 1991;73:118–124.

175. Johnell O, Nilsson BE, Wiklund PE. Bone morphometry in alcoholics. Clin Orthop 1982;165:253–258.

176. Saville PD, Lieber CS. Increases in skeletal calcium and femur cortex thickness in undernutrition. J Nutr 1969;99: 141–144.

177. Territo MC, Tanaka KR. Hypophosphatemia in chronic alcoholism. Arch Intern Med 1974;134:445–447.

178. Laitinen K, Lamberg-Allardt C, Tunnninen R, et al. Transient hypoparathyroidism during acute alcohol intoxication. N Engl J Med 1991;324:721–727.

179. Verbanck MZ, Verbanck J, Brauman J, Mullier JT. Bone histology and 25 OH-vitamin D plasma levels in alcoholics without cirrhosis. Calcif Tissue Res 1977;22(suppl):538–541.

180. Sorensen OH, Lund B, Hilden M, Lund B. 25-Hydroxylation in chronic alcoholic liver disease. In: Norman AW, Schaefer K, Coburn JW, et al., eds. Vitamin D: biochemical, chemical and clinical aspects related to calcium metabolism. Hawthorne, NY: Walter de Guyter, 1977, 843–845.

181. Posner DB, Russell RM, Absood S, et al. Effective 25-hydroxylation of vitamin D in alcoholic cirrhosis. Gastroenterology 1978;74:866–870.

182. Bikle DD, Gee E, Halloran B, Haddad JG. Free 1,25-dihydroxyvitamin D levels in serum from normal subjects, pregnant subjects and subjects with liver disease. J Clin Invest 1984;74:1966–1971.

183. Bikle DD, Halloran BP, Gee E, et al. Free 25-hydroxyvitamin D levels are normal in subjects with liver disease and reduced total 25-hydroxyvitamin D levels. J Clin Invest 1986;78:748–752.

184. Valimaki M, Salaspuro M, Ylikahri R. Liver damage and sex hormones in chronic male alcoholics. Clin Endocrinol 1982;17:469–477.

185. Friday K, Howard GA. Ethanol inhibits human bone cell proliferation and function in vitro. Metabolism 40:562–565.

186. Garcia-Carrasco M, Gruson M, de Vernejoul C, et al. Osteocalcin and bone histomorphometric parameters in adults without bone disease. Calcif Tissue Int 1988;42:13–17.

187. Delmas PD, Malaval L, Arlot ME, Meunier PJ. Serum bone Gla-protein compared to bone histomorphometry in endocrine diseases. Bone 1985;6:339–341.

188. Labib M, Abdel-Kader M, Ranganath L, Teale D, Marks V. Bone disease in chronic alcoholism: the value of plasma osteocalcin measurement. Alcohol Alcohol 1989;24:141–144.

189. Rico H, Cabranes JA, Cabello J, Gomez-Castresana F, Hernandez ER. Low serum osteocalcin in acute alcohol intoxication: a direct effect of alcohol on osteoblasts. Bone Miner 1987;2:221–225.

190. Nielsen HK, Lundby L, Rasmussen K, et al. Alcohol decreases serum osteocalcin in a dose-dependent way in normal subjects. Calcif Tissue Int 1990;46:173–178.

191. Mossberg D, Liljeberg P, Borg S. Clinical conditions in alcoholics during long term abstinence: a descriptive longitudinal study. Alcohol 1985;2:551–553.

192. Tovey FI, Godfrey JE, Lewin MR. A gastrectomy population: 25-30 years on. Postgrad Med J 1990;66:450–456.

193. Morgan DB, Paterson CR, Woods CG, Pulvertaft CN, Fourman P. Search for osteomalacia in 1228 patients after gastrectomy and other operations on the stomach. Lancet 1965;ii:1085–1088.

194. Garrick R, Ireland AW, Posen S. Bone abnormalities after gastric surgery: a prospective histological study. Ann Intern Med 1971;75:221–225.

195. Sitrin M, Meredith S, Rosenberg IH. Vitamin D deficiency and bone disease in gastrointestinal disorders. Arch Intern Med 1978;138:886–888.

196. Rao DS. Metabolic bone disease in gastrointestinal and biliary disorders. In: Favus MJ, ed. Primer on the metabolic bone diseases and disorders of mineral metabolism. Kelseyville, Calif: American Society for Bone and Mineral Research, 1990:175–178.

197. Inoue K, Shiomi K, Higashide S, et al. Metabolic bone disease following gastrectomy: assessment by dual energy x-ray absorptiometry. Br J Surg 1992;79:321–324.

198. Kaufman JM, Giri M, Deslypere JM, Thomas G, Vermeulen A. Influence of age on the responsiveness of the gonadotrophs to luteinizing hormone-releasing hormone in males. J Clin Endocrinol Metab 1991;72:1255–1260.

199. Kaye JM, Lawton MP, Gitlin LN, Kleban MH, Windsor LA, Kaye D. Older people's performance on the profile of mood states (POMS). Clin Gerontol 1988;7:35–36.

200. Keenan E, Stribrska L, Ramsay E, Orwoll E. Dihydrotestosterone regulation

of androgen receptor expression in skeletal (osteoblastic) cells. Endocrine Society 74th Annual Meeting, Programs and Abstracts (Abstract #1010), June 1992, San Antonio, Tex, 1992;304.

201. Keibzak GM, Smith R. Bone mineral content in the senescent rat femur: an assessment using single photon absorptiometry. J Bone Miner Res 1988;3:311–317.

202. Keibzak GM, Smith R. Bone status of secescent male rats: chemical morphometric, and mechanical analysis. J Bone Miner Res 1988;3(1):37–45.

203. Kellie SE. Measurement of bone density with dual-energy x-ray absorptiometry (DEXA). JAMA 1992;267:286–294.

204. Morgan DB, Hunt G, Paterson CR. The osteomalacia syndrome after stomach operations. Q J Med 1970;39:395–410.

205. Gertner JM, Lilburn M, Domenech M. 25-Hydroxycholecalciferol absorption in steatorrhoea and postgastrectomy osteomalacia. BMJ 1977;1:1310–1312.

206. Deller DJ, Begley MD. Calcium metabolism and the bones after partial gastrectomy: I. Clinical features and radiology of the bones. Australas Ann Med 1963; 12:282–294.

207. Ekbom K, Hed R. Calcium studies in partially gastrectomized patients, with special reference to the oral intake of calcium. Acta Med Scand 1965;178:193–201.

208. Kaplan MM. Metabolic bone disease associated with gastro-intestinal diseass. Viewponts Dig Dis 1983;15:9–12.

209. Jensen J, Oftebro H, Breigan B. Comparison of changes in testosterone concentrations after strength and endurance exercise in well-trained men. Eur J Appl Physiol 1991;63:467–471.

210. Kertzman C, Robinson DL, Sherins RJ, Schwankhaus JS, McClurkin JW. Abnormalities in visual spatial attention in men with mirror movements associated with isolated hypogonadotropic hypogonadism. Neurology 1990;40:1057–1063.

211. Chalmers J, Conacher WDH, Gardner DL, Scott PJ. Osteomalacia—a common disease in elderly women. J Bone Joint Surg 1967;49B:403–423.

212. Compston JE, Horton LWL, Ayers AB, Tighe JR, Creamer B. Osteomalacia after small-intestinal resection. Lancet 1978;i:9–12.

213. Jones CT, Williams JA, Nicholson G. Disturbances of bone metabolism after partial gastrectomy. In: Stammer FAR, Williams JA, eds. Partial gastrectomy: complications and metabolic consequences. London: Butterworths, 1963:190–226.

214. Hall GD, Neale G. Bone rarefaction after partial gastrectomy. Ann Intern Med 1963;59:455–463.

215. Thompson GR, Lewis B, Booth CC. Vitamin D absorption after partial gastrectomy. Lancet 1966;i:457–458.

216. Eddy RL. Metabolic bone disease after gastrectomy. Am J Med 1971;50:442–449.

217. Klein KB, Orwoll ES, Lieberman DA, Meier DE, McClung MR, Parfitt AM. Metabolic bone disease in asymptomatic men after partial gastrectomy with Billroth II anastomosis. Gastroenterology 1987;92:608–616.

218. Bisballe S, Eriksen EF, Melsen F, Mosekilde L, Sorensen OH, Hessov I. Osteopenia and osteomalacia after gastrectomy: interrelations between biochemical markers of bone remodelling, vitamin D metabolites, and bone histomorphometry. Gut 1991;21:1303–1307.

219. Parfitt AM. Osteomalacia and related disorders. In: Krane SM, ed. Metabolic bone disease. 2d ed. New York: Grune & Stratton, 1990:329–396.

220. Hessov I, Mosekilde L, Melsen F, et al. Osteopenia with normal vitamin D metabolites after small-bowel resection for Crohn's disease. Scand J Gastroenterol 1984;19:691–696.

221. Friedman HZ, Langman CB, Favus MJ. Vitamin D metabolism and osteomalacia in cystic fibrosis. Gastroenterology 1985;88:808–813.

222. Parfitt AM, Miller MJ, Frame B, et al. Metabolic bone disease after intestinal bypass for treatment of obesity. Ann Intern Med 1978;89:193–199.

223. McKenna MJ, Freaney R, Casey OM, Towers RP, Muldowney FP. Osteomalacia and osteoporosis: evaluation of a

diagnostic index. J Clin Pathol 1983; 36:245–252.

224. Bordier P, Ryckewart A, Gueris J. On the pathogenesis of so-called hypercalciuria. Am J Med 1977;63:398–409.

225. Alhava EM, Juuti M, Karjalainen P. Bone mineral density in patients with urolithiasis. Scand J Urol Nephrol 1976;10: 154–156.

226. Lawoyin S, Sismilich S, Browne R. Bone mineral content in patients with calcium urolithiasis. Metabolism 1979;28: 1250–1254.

227. Wilson DR, Barkin J, Strauss AL. Bone mineral content in calcium urolithiasis. Urol Res 1984;12:37.

228. Smith LH. The medical aspects of urolithiasis. J Urol 1989;141:707–710.

229. Sakhaee K, Nicar MJ, Glass K, Pak CYC. Postmenopausal osteoporosis as a manifestation of renal hypercalciuria with secondary hyperparathyroidism. J Clin Endocrinol Metab 1985;61:368–373.

230. Sutton RAL, Walker VR. Bone resorption and hypercalciuria in calcium stoneformers. Metabolism 1986;35:485–488.

231. Zerwekh JE, Sakhaee K, Breslau NA, Gottschalk F, Pak CYC. Impaired bone function in male idopathic osteoporosis: further reduction in the presence of concomitant hypercalciuria. Osteoporosis Int 1992;2:128–134.

232. Coe FL, Canterbury JM, Firpo JJ, Reiss E. Evidence for secondary hyperparathyroidism in idiopathic hypercalciuria. J Clin Invest 1973;52:134–142.

233. Lemann JJ, Worcester EM, Gray RW. Hypercalciuria and stones. Am J Kid Dis 1991;XVII:386–391.

234. Fuss M, Pepersack T, Van Geel J, et al. Involvement of low-calcium diet in the reduced bone mineral content of idiopathic renal stone formers. Calcif Tissue Int 1990; 46:9–13.

235. Branner RJ, Spring DB, Sebastian A, et al. Incidence of radiographically evident bone disease, nephrocalcinosis, and nephrolithiasis in various types of renal tubular acidosis. New Engl J Med 1982; 307:217–221.

236. Tieder M, Modai D, Shaked U, et al. "Idiopathic" hypercalciuria and hereditary hypophosphatemic rickets. N Engl J Med 1987;316:125–129.

237. Rao DS, Frame B, Block MA. Primary hyperparathyroidism: a cause of hypercalciuria and renal stones in patients with medullary sponge kidney. JAMA 1977;237:1353–1355.

238. Dlabal PW, Jordan RM, Dorfman SG. Medullary sponge kidney and renal-leak hypercalciuria: a link to the development of parathyroid adenoma? JAMA 1979; 241:1490–1491.

239. O'Neill M, Breslau NA, Pak CYC. Metabolic evaluation of nephrolithiasis in patients with medullary sponge kidney. JAMA 1981;245:1233–1236.

240. Perry HMI, Fallon MD, Bergfeld M, Teitelbaum SL, Avioli LV. Osteoporosis in young men—a syndrome of hypercalciuria and accelerated bone turnover. Arch Intern Med 1982;142:1295–1298.

241. Malluche HH, Tschoepe W, Ritz E, Meyer-Sabellek W, Massry SG. Abnormal bone histology in idiopathic hypercalciuria. J Clin Endocrinol Metab 1980;50:654–658.

242. Jackson W. Osteoporosis of unknown cause in younger people. J Bone Joint Surg 1958;40B:420–441.

243. Krall EA, Dawson-Hughes B. Smoking and bone loss among postmenopausal women. J Bone Miner Res 1991; 6:331–338.

244. Jensen J, Christiansen C. Effects of smoking on serum lipoproteins and bone mineral content during postmenopausal hormone replacement therapy. Am J Obstet Gynecol 1988;159:820–825.

245. Lindsay R, Fogelman I, Hart DM. Prevention of postmenopausal bone loss using sex steroids. In: DeLuca HF, Frost HM, Jee WSS, Johnston CC, Parfitt AM, eds. Osteoporosis: recent advances in pathogenesis and treatment. Baltimore: University Park Press, 1981:399–406.

246. Daniell HW. Osteoporosis of the slender smoker. Arch Intern Med 1976; 136:298–304.

247. Jensen J, Christiansen C, Rodbro P. Cigarette smoking, serum estrogens, and bone loss during hormone-replacement therapy early after menopause. New Engl J Med 1985;313:973–975.

248. Hahn TJ. Drug-induced disorders of vitamin D and mineral metabolism. Clin Endocrinol Metab 1980;9:107–129.

249. Bornemann M, Saxon JR, Kidd GSI. Osteoporosis unmasked by hyperthyroidism in a young man with osteogenesis imperfecta. Arch Intern Med 1987;147:1947–1948.

250. Anderson RA, Bancroft J, Wu FCW. The effects of exogenous testosterone on sexuality and mood of normal men. J Clin Endocrinol Metab 1992;75:1503–1507.

251. Parfitt AM, Duncan H. Metabolic bone disease affecting the spine. In: Rothman R, ed. The spine. 2d ed. Philadelphia: WB Saunders, 1982:775–905.

252. Hills E, Dunstan CR, Wong SYP, Evans RA. Bone histology in young adult osteoporosis. J Clin Pathol 1989;42:391–397.

253. Bordier PJ, Miravet L, Hioco D. Young adult osteoporosis. Clin Endocrinol Metab 1973;2:277–292.

254. Nordin BEC, Aaron J, Speed R, Francis RM, Makins N. Bone formation and resorption as the determinants of trabecular bone volume in normal and osteoporotic men. Scot Med J 1984;29:171–175.

255. Aaron JE, Francis RM, Peacock M, Nakins NB. Contrasting microanatomy of idiopathic and corticosteroid-induced osteoporosis. Clin Orthop Rel Res 1989; 243:294–305.

256. Eastell R, Riggs BL. Diagnostic evalution of osteoporosis. Endocrinol Metab Clin 1980;17:547–571.

257. Lane JM, Vigorita VJ. Osteoporosis. Orthop Clin North Am 1984;15:711–728.

258. Seeley DG, Browner WS, Nevitt MC, Genant HK, Scott JC, Cummings SR. Which fractures are associated with low appendicular bone mass in elderly women? Ann Intern Med 1991;115:837–842.

259. Mann T, Oviatt SK, Wilson D, Orwoll ES. Vertebral deformity in men. J Bone Miner Res 1992;7:1259–1265.

260. Laredo JD, Bard M. Thoracic spine: percutaneous trephine biopsy. Radiology 1986;160:485–489.

261. McHenry MC, Duchesneau PM, Keys TF, Rehm SJ, Boumphrey RS. Vertebral osteomyelitis presenting as spinal compression fracture. Arch Intern Med 1988;148:417–423.

262. Fornasier VL, Czitrom AA. Collapsed vertebrae—a review of 659 autopsies. Clin Orthop Rel Res 1978;131:261–265.

263. Johnston CCJ, Melton LJI, Lindsay R, Eddy DM. Clinical indications for bone mass measurements—a report from the scientific advisory board of the national osteoporosis foundation. J Bone Miner Res 1989;4:1–28.

264. Campbell GA, Hosking DJ. How common is osteomalacia in the elderly? Lancet 1984; August 18:386–388.

265. Aaron JE, Stasiak L, Gallagher JC, et al. Frequency of osteomalacia and osteoporosis in fractures of the proximal femur. Lancet 1974; February 16:229–233.

266. Hordon LD, Peacock M. Osteomalacia and osteoporosis in femoral neck fracture. Bone 1990;11:247–259.

267. Sokoloff L. Occult osteomalacia in America (USA) patients with fracture of the hip. Am J Surg Pathol 1978;2:21–30.

268. Wilton TJ, Hosking DJ, Pawley E, Stevens A, Harvey L. Osteomalacia and femoral neck fractures in the elderly patient. J Bone Joint Surg 1987;69B:388–390.

269. Marel GM, McKenna MJ, Frame B. Osteomalacia. In: Peck WA, ed. Bone and Mineral Research. Vol 4. Amsterdam: Elsevier Science Publishers, 1986:335–413.

270. Singer FR. Metabolic bone disease. In: Felig P, Baxter JD, Broadus AE, Frohman LA, eds. Endocrinology and metabolism, ed. 2. New York: McGraw-Hill, 1987:1454–1499.

271. Klein RF, Gunness M. The transiliac bone biopsy: when to get it and how to in-

▶ 199

terpret it. The Endocrinologist 1992; 2:158–168.

272. Chines A, Pacifici R, Avioli LA, Korenblat PE, Teitelbaum SL. Systemic mastocytosis and osteoporosis. Osteoporosis Int 1993;1:S147–S149.

273. Chines A, Pacifici R, Avioli LV, Teitelbaum SL, Korenblat PE. Systemic mastocytosis presenting as osteoporosis: a clinical and histomorphometric study. J Clin Endocrinol Metab 1991;72:140–144.

274. Civitelli R, Gonnelli S, Zacchei F, et al. Bone turnover in postmenopausal osteoporosis: effect of calcitonin treatment. J Clin Invest 1988;82:1268–1274.

275. Demiaux B, Arlot ME, Chapuy M-C, Meunier PJ, Delmas PD. Serum osteocalcin is increased in patients with osteomalacia: correlations with biochemical and histomorphometric findings. Clin Endocrinol Metab 1992;74:1146–1151.

276. Rubenstein L, Josephson K. Causes and prevention of falls in elderly people. In: Vellas B, Toupet M, Rubenstein L, Albarede J, Christen Y, eds. Falls, balance and gait disorders in the elderly. Paris: Elsevier, 1992;21–38.

277. Curhan GC, Willett WC, Rimm EB, Stampfer MJ. A prospective study of dietary calcium and other nutrients and the risk of symptomatic kidney stones. N Engl J Med 1993;328:833–838.

278. Agrawal R, Wallach S, Cohn S, et al. Calcitonin treatment of osteoporosis. In: Pecile A, ed. Calcitonin 1980. Vol 540. Amsterdam: Exerpta Medica, 1981: 237.

279. Burckhardt P, Burnand B. The effect of treatment with calcitonin on vertebral fracture rate in osteoporosis. Osteoporosis Int 1993;3:24–30.

280. McDermott MT, Kidd GS. The role of calcitonin in the development and treatment of osteoporosis. Endocr Rev 1987; 8:377–390.

281. Montemurro L, Schiraldi G, Farioli P, Tosi G, Riboldi A, Rizzato G. Prevention of corticosteroid-induced osteoporosis with salmon calcitonin in sarcoid patients. Calcif Tissue Int 1991;49:71–76.

282. Valkema R, Vismans F-JFE, Papapoulos SE, Pauwels EKJ, Bijvoet OLM. Maintained improvement in calcium balance and bone mineral content in patients with osteoporosis treated with the bisphosphonate APD. Bone Miner 1989;5:183–192.

283. Reid IR, Alexander CJ, King AR, Ibbertson HK. Prevention of steroid-induced osteoporosis with (3-amino-1-hydroxypropylidene)-1, 1-bisphosphonate (APD). Lancet 1988; January 23:143–146.

284. Papapoulos SE, Landman JO, Bijvoet OLM, et al. The use of bisphosphonates in the treatment of osteoporosis. Bone 1992;13:S41–S49.

285. Reeve J, Meunier PJ, Parsons JA, et al. Anabolic effect of human parathyroid hormone fragment on trabecular bone in involutional osteoporosis: a multicentre trial. BMJ 1980; June 7:1340–1344.

286. Slovik DM, Neer RM, Potts JTJ. Short-term effects of synthetic human parathyroid hormone (1-34) administration on bone mineral metabolism in osteoporotic patients. J Clin Invest 1981; 68:1261–1271.

287. Reeve J, Bradbeer JN, Arlot M, et al. hPTH 1-34 treatment of osteoporosis with added hormone replacement therapy: biochemical, kinetic and histological responses. Osteoporosis Int 1991;1:162–170.

288. Slovik DM, Rosenthal DI, Doppelt SH, et al. Restoration of spinal bone in osteoporotic men by treatment with human parathyroid hormone (1-34) and 1,25-dihydroxyvitamin D. J Bone Miner Res 1986;1:377–381.

289. Marcus R, Butterfield G, Holloway L, et al. Effects of short term administration of recombinant human growth hormone to elderly people. J Clin Endocrinol Metab 1990;70:519–527.

290. Mann DR, Rudman CG, Akinbami MA, Gould KG. Preservation of bone mass in hypogonadal female monkeys with recombinant human growth hormone administration. J Clin Endocrinol Metab 1992;74:1263–1269.

291. Ljunghall S, Johansson AG, Burman P, Kampe O, Lindh E, Karlsson FA.

Low plasma levels of insulin-like growth factor 1 (IGF-1) in male patients with idiopathic osteoporosis. J Intern Med 1992; 232:59–64.

292. Rudman D, Feller AG, Nagraj HS, et al. Effects of human growth hormone in men over 60 years old. N Engl J Med 1990; 323:1–6.

293. Kelly PJ, Twomey L, Sambrook PN, Eisman JA. Sex differences in peak adult bone mineral density. J Bone Miner Res 1990;5:1169–1175.

8 ▸ Glucocorticoid-Induced Osteoporosis

▶ ▶ ▶ Lorraine A. Fitzpatrick

Skeletal decalcification was recognized as a clinical feature of Cushing's disease as early as 1932 (1). With the isolation of cortisol, the anti-inflammatory, antineoplastic, and immunosuppressive properties of glucocorticoids have become useful in the treatment of a variety of diseases. Patients exposed to long-term glucocorticoid therapy have distinctive clinical features associated with suppression of the hypothalamic-pituitary-adrenal axis: centripetal obesity; striae; thin, fragile skin; increased bruisability; fluid retention; proximal muscle weakness; glucose intolerance or frank hyperglycemia; posterior subcapsular lens opacities; and vertebral compression fractures. In children, glucocorticoids interfere with normal linear growth and retardation of height (2). Glucocorticoid-induced osteoporosis is probably the most common cause of "secondary" osteoporosis. Although the true incidence of osteoporosis in this patient population is unknown, patients on high-dose glucocorticoid therapy experience rapid loss of bone and vertebral compression fractures can occur within weeks to months of initiation of therapy (3). Overall, 30% to 35% of patients on glucocorticoid therapy experience vertebral crush fractures and the risk of hip fracture is increased by 50%.

The bone loss caused by excess glucocorticoids is diffuse and affects both the cortical and axial skeleton. Glucocorticoids damage trabecular bone to a greater extent than cortical bone, perhaps due to the greater surface area of trabecular bone. This osteopenia is caused by several mechanisms: suppression of osteoblast function, inhibition of intestinal calcium absorption leading to secondary hyperparathyroidism, and increased osteoclast-mediated bone resorption. Bone loss is also promoted by the direct stimulation of renal excretion of calcium by glucocorticoids and hypogonadism associated with the suppressive effects of glucocorticoids.

Epidemiology of Glucocorticoid-Induced Osteoporosis

In patients with endogenous glucocorticoid excess, retrospective studies have demonstrated reduced bone density in 40% to 60% and pathologic fractures in 16% to 67% of patients (4–11). It is more difficult to assess incidence and fracture rates in patients with excessive amounts of exogenous glucocorticoids although several studies have suggested that bone loss is greatest in the first 6 months after introduction of therapy.

Few prospective studies comparing bone loss in patients on glucocorticoid therapy have been completed. Often confounding variables such as additional immunosuppressive therapy, altered drug clearance rates, changes in the dose of the corticosteroid or autoimmune disease are present. The incidence of glucocorticoid-induced osteoporosis has been estimated at 30% to 50% (12,13). Further problems in the assessment of the extent of disease lie in the cross-sectional design of many studies. In these studies, bone mineral density (BMD) prior to the initiation of glucocorticoid therapy is not available, limiting the comparisons between individuals. In short-term studies, glucocorticoid-induced bone loss appears to be greater in the first 6 to 12 months of therapy (14–16). These studies suggest that bone loss is related to both duration of therapy and total cumulative dose (17). The minimal dose of glucocorticoids associated with rapid bone loss is not well established. One study observed vertebral fractures in patients ingesting a cumulative dose of 5 g prednisone (18). In a prospective one-year study, patients receiving 2 days of 34 to 51 mg lost up to 17.5% BMD per year (13). Patients receiving less than 17 mg over 2 days lost an insignificant amount of bone, and patients receiving an intermediate dose, 17 to 34 mg over 2 days, lost 0% to 8% BMD per year. In this study, BMD was measured by quantitative computerized tomography at the distal tibia and radius. Studies that evaluate mineral density of trabecular bone indicate significantly increased bone loss compared to loss in the radius, probably due to the differential effect of glucocorticoid therapy on trabecular versus cortical bone.

Traditional risk factors associated with osteoporosis are thought to influence glucocorticoid-induced osteoporosis. The relative risk of each factor, however, remains enigmatic. Retrospective analysis suggests that certain factors are associated with an increased risk of glucocorticoid-induced bone loss. Osteoporosis is more severe in patients less than 15 years or greater than 50 years and in postmenopausal women (18,19). In the older, immobilized or postmenopausal patient, a preexisting low level of bone mass may lead to rapid development of clinically significant osteopenia. In the younger individual, a higher rate of bone turnover results in more rapid bone loss.

Improved longevity in transplant patients has raised the issue of glucocorticoid-associated bone loss in a different patient population. Often these patients are taking additional immunosuppressive agents, and the relative contribution of each therapeutic agent to bone loss is difficult to assess. In one study of 40 cardiac transplant recipients, osteopenia as determined by dual-energy x-ray absorptiometry was present in 28% of patients at the lumbar spine and 20% of patients at femoral neck (20). Vertebral fractures were noted in 35% of individuals. All patients were receiving prednisone and cyclosporin A. Cyclosporin A may have altered calcium kinetics by its direct effects on bone (21,22). In contrast to patients ingesting prednisone alone, 60% of these transplant recipients had elevated levels of osteocalcin. This elevation may reflect an increase in bone formation or turnover (20).

Pathophysiology

A variety of interrelated factors affect mineral metabolism in the patient on glucocorticoid therapy. Glucocorticoids have a direct effect on bone, alter calcium absorption from the intestine, change the ability of the kidney to reabsorb calcium, and alter gonadal hormone secretion.

The Effect of Glucocorticoids on Bone Remodeling

Bone constantly undergoes remodeling and can be greatly affected by administration of this class of steroid hormones. There is tight regulation of bone formation and resorption, and this process is under the influence of myriad factors. Although the role of systemic factors has been studied in some detail, we are just beginning to appreciate the numerous and complex interactions between bone and locally produced cytokines. The autocrine/paracrine relationships between osteoblasts and osteoclasts are poorly defined. In general, coupling between formation and resorption maintains bone mass at a steady-state level until the tissue is influenced by endogenous (such as aging or menopause) or exogenous (such as drug administration) perturbations.

Remodeling begins by the recruitment and activation of the osteoclast, which resorbs matrix and mineral to form Howship's lacunae. After detachment of the osteoclast, osteoblasts are recruited to the surface to deposit matrix proteins (osteoid). Over several weeks, the new matrix mineralizes, filling in the defect. Glucocorticoids uncouple the formation/resorption cycle, resulting in net bone loss. Overall, the depressive effect of glucocorticoids on osteoblasts directly uncouples remodeling and accelerates bone loss.

Suppression of bone formation is the major impairment in bone physiology caused by glucocorticoids. Glucocorticoids exert a direct effect on osteoblasts in inhibiting differentiation of preosteoblasts (23,24). Feldman and colleagues (25) demonstrated glucocorticoid receptors on bone cells, and direct effects have been analyzed in cell culture systems (26). Glucocorticoids inhibit osteoblast-like cell growth, citrate decarboxylation, alkaline phosphatase activity, and synthesis of collagen and noncollagenous proteins (26–33). In human osteoblast-like cell culture systems, pharmacologic concentrations of glucocorticoids cause similar effects, although low-dose, short-term exposure may stimulate cell growth and collagen synthesis (33,34). In human osteoblast-like cells, dexamethasone caused an increase in steady-state levels of c-myc, c-fos and c-jun mRNAs, indicating that glucocorticoids may induce the oncoproteins that subsequently regulate the genes encoding for alkaline phosphatase, osteocalcin, and possibly other growth factors (26). Shalhoub and coworkers have demonstrated that glucocorticoids exert both transcriptional and posttranscriptional effects on fetal rat calvaria-derived osteoblasts (34). The authors propose that glucocorticoids alter gene expression which in turn regulates cell-cell and cell-extracellular matrix signaling mechanisms that support osteoblast-like cell growth and differentiation.

▶ 205

Recent investigations have explored the influence of glucocorticoids on the role of transforming growth factor-β (TGF_β), a multifunctional growth factor that influences bone cell activity. In human osteoblast-like cells, dexamethasone activated multiple latent forms of TGF_β. In addition, treatment of human osteoblast-like cells with dexamethasone resulted in a dose-dependent increase in the mRNA levels of cathepsin B and cathepsin D, suggesting that these lysosomal proteases may be the mechanisms by which activation of latent TGF_β occurs (35).

Histomorphometrically, dynamic measures of bone formation are profoundly reduced, indicating that remodeling has been uncoupled. These studies strongly support the results of in vitro studies indicating a decrease in osteoblast function. There is a reduction in the number of osteoid seams and a low mineral apposition rate as determined by tetracycline labeling. The mean wall thickness of trabecular osteons is decreased in steroid-treated patients, which has been hypothesized to reflect decreased longevity of active osteoblasts within each remodeling unit (12,23). Overall, there is a reduction in cancellous bone volume (12,23,36,37,38,39,40). In one study, cancellous bone volume was less than 11% in over 60% of glucocorticoid-treated patients, which has been interpreted as at the threshold for fracture susceptibility (12). The larger surface area of trabecular bone suggests it is affected to a greater extent than cortical bone by glucocorticoids; however, several studies have confirmed a reduction in cortical bone volume (41,42). It has been estimated that a 30% loss of bone occurs during each remodeling cycle in patients on glucocorticoid therapy (23).

Osteocalcin, a noncollagenous, vitamin K–dependent protein, is synthesized by osteoblasts, and serum levels of osteocalcin have been used as a marker of bone formation. Acute administration of 10 mg prednisone suppresses osteocalcin levels by 50% to 80% (44,45), and several studies have documented low levels of circulating osteocalcin in patients receiving long-term glucocorticoid therapy (46). In human beings and in rats, administration of 1,25–dihydroxyvitamin D (1,25(OH)$_2$D) abrogates the suppression of osteocalcin levels during glucocorticoid administration (44,47,48).

Calcium kinetic studies and histomorphometric analyses support the hypothesis that glucocorticoids enhance bone resorption (38,49). An increased prevalence of resorption lacunae and osteoclasts is frequently observed in corticosteroid-treated patients, and overall, bone turnover is increased. It is unclear if the effect of glucocorticoids on bone resorption in vivo is in response to increased levels of parathyroid hormone (PTH). In bone organ culture, diverse results have been published regarding the direct effect(s) of glucocorticoids on bone resorption. One explanation for these divergent results is a possible biphasic dose effect of glucocorticoids on differentiation and function of osteoclasts. Generation of new osteoclasts may be inhibited by high doses (32) and in other studies, glucocorticoids enhance the attachment of macrophages to bone by altering cell surface oligosaccharides (50). In the mouse calvaria resorption assay, glucocorticoids have been demonstrated to have a direct stimulatory effect on osteoclasts (51). In animal studies, bone resorption is reduced after steroid therapy although Jee and coworkers demonstrated that supraphysiologic doses of glucocorticoids stimulate bone resorption in rats (52). A recent study further explained the potential role of bone matrix proteins in resorption as influenced by hydrocortisone. Devitalized, mineralized bone particles were implanted subcutaneously in rats, and treatment with hydrocortisone or dexamethasone was initiated. Recruitment of bone-resorbing cells was impaired, and resorption of the implanted bone particle was reduced. If bone particles were implanted in the animals and treatment with glucocorticoids was delayed for 7 days allowing osteoclast-like cell recruitment, overall resorption was increased. Glucocorticoids may therefore have distinct effects at varying stages of bone resorption in that these pharmaceutical agents may inhibit recruitment of osteoclast progenitor cells and stimulate the activity of differentiated osteoclasts. Resorption of bone particles deficient in osteocalcin was enhanced by the addition of hydrocortisone (53).

Glucocorticoid Effects on Intestinal Calcium Absorption

Intestinal absorption of calcium determines the substrate supply available to meet the needs of bone remodeling. The amount of calcium absorbed is determined by the dietary intake and the capacity of the intestines. Mineral absorption is accompanied by two mechanisms: physiologically regulated, saturable transcellular absorption and nonsaturable pericellular absorption. Calcitriol, or 1,25 $(OH)_2D$ is the hormonal stimulus of active calcium absorption in the duodenum and jejunum.

Glucocorticoids decrease net intestinal calcium absorption (36,54–56) by an unknown mechanism. Other studies have provided divergent results that may reflect the differential rates of absorption in the small intestine versus the colon and differences in the doses studied. Only active intestinal absorption is inhibited: passive diffusion of calcium is not altered.

▶ 207

Animal studies have attempted to explain the mechanisms responsible for glucocorticoid-induced inhibition of active transcellular transport of calcium. Several possible mechanisms have been proposed. In mice, the number of 1,25 $(OH)_2D$ receptors is downregulated by glucocorticoids (58). In chickens, glucocorticoids decrease the amount of soluble calcium-binding protein and alkaline phosphatase activity (58). Other investigators have demonstrated that glucocorticoids depress vitamin D-dependent calcium absorption and increase vitamin D-dependent backflux into the gut lumen in rats (59).

At the cellular level, glucocorticoids deplete adenosine triphosphate (ATP) which inhibits mitochondrial calcium release (60). Stimulation of the sodium–potassium ATPase by glucocorticoids may lead to pericellular back flux of calcium (61). Synthesis of calcium-binding protein is decreased, and this limitation of available substrate may be important (62). The contribution of each of these possible alterations in calcium transport to glucocorticoid-induced inhibition of calcium absorption is unknown.

Initially it was proposed that glucocorticoids may alter vitamin D metabolism, and some clinical studies supported this hypothesis. Circulating levels of 1,25 $(OH)_2D$ are higher in patients acutely ingesting glucocorticoids (63,64) but normalize with chronic administration despite the persistent defect in calcium absorption (65,66). Serum concentrations of 25-hydroxyvitamin D_3 ($25(OH)D_3$) are normal or decreased (42,63,67). Such studies are difficult to interpret due to limitations imposed by the glucocorticoid-requiring disorder.

It was further proposed that the decrease in intestinal calcium absorption was due to defective conversion of vitamin D to its active metabolites. Synthesis and clearance rates of $1,25(OH)_2D$ have been reported as low (68), normal (69), or increased (64,70). Administration of 1,25(OH)$_2$D to patients does not abrogate completely the abnormal calcium transport (55). A high sodium (72) or low calcium (70,72,73) dietary intake exacerbates the defect in intestinal calcium transport. Animal studies, however, do not support an important role for aberrant vitamin D metabolism in glucocorticoid action.

In a recently published study, 22 subjects under treatment with prednisone for chronic obstructive pulmonary disease were compared to 14 patients who were not on glucocorticoid therapy. Bone density measurements were reduced in prednisone-treated patients and correlated with pulmonary impairment independent of glucocorticoid use. Serum levels of 1,25(OH)$_2$D and PTH were significantly higher in prednisone-treated patients (147 ± 50 versus 95 ± 30 pmol/L for 1,25(OH)$_2$D) as compared to controls. The investigators suggest that the lack of correlation between 1,25(OH)$_2$D levels and serum phosphorus or PTH levels provides evidence that alterations in 1,25(OH)$_2$D production are brought about by a mechanism other than secondary hyperparathyroidism (74).

Regardless of the mechanism of glucocorticoid-induced inhibition of calcium absorption, several important clinical features are present in patients on therapy. Inhibition of intestinal calcium absorption has been documented as early as 2 weeks after initiation of therapy. The effect appears to be dose related (75). To date, the mechanism by which glucocorticoids interfere with intestinal calcium absorption remains controversial, but the net effect of reduced calcium absorption is the development of secondary hyperparathyroidism.

Association of Glucocorticoids with Secondary Hyperparathyroidism

Secondary hyperparathyroidism has been documented in patients on glucocorticoid therapy (42,65,66). The etiology is not completely certain and often attributable to the decrease in calcium absorption that occurs at the intestinal level. Transient hypocalcemia may cause compensatory stimulation of PTH release. Direct action of glucocorticoids on the parathyroid gland has been documented. In normal subjects, infusion of cortisol results in increased serum levels of PTH within an hour (76,77). In isolated rat parathyroid cells, glucocorticoids have a stimulatory effect (78).

Other investigators have demonstrated an increased sensitivity of osteoblasts to PTH in the presence of glucocorticoids. Glucocorticoid receptors are present on bone cells (25,28), and potentiation of the cyclic AMP response to PTH occurs (79–81). Other findings include potentiation of PTH-mediated inhibition of collagen synthesis and alkaline phosphatase activity in bone cells (82).

Osteoporosis

Gonadal Dysfunction

Glucocorticoids can alter levels of gonadal hormones in both men and women. Two distinct mechanisms of glucocorticoid-induced gonadal dysfunction have been described. Glucocorticoids reduce testosterone levels in men (83–86) and interfere with normal ovulation in women (87,88). Studies indicate that these effects are due, in part, to direct suppression of gonadal steroid secretion.

Chronic glucocorticoid therapy lowers serum testosterone levels in men receiving doses of methylprednisolone as low as 15 mg/dL (86,87). Glucocorticoid therapy reduces the level of sex hormone-binding globulin (86) and with the concurrent reduction in total testosterone, this therapy also reduces the bio-active free testosterone levels. In these patients, serum follicle-stimulating hormone and luteinizing hormone (LH) levels were inappropriately low, suggesting that glucocorticoid therapy directly suppressed gonadotropin release from the pituitary (85). Exogenous synthetic gonadotropin-releasing hormone stimulation was not altered in male patients versus controls. In women, inhibition of LH secretion induced by synthetic LH-releasing hormone was present with long-term glucocorticoid therapy (87). In animal studies, bone loss is augmented in oophorectomized rats receiving glucocorticoids as compared to rats with intact ovaries (89).

▶ 209

Additional alterations in sex steroid hormone levels may be due to the glucocorticoid-induced suppressive effects on the adrenal. Circulating levels of estrone and androstenedione are reduced due to suppression of ACTH and adrenal atrophy (90). Although the primary source of testosterone is from the testes, a small contribution from the adrenals may also be altered by glucocorticoid administration.

Estrogen deficiency due to ovariectomy and glucocorticoid administration had additive effects on bone loss (88). Several studies have demonstrated the efficacy of estrogen replacement therapy in reducing, in part, glucocorticoid-mediated bone loss (91).

Clinical Presentation

The true incidence of osteoporosis in patients receiving glucocorticoid therapy is unknown, and as defined, has been estimated at 30% to 50%. Several studies have suggested that bone loss is greatest in the first 6 months after institution of glucocorticoid therapy. Major risk factors for glucocorticoid-induced osteopenia include high total cumulative dose of glucocorticoids, age less than 15 years or greater than 50 years, and postmenopausal status. Secondary risk factors include duration of glucocorticoid therapy, disorders associated with increased interleukin-1(IL-1) production (ie, rheumatoid arthritis), and general osteoporosis risk factors (age, race, sex, menopausal state, and parity).

Serum and urine biochemical parameters in patients with glucocorticoid-induced osteopenia are generally normal. Fasting serum calcium, phosphate, and vitamin D metabolite levels are within normal limits. Serum immunoreactive PTH concentrations may be normal or mildly elevated. Serum alkaline phosphatase and osteocalcin levels decline progressively after the initiation of glucocorticoid therapy. Urinary calcium excretion may be increased during the first several months to years of steroid therapy and is due to the direct calciuric effect of glucocorticoids on the kidney. After several years of glucocorticoid therapy, urinary calcium excretion is usually within the normal range.

Adverse Effects of Inhaled Glucocorticoids

The effects of inhaled glucocorticoids on mineral homeostasis remain controversial. Recently, this mode of administration has gained widespread acceptance as a first-line treatment to avoid the systemic effects of oral glucocorticoids. However, few data exist that clearly define the clinical relevance of inhaled glucocorticoids and their effect on bone metabolism (92). Aerosolized glucocorticoids are rapidly absorbed from the respiratory tract and usually biotransformed to less active metabolites. However, daily doses of greater than 1500 mg have been associated with adrenal suppression (93,94).

In normal volunteers, high-dose beclomethasone decreases serum osteocalcin levels (95) but does not alter the diurnal variation of osteocalcin (96). Changes in serum alkaline phosphatase, a relatively insensitive marker of bone formation, were not noted. Ali and coworkers demonstrated that healthy, normal volunteers taking 2000 µg beclomethasone daily had a significant rise in urinary hydroxyproline, suggesting increased breakdown of the osteoid matrix. Although these studies contained a small number of subjects and a prospective longitudinal study with bone density measurements has not been accomplished to date, most clinicians suggest that inhaled glucocorticoids may be associated with some risk of long-term skeletal loss (92).

Evaluation of the Patient

In all patients suspected of steroid-induced osteopenia, other causes of osteopenia must be excluded. A bone biopsy may be helpful in this differential diagnosis. Patients who have the lowest initial bone mass and strength, the most serious impairment of calcium absorption, the highest urinary loss of calcium, and the greatest degree of secondary hyperparathyroidism are most likely to develop osteoporosis. Measurement of 24-hour urinary calcium concentration is helpful to assess calcium balance. Baseline measurements of serum calcium, phosphorus, creatinine, and PTH levels are warranted. Vitamin D deficiency augments the adverse effects of glucocorticoids. Serum 25 hydroxyvitamin D concentrations should be measured to assess vitamin D status. Gonadal steroid levels are useful to assess the need for replacement therapy. Urinary hydroxyproline levels, an insensitive measure of bone resorption, will most likely be replaced by measurement of urinary pyridinoline cross-links, once prospective studies concerning the clinical utility of this test in the assessment of glucocorticoid-induced bone loss are accomplished.

Bone loss is most rapid in areas of the skeleton containing the greatest proportion of trabecular bone. Earliest changes in bone density can be detected in the spine and femoral neck. Some patients who are on glucocorticoid therapy do not develop osteoporosis, making it important to identify patients at risk for closer follow-up and prevention. Early changes of BMD can be detected by x-ray or dual photon absorptiometry (97,98). The features of glucocorticoid-induced bone disease on a roentgenogram are distinctive. Vertical and horizontal trabeculae tend to be equally thin, producing a uniformly translucent appearance of the vertebrae, ribs, and pelvis. Pseudocallous formation at sites of stress fracture is another hallmark of glucocorticoid-induced osteoporosis. Pseudocallous formation may also be seen at the endplates of collapsed vertebrae or around stress fractures in the pelvis or ribs.

Sudden pain or weakness in a joint could be the first presenting complaint of osteonecrosis. Osteonecrosis, or aseptic necrosis, is a serious complication of steroid therapy that can occur in patients who are otherwise asymptomatic from bone loss. Several theories about ischemia have been proposed and include the presence of microscopic fat emboli or mechanical problems resulting in fatigue fractures and collapse of ischemic bone. Radiographically, an isolated epiphyseal compression or subchondral fracture of the symptomatic epiphysis is present. Early diagnosis is difficult and may require a bone scan or magnetic resonance imaging for confirmation (98).

Therapeutic Recommendations

Sufficient data do not exist to allow definitive recommendations for prevention and treatment of steroid-induced osteoporosis. As a result, the treatment of established steroid osteoporosis may be a frustrating experience to the clinician. In general, treatment is directed toward reversing disordered osteoblastic and osteoclastic activity.

Studies suggest that steroid dose is the major determinant of bone loss, and the mainstay of therapy is usually reduction of dose to the lowest effective dose possible (3,98–102). Significant osteopenia has been observed in patients treated chronically with doses as low as 7.5 to 10 mg prednisone per day. Alternate-day therapy may preserve the pituitary-adrenal axis but does not prevent bone loss (103,104). Topical steroid preparations are recommended when possible, although prospective studies regarding bone loss have not been completed.

Development of Synthetic Glucocorticoid Derivatives

The development of glucocorticoids that are less toxic to bone would be helpful. Ideally, the compound would need to have equivalent immunosuppressive and anti-inflammatory actions without the other toxic effects. Deflazacort, an ox-azoline derivative of prednisolone with lower lipid solubility, has been reported to be less potent than prednisone in altering calcium metabolism. Specifically, less secondary hyperparathyroidism is associated with the use of deflazacort (16,105,106). Although long-term clinical trials comparing deflazacort and prednisone are not available, an initial study suggests that trabecular bone loss is less with deflazacort compared to prednisone (107). Recent trials of one-year duration suggest that impairment of calcium absorption is less with deflazacort (108). In 29 patients with nephrotic syndrome, bone decay rate determined at the radius and lumbar spine were significantly reduced in deflazacort-treated patients compared to prednisone-treated patients over 12 months (107). Serum osteocalcin levels drop rapidly after administration of deflazacort (107) but to a lesser extent than after treatment with prednisone. Currently, this drug is not available for general use in the United States, and it is unclear if it contains adequate therapeutic anti-inflammatory and immunosuppressive actions as compared to prednisone.

Recent findings have demonstrated that even alternate-day prednisone therapy results in bone loss (103,104). Few studies have addressed the issue of whether therapeutically equivalent doses of different glucocorticoids result in differing metabolic side effects. The development of cloprednol (6-chloro-11,17,21-trihydroxypregna-1,4,6,triene-3,20-dione), a synthetic glucocorticoid with twice the inflammatory potency of prednisone, led to the hope that this synthetic derivative, used on alternate days would preserve BMD. Cloprednol causes less excretion of calcium and minimally alters hypothalamic-pituitary-adrenal axis function as compared to prednisolone. A prospective, double-blind, randomized study with 49 patients compared cloprednol (2.5 mg) with prednisone (5 mg) every other day for one year. Both systemically administered drugs and inhaled beclomethasone (used as one control population) induced bone loss. The decreases in trabecular bone loss, however, were greater in the prednisone-treated postmenopausal patients. No differences in cortical bone loss were noted between the two groups (109).

Physical Activity

One way to stimulate osteoblastic bone forming activity directly is to increase weight-bearing physical activity. Conversely, inactivity increases urinary calcium output and bone mineral loss (110). Resistance exercise can attenuate or prevent the steroid-dependent muscle loss in animals and human beings; however, there may be limits to the use of this modality in chronically ill individuals. In a group of subjects with chronic obstructive pulmonary disease, the limited activity associated with reduced forced expired volume in one second breathing mechanics in these patients appeared to have an impact on the development of osteoporosis that was independent of glucocorticoid therapy (74).

▶ 213

Use of Supplemental Calcium, Vitamin D and Diuretics

Most regimens have attempted to maximize calcium absorption and decrease urinary calcium excretion. Stimulation of intestinal calcium absorption should suppress PTH secretion and reduce osteoclastic bone resorption. Many clinicians have used pharmacologic doses of vitamin D to prevent and treat glucocorticoid-induced osteoporosis even though study results are equivocal. One study (111) indicated that calcitriol and 500 mg calcium daily prevented bone loss over a 2-year period. Trials have attempted treatment with vitamin D plus 500–1000 mg elemental calcium per day with less positive results; occasionally partial reversal of glucocorticoid-induced bone loss has been achieved. Frequently, the response to vitamin D and calcium is rapid initially and then plateaus. Histologic data indicate that bone formation is increased, and bone resorption is suppressed (112). Vitamin D toxicity in the form of hypercalciuria and hypercalcemia is present in the majority of patients and suggests that patients must be closely monitored while on steroid therapy. Patients with low levels of vitamin D should be placed on replacement therapy. In one study, the administration of calcium alone (1 g/d) was associated with a fall in urinary hydroxyproline levels without alterations in urine or serum calcium values or osteocalcin concentrations (113).

Recently, a randomized, double-blind, prospective study involved 103 patients on chronic glucocorticoid therapy who were randomized to receive oral calcium supplement and calcitriol with or without calcitonin (114). Patients were selected who had a variety of immunologic, rheumatologic, or respiratory diseases and had recently (within 4 weeks) initiated glucocorticoid therapy. Patients were randomized with stratification for age, sex, initial dose of prednisone or prednisolone, and underlying disease, and treatment for the first year was initiated. Physical activity was not controlled and all patients received 1000 mg elemental calcium daily. One group received calcitriol, 1.0 μg/d, and a placebo nasal spray. A second group received calcitriol and 400 IU salmon calcitonin nasal spray per day. The third group received placebo calcitriol tablets and placebo nasal spray. Bone density was measured by dual photon absorptiometry every 4 months for the 2 years of the study. Lateral thoracic and lumbar spine radiographs were obtained to determine the occurrence of vertebral fracture. The mean daily dose of corticosteroid was 13.5 mg for the first year and 7.5 mg for the second year.

Loss of bone from the lumbar spine was greater in patients treated with calcium alone, and an inverse dose–response relationship was noted in patients receiving calcitriol; those taking more calcitriol lost less bone. No statistically significant differences were noted in BMD measurements of the radius or femoral neck among the groups in the first year of therapy. However, glucocorticoid-induced bone loss from the lumbar spine was abrogated in the first year by treatment with calcium plus calcitriol, with or without calcitonin.

In the second year, therapies directed toward prevention of bone loss were discontinued despite continued glucocorticoid administration. Bone loss from the femoral neck and distal radius occurred in all groups. Mean bone loss from the lumbar spine continued in patients who had been treated with calcium alone or calcium and calcitriol.

The small number of subjects prevented any conclusions regarding fracture efficacy during the trial. Side effects of therapy included hypercalciuria in all patient groups suggesting the common etiology of corticosteroid therapy; renal function was not altered in these patients. Hypercalcemia occurred in 25% of patients; headaches in two patients and nasal symptoms in one patient prevented continuation of therapy.

Conclusions from this study include the fact that calcium and calcitriol may reduce corticosteroid bone loss, and the rate of lumbar spine mineral loss was less in patients treated with calcium and calcitriol as compared to controls. Bone loss from the lumbar spine was prevented by administration of calcium and calcitriol. Calcitonin may have longer-term effects, as in the second year of the study, patients treated in the first year with calcium, calcitriol, and calcitonin appear to have a persistent benefit from their treatment. With the high incidence of hypercalcemia in these patients, the risk–benefit ratio may need further evaluation (114).

The use of calcium and vitamin D supplementation appears warranted in view of the data presented thus far. In theory, the additional calcium and vitamin

D reverse the negative calcium balance resulting in increased calcium absorption, decreased calcium excretion, and a reduction in the presence of secondary hyperparathyroidism. The risk of hypercalcemia and hypercalciuria with attendant nephrocalcinosis or nephrolithiasis suggests that close monitoring of these patients is necessary.

Despite reduced intestinal calcium absorption, 24-hour urinary calcium concentration is increased in the first few months of glucocorticoid administration (115). A complementary approach is to reduce urinary calcium loss with hydrochlorothiazide, 25–50 mg twice daily. Thiazide therapy can reduce serum immunoreactive PTH levels in steroid-treated patients, and the use of thiazides with vitamin D and calcium therapy may reduce the risk of hypercalciuria (116,117). The efficacy of thiazide therapy in reducing bone loss in steroid-treated patients has not been examined. Thiazide diuretics may aggravate hypercalcemia in glucocorticoid-treated patients, and a combination of thiazide and amelioride, a potassium-sparing diuretic that also diminishes hypercalciuria, may be warranted. Serum calcium and potassium and urinary calcium concentrations must be monitored closely in these patients.

Clinical Studies of Bisphosphonate Use in Glucocorticoid-Induced Osteoporosis

Few studies have addressed the use of the bisphosphonates as a pharmacologic approach to the treatment of steroid-induced osteoporosis. An initial study using a new bisphosphonate pamidronate (APD) [(3-amino-1-hydroxy-propylidene)-1, 1 biphosphonate] indicated an increase in bone mineral at the lumbar spine as compared to controls (118). No significant side effects of this medication and no evidence for osteomalacia were noted. An additional study evaluated 150 mg APD administered daily to 16 glucocorticoid-treated patients and 19 steroid-treated controls (102). There was an early and sustained decrease in hydroxyproline excretion, consistent with the known inhibitory effects of APD on bone resorptive indices.

Calcitonin for the Treatment of Steroid-Induced Bone Loss

Treatment of glucocorticoid-induced osteoporosis with calcitonin has been attempted in glucocorticoid-treated patients. Calcitonin is a potent inhibitor of bone resorption, and most studies using this agent in glucocorticoid-induced osteoporosis are short term. In 18 patients receiving 100 IU of salmon calcitonin every other day for 6 months, increases in forearm BMD were noted (119). The disadvantage of parental administration limits its acceptability. In another prospective study, administration of intranasal calcitonin over 24 months protected the patients from glucocorticoid-induced osteoporosis (121). Calcitonin caused a 2.1% increase in bone mineral content (BMC) in the spine and an increase of 0.9% in the femoral neck compared to a decrease of 4.9% and 3.7%, respectively, in the placebo-controlled group. The most recent study suggests that calcitonin may provide long-term augmentation of the preventive effects of vitamin D and calcium supplementation (114).

Gonadal Hormone Replacement Therapy

The use of gonadal hormones to prevent and treat glucocorticoid-induced osteoporosis has not been adequately studied. A retrospective study of 15 postmenopausal or amenorrheic women (aged 34 to 78 years) who were on chronic prednisone therapy were compared to 17 age-matched women. Women were divided into those taking estrogen replacement therapy (ERT) (0.625 mg Premarin daily for 25 days and 5 mg medroxyprogesterone daily for 10 days) and those without ERT. Loss of bone from the lumbar spine was significant in the group that did not take ERT. The amount of bone loss was significantly correlated with the cumulative dose of prednisone in patients who were not given ERT. No relationship was obtained in glucocorticoid-treated patients receiving ERT. The authors concluded that ERT was protective against glucocorticoid-induced bone loss in this year-long study (91). Evidence suggests estrogen supplementation may be helpful in postmenopausal women or in women with glucocorticoid-induced amenorrhea. Men receiving glucocorticoid therapy should be evaluated for hypogonadism. In one study, serum levels of testosterone were reduced by 40% in steroid-treated patients (121). Testosterone replacement is appropriate for men with low serum testosterone levels. The anabolic steroid, nandrolone decanoate, given every 3 weeks intramuscularly, has been shown to increase forearm BMD in glucocorticoid-treated patients. Overall, experience with anabolic steroids has been limited.

In both sexes, the role of adrenal androgens in the maintenance of bone mass remains unknown. Recent data suggest the importance of the adrenal steroids in the maintenance of adequate bone mass (122). Concurrent suppression of the gonads and adrenal glands by glucocorticoids may aggravate the osteopenia in men and women. Most clinicians agree that hormone supplementation of the hypogonadal patient is an important therapeutic intervention in the prevention and treatment of glucocorticoid-induced osteopenia.

Progesterone may function as a glucocorticoid antagonist as it competes with cortisol and dexamethasone for glucocorticoid receptor occupancy on bone cells (25,28). In vitro, progesterone stimulates secretion of calcitonin from thyroid C cells (123). Because calcitonin may abrogate bone loss, this additional effect of progesterone may aid in the prevention of bone loss. Others have suggested a direct effect of synthetic progestins to increase bone formation (124,125). Several studies have advocated the administration of long-acting medroxyprogesterone acetate to patients on glucocorticoid therapy.

Sodium Fluoride for the Treatment of Glucocorticoid-Induced Osteoporosis

Fluoride has been used as an osteoblast stimulator. It increases osteoid surface and thickness and increases mineral apposition rate (126). In glucocorticoid-induced osteoporosis, fluoride treatment has produced inconsistent results (127–129). Rickers and colleagues found that sodium fluoride, administrated in combination with calcium, phosphate and vitamin D, did not decrease bone loss over a 6-month period (127). This period of observation may not have allowed full assessment of the therapeutic potential of fluoride. Common side effects of fluoride, such as gastrointestinal manifestations and lower extremity stress fractures, can be obviated by reduction of the therapeutic dose or administration of a slow-release preparation (126). The debate regarding appropriate dose and formulation suggests that this pharmacologic therapy should be restricted to well-controlled clinical trials.

▶ 217

Cytokines and Glucocorticoid Administration

Many paracrine and autocrine factors are responsible for the cellular interactions that occur during bone remodeling. In addition, both local and systemic factors have been found to alter bone cell proliferation or differentiation, singly or synergistically. For example, IL-1 (α and β) and tumor necrosis factor (α and β) stimulate bone resorption and prostaglandin production and inhibit collagen synthesis. Glucocorticoids alter the actions of these cytokines by direct inhibition of synthesis and interference with actions at the target site. Blockade of endogenous prostaglandins, for example, may abrogate the effects of epidermal growth factor, fibroblast growth factor, and platelet-derived growth factor, which promote bone resorption via prostaglandins.

Insulin-like growth factor I (IGF-I) and growth hormone (GH) are known stimulators of skeletal growth. Serum concentrations of IGF-I and GH are normal in glucocorticoid-treated patients (130,131). Some investigators have hypothesized that an inhibitor of GH is present in the sera of children receiving glucocorticoids (132).

TABLE 8-1 Prevention of Glucocorticoid-Induced Osteopenia

Prophylaxis
  Maintain lowest possible glucocorticoid dose.
  General measures:
    Regular program of weight-bearing physical activity.
    Eliminate adverse health habits—smoking, alcohol excess.
    Adequate calcium intake (800 mg/d premenopausal and 1500 mg/d postmenopausal).
  Reduce urinary calcium loss during the initial 6–24 month calciuric phase of steroid
    therapy with hydrochlorothiazide 25–50 mg twice daily.
  When 24-h urine calcium returns to normal, cautiously treat with vitamin D 50,000 units
    1–3 times per week (or 25-(OH)D 50 μg 3–5 times per week) plus calcium supplemen-
    tation to maintain serum 25-(OH)D at 1.5–2 times upper limits of normal, iPTH sup-
    pressed, and 24-h urine calcium at 2.5–3.5 mg/kg body weight. Alternatively, calcitriol
    0.5–1.0 μg/d and 1000 mg elemental calcium per day can be administered.

Therapeutic Recommendations

Vitamin D metabolite and calcium therapy are current therapeutic modalities used for the treatment of glucocorticoid-induced osteoporosis. The timing of initiation of such treatment is important, and high-risk individuals should be started early in their course of steroid therapy to prevent significant bone loss (Tables 8-1 and 8-2; 133). Because the initial phase of glucocorticoid therapy is characterized by increased urinary calcium excretion and the risk of nephrocalcinosis is increased in steroid-treated patients who have not received vitamin D or calcium supplementation, early initiation of vitamin D and calcium therapy could theoretically increase the risk of harmful effects of hypercalciuria. Therefore, the use of hydrochlorothiazide, 25 to 50 mg twice daily, to reduce urinary calcium excretion is recommended. After 12 to 18 months, when urinary calcium excretion returns to normal, vitamin D and calcium supplementation can be initiated. Vitamin D, 50,000 units, two to three times weekly, (or 25-(OH)D,

TABLE 8-2 Treatment of Established Glucocorticoid-Induced Osteopenia

Exclude secondary causes of osteoporosis.
Maintain lowest possible glucocorticoid dose.
General measures as for prevention of glucocorticoid-induced osteoporosis.
If 24-h urine calcium ≥4 mg/kg/d use hydrochlorothiazide to reduce urinary calcium
  excretion.
If 24-h urine calcium <3.5 mg/kg/d treat with vitamin D metabolites and calcium
  (± hydrochlorothiazide) as above.
Estrogen therapy may reduce bone loss in postmenopausal women.
Hypogonadism in men warrants testosterone administration.

Adapted from Hahn TJ. Steroid and drug induced osteopenia. In: Favus MJ, ed. Primer on metabolic bone diseases and disorders of mineral metabolism. Kelseyville, CA: American Society for Bone and Mineral Research, 1990;158–162.

50 μg 5 days per week), plus 1000 mg elemental calcium per day, may prevent glucocorticoid-induced bone loss. The serum 25-(OH)D concentration should be maintained at 1.5 to 2 times the upper limit of normal, and serum PTH levels should be normal to suppressed. At the same time, hypercalciuria and hypercalcemia should be avoided. Serum and 24-hour urinary calcium values should be monitored at 1- to 2-month intervals.

Monitoring the Cushingoid Patient

The extent of bone loss in patients with Cushing's disease is difficult to evaluate ▶ 219
because many of the studies are cross-sectional. This makes it unfeasible to determine the condition of the patient's skeleton before the advent of Cushing's disease and whether bone loss was linear over time. Bone loss in patients with Cushing's disease has been shown to be partially reversible (134,135). Therefore, the surgical treatment of Cushing's disease is important in the prevention of further bone loss. In young patients (less than 50 years of age), up to 20% increase in bone density of the lumbar spine has been noted after surgical correction of Cushing's syndrome. Bone density should be measured every 6 months during this phase of rapid bone loss.

Summary

The pathogenesis of glucocorticoid-induced osteoporosis is poorly understood. The interactions between glucocorticoids, bone, and growth factors are being explored and may lead to direct clinical recommendations regarding the prevention of this disorder. Assessment of other risk factors for osteoporosis and prevention of negative calcium balance in each individual patient are the current recommendations for the management of this clinically vexing problem. The initiation of well-designed, prospective clinical trials is necessary to evaluate fully the efficacy of various treatments to prevent glucocorticoid-associated bone loss.

References

1. Cushing H. The basophil adenomas of the pituitary body and their clinical manifestations (pituitary basophilism). Bull Johns Hopk Hosp 1932;50:137–142.

2. Ansell BM. Bywaters EGL. Growth in Still's disease. Ann Rheum Dis 1956;15:295–319.

3. Baylink DJ. Glucocorticoid-induced osteoporosis. N Engl J Med 1983;309:306–308.

4. Carpenter PC. Diagnostic evaluation of Cushing's syndrome. Endocrinol Metab Clin North Am 1988;17(3):445–472.

5. Cryer PE, Kissane JM, eds. Vertebral compression fractures with accelerated bone turnover in a patient with Cushing's disease (clinicopathologic conference). Am J Med 1980;68(6):932–940.

6. Greenberger PA, Hendrix RW, Patterson R, et al. Bone studies in patients on prolonged systemic corticosteroid therapy for asthma. Clin Allergy 1982;12(4): 363–368.

7. Hough S, Teitelbaum SL, Bergfeld MA, et al. Isolated skeletal involvement in Cushing's syndrome: response to therapy. J Clin Endocrinol Metab 1981;52(5):1033–1038.

8. Howland WJ Jr, Pugh DG, Sprague RG. Roentgenologic changes of the skeletal system in Cushing's syndrome. Radiology 1958;71:69–78.

9. Need AG. Corticosteroids and osteoporosis. Aust N Z J Med 1987;17(2): 267–272.

10. Petersen P, Jacobsen SEH. Cushing's disease presenting with severe osteoporosis. Acta Endocrinol (Copenh) 1986; 111(2):168–171.

11. Sprague RG, Randall RV, Salassa RM, et al. Cushing's syndrome: a progressive and often fatal disease: a review of 100 cases seen between July 1945 and July 1954 Arch Intern Med 1956;98:389–397.

12. Bressot C, Meunier PJ, Chapuy MC, Lejeune E, Edourd C, Darby AJ. Histomorphometric profile, pathophysiology and reversibility of corticosteroid-induced osteoporosis. Metab Bone Dis Rel Res 1979;1:303–319.

13. de Deuxchaisnes CN, Devogelaer JP, Esselinckx W, et al. The effect of low dosage glucocorticoids on bone mass in rheumatoid arthritis: a cross-sectional and a longitudinal study using single photon absorptiometry. Adv Exp Med Biol 1984; 171:210–239.

14. Sambrook PN, Birmingham, J, Kempler S, et al. Corticosteroid effects on proximal femur bone loss. J Bone Miner Res 1990:5:1211–1216.

15. Gennari C, Civitelli R. Glucocorticoid-induced osteoporosis. Clin Rheum Dis 1986;12:637–654.

16. LoCascio V, Bonucci E, Imbimbo B, et al. Bone loss in response to long-term glucocorticoid therapy. Bone Miner 1990; 8:39–51.

17. Reed IR, Heap SW. Determinants of vertebral mineral density in patients receiving long-term glucocorticoid therapy. Arch Intern Med 1990;150:2545–2548.

18. Varanos S, Ansell BM, Reeve J. Vertebral collapse in juvenile chronic arthritis: its relationship with glucocorticoid therapy. Calcif Tissue Int 1987;41(2):75–78.

19. Als OS, Gotfredsen A, Christiansen C. The effect of glucocorticoids on bone mass in rheumatoid arthritis patients: influence of menopausal state. Arthritis Rheum 1985;28(4):369–375.

20. Shane E, Rivas MDC, Silverberg SJ, Kim TS, Staron RB, Bilezikian JP. Osteoporosis after cardiac transplantation. Am J Med 1993;94:257–264.

21. Schlosberg M, Movsowitz C, Epstein S, Ismall F, Fallon MD, Thomas S. The effect of cyclosporin A administration and its withdrawal on bone mineral metabolism in the rat. Endocrinology 1989; 124:2179–2184.

22. Movsowitz C, Epstein S, Ismall F, Fallon M, Thomas S. Cyclosporin A in the oophorectomized rat: unexpected severe bone resorption. J Bone Miner Res 1989;4:393–398.

23. Dempster DW, Arlot MA, Meunier PJ. Mean wall thickness formation periods of trabecular bone packets in corticosteroid-induced osteoporosis. Calcif Tissue Int 1983;35:410–417.

24. Peck WA, Brandt J, Miller I. Hydrocortisone-induced inhibition of protein synthesis and uridine incorporation in isolated bone cells in vitro. Proc Natl Acad Sci USA 1987;57:1599–1606.

25. Feldman D, Dziak R, Koehler R, Stern P. Cytoplasmic glucocorticoid binding proteins in bone cells. Endocrinology 1975;96(1):29–36.

26. Subramaniam M, Colvard D, Keeting P, Rasmussen K, Riggs BL, Spelsberg

TC. Glucocorticoid regulation of alkaline phosphatase, osteocalcin and proto-oncogenes in normal human osteoblast-like cells. J Cell Biochem 1992;50(4):411–424.

27. Canalis E. Effect of glucocorticoids on type I collagen synthesis, alkaline phosphatase activity and deoxyribonucleic acid content in cultured rat calvariae. Endocrinology 1983;112(3):931–939.

28. Chen TL, Aronow L, Feldman D. Glucocorticoid receptors and inhibition of bone cell growth in primary culture. Endocrinology 1977;100(3):619–628.

29. Haussler MR, Manolagas SC, Deftos LJ. Glucocorticoid receptor in clonal osteosarcoma cell lines: a novel system for investigating bone active hormones. Biochem Biophys Res Commun 1980;94(1):373–380.

30. Manolagas SC, Anderson DC. Detection of high-affinity glucocorticoid binding in rat bone. J Endocrinol 1978;76(2):379–380.

31. Rath NC, Reddi AH. Influence of adrenalectomy and dexamethasone on matrix-induced endochondral bone differentiation. Endocrinology 1979;104(6):1698–1704.

32. Wong GL. Basal activities and hormone responsiveness of osteoclast-like and osteoblast-like bone cells are regulated by glucocorticoids. J Biol Chem 1979;254(14):6337–6340.

33. Gallagher JA, Beresford JN, MacDonald BR, Russell RGG. Hormone target cell interactions in human bone. In: Christiansen C, ed. Osteoporosis. Glostrup Hospital, 1984;431–439.

34. Shalhoub V, Conlon D, Tassinari M, Quinn C, Partridge N, Stein GS. Glucocorticoids promote development of the osteoblast phenotype by selectively modulating expression of cell growth and differentiation associated genes. J Cell Biochem 1992;50:425–440.

35. Oursler MJ, Riggs BL, Spelsberg TC. Glucocorticoid induced activation of latent transforming growth factor-β by normal human osteoblast-like cells. Endocrinology 1993;133:2187–2196.

36. Gallagher JC, Aaron J, Horsman A, Wilkinson R, Nordin BE. Corticosteroid osteoporosis. Clin Endocrinol Metab 1973;2:355–368.

37. Lo Cascio V, Bonucci E, Imbimbo B, et al. Bone loss after glucocorticoid therapy. Calcif Tissue Int 1984;36(4):435–438.

38. Lund B, Storm TL, Lund B, et al. Bone mineral loss, bone histomorphometry and vitamin D metabolism in patients with rheumatoid arthritis on long-term glucocorticoid treatment. Clin Rheumatol 1985;4:143–149.

39. Meunier PJ, Dempster DW, Edouard C, et al. Bone histomorphometry in corticosteroid-induced osteoporosis and Cushing's syndrome. Adv Exp Med Biol 1984;171:191–200.

40. Stellon AJ, Davies A, Compston J, et al. Bone loss in autoimmune chronic active hepatitis on maintenance corticosteroid therapy. Gastroenterology 1985;89(5):1078–1083.

41. Adinoff AD, Hollister JR. Steroid-induced fractures and bone loss in patients with asthma. N Engl J Med 1983;309(5):265–268.

42. Hahn TJ, Halstead LR, Teitelbaum ST, et al. Altered mineral metabolism in glucocorticoid-induced osteopenia: effect of 25-hydroxyvitamin D administration. J Clin Invest 1979;64(2):655–665.

43. Mitchell DR, Lyles KW. Glucocorticoid-induced osteoporosis: mechanisms for bone loss; evaluation of strategies for prevention. J Gerontol 1990;45:M153-158.

44. Nielsen HK, Charles P, Mosekilde L. The effect of single oral doses of prednisone on the circadian rhythm of serum osteocalcin in normal subjects. J Clin Endocrinol Metab 1988;67:1025–1030.

45. Gosschalk MF, Downs RW. Effect of short-term glucocorticoids on serum osteocalcin in healthy young men. J Bone Min Res 1988;3:113–115.

46. Nielsen HK, Brixen D, Kassem M, Mosekilde L. Acute effect of 1,25-dihydroxyvitamin D_3, prednisone, and 1,25-dihydroxyvitamin D_3 plus prednisone on serum osteocalcin in normal individuals. J Bone Miner Res 1991;6:435–441.

47. Jowell PS, Epstein S, Fallon MD, Reinhardt TA, Ismail F. 1,25-dihydroxyvitamin D_3 modulates of glucocorticoid-induced alteration in serum bone Gla protein and bone histomorphometry. Endocrinology 1987;120:531–536.

48. Reid IR, Chapman GE, Fraser TRC, Davis AD, Surus AS, Meyer J. Low serum osteocalcin levels in glucocorticoid treated asthmatics. J Clin Endocrinol Metab 1986;62:379–383.

49. Meunier PJ, Bressot C. Endocrine influences on bone cells and bone remodeling evaluated by clinical histomorphometry. In: Parsons JA, ed. Endocrinology of Calcium Metabolism. New York: Raven Press, 1982;445–465.

50. Bar-Shavit Z, Kahn AJ, Pegg LE, Stone KR, Teitelbaum SL. Glucocorticoids modulate macrophage surface of oligosaccharides and their bone binding activity. J Clin Invest 1984;73:1277–1283.

51. Reid IR, Katz JM, Ibbertson HK, Gray DH. The effects of hydrocortisone, parathyroid hormone, and the bisphosphonate, APD, on bone resorption in neonatal mouse calvaria. Calcif Tissue Int 1986; 38:38–43.

52. Jee WSS, Roberts WI, Park HZ, Julian G, Kramer M. Interrelated effects of glucocorticoid and parathyroid hormone upon bone remodeling. In: Talmage RV, Munson PL, eds. Calcium, parathyroid hormone and the calcitonins. Amsterdam: Excerpta Medica, 1972:430.

53. De Franco DJ, Lian JB, Glowacki J. Differential effects of glucocorticoid on recruitment and activity of osteoclasts induced by normal and osteocalcin–deficient bone implanted in rats. Endocrinology 1992;131:114–121.

54. Caniggia A, Gennari C. Effect of 25-hydroxycholecalciferol (25-OHCC) on intestinal absorption of [47]Ca in four cases of iatrogenic Cushing's syndrome. Helv Med Acta 1973;37:221–225.

55. Colette C, Monnier L, Pares Herbute N, Blotman F, Mirouze J. Calcium absorption in corticoid-treated subjects: effects of a single oral dose of calcitriol. Horm Metabol Res 1987;19:335–338.

56. Klein RG, Arnaud SB, Gallagher JC, DeLuca HF, Riggs BL. Intestinal calcium absorption in exogenous hypercortisonism. Role of 25-hydroxyvitamin D and corticosteroid dose. J Clin Invest 1977;60:253–259.

57. Hirts M, Feldmen D. Glucocorticoids down-regulate the number of 1,25-dihydroxyvitamin D receptors in mouse intestine. Biochem Biophys Res Commun 1982;105:1590–1596.

58. Kimberg DV, Baeig RD, Gershon E, Graudusius RT. Effect of cortisone treatment on the active transport of calcium by the small intestine. J Clin Invest 1971; 50:1309–1321.

59. Yeh JK, Aloia JF, Semla HM. Interrelation of cortisone and 1,25-dihydroxycholecalciferol on intestinal calcium and phosphate absorption. Calcif Tissue Int 1984;36:608–614.

60. Kimura S, Rasmussen H. Adrenal glucocorticoids, adenine nucleotide translocation and mitochondrial calcium accumulation. J Biol Chem 1977;252:1217–1225.

61. Charney AN, Kinsey MD, Myers L, Giannella RA, Gots RE. Na^+-K^+-activated adenosine triphosphatase and intestinal electrolyte transport. Effect of adrenal steroids. J Clin Invest 1975;56:653–660.

62. Feher JJ, Wasserman RH. Intestinal calcium binding protein and calcium absorption in cortisol treated chicks, effects of vitamin D_3 and 1,25-dihydroxyvitamin D_3. Endocrinology 1979;104:547–551.

63. Hahn TJ, Halstead LR, Baran DT. Effect of short-term glucocorticoid administration on intestinal calcium absorption and circulating vitamin D metabolite concentrations in man. J Clin Endocrinol Metab 1981;52:111–115.

64. Nielsen HK, Thomsen K, Eriksen EF, et al. The effects of high-dose glucocorticoid administration on serum bone gamma carboxyglutamic acid-containing protein, serum alkaline phosphatase and vitamin D metabolites in normal subjects. Bone Miner 1988;4(1):105–113.

65. Lukert BP, Adams JS. Calcium and phosphorus homeostasis in man: effect of corticoteroids. Arch Intern Med 1976; 136(11):1249–1253.

Osteoporosis

66. Gennari C, Imbimbo B, Montagnani M, et al. Effects on prednisone and deflazacort on mineral metabolism and parathyroid hormone activity in humans. Calcif Tissue Int 1984;36(3):245–252.

67. Aloia JF, Roginsky M, Ellis K, et al. Skeletal metabolism and body composition in Cushing's syndrome. J Clin Endocrinol Metab 1974;39(6):981–985.

68. Chesney RW, Mazess RB, Hamstra AJ, DeLuca HF, O'Reagan S. Reduction of serum-1, 25-dihydroxyvitamin D_3 in children receiving glucocorticoids. Lancet 1978;2:1123–1125.

69. Adams JS, Lukert BP. Effects of sodium restriction of ^{45}Ca and ^{22}Na transduodenal flux in corticosteroid-treated rats. Miner Electrolyte Metab 1980;4:216–226.

70. Lukert BP, Stanbury SW, Mawer EB. Vitamin D and intestinal transport of calcium: effects of prednisolone. Endocrinology 1973;93:718–722.

71. Adams JS, Wahl TO, Lukert BP. Effect of hydrochlorothiazide and dietary sodium restriction on calcium metabolism in corticosteroid treated patients. Metabolism 1981;30:217–221.

72. Favus MJ, Walling MW, Kimberg DV. Effects of 1,25-dihydroxycholecalciferol on intestinal calcium transport in cortisone-treated rats. J Clin Invest 1973,52.1800 1805.

73. Fox J, Care AD, Blahos J. Effects of low calcium and low phosphorus diets on the duodenal absorption of calcium in betamethasone-treated chicks. J Endocrinol 1978;78:255–260.

74. Bikle DD, Halloran B, Fong L, Steinbach L, Shellito J. Elevated 1,25-dihydroxyvitamin D levels in patients with chronic obstructive pulmonary disease treated with prednisone. J Clin Endocrinol Metab 1993;76:456–461.

75. Milsom S, Ibbertson K, Hannan S, Shaw D, Pybus J. Simple test of intestinal calcium absorption measured by stable strontium. BMJ 1987;295:231–234.

76. Findling JW, Adams ND, Lemann J Jr, et al. Vitamin D metabolites and parathyroid hormone in Cushing's syndrome: relationship to calcium and phosphorus homeostasis. J Clin Endocrinol Metab 1982;54(5):1039–1044.

77. Fucik RF, Kukreja SC, Hargis GK, et al. Effect of glucocorticoids on function of the parathyroid glands in man. J Clin Endocrinol Metab 1975;40(1):152–155.

78. Au WYW. Cortisol stimulation of parathyroid hormone secretion by rat parathyroid glands in organ culture. Science 1976;193(4257):1015–1017.

79. Chen TL, Feldman D. Glucocorticoid receptors and actions in subpopulations of cultured rat bone cells. Mechanism of dexamethasone potentiation of parathyroid hormone-stimulated cyclic AMP production. J Clin Invest 1979;63:750–758.

80. Catherwood BD. 1,25-dihydrocholecalciferol and glucocorticoid regulation of adenylate cyclase in an osteoblast-like cell line. J Biol Chem 1985;160:736–743.

81. Ng B, Hekkelman JW, Heersche JN. The effect of cortisol on the adenosine 3,5-monophosphate response to parathyroid hormone in cultured rat bone cells. Endocrinology 1979;102:589–596.

82. Heersche JN, Jez DH, Aubin J, Sodek J. Regulation of hormone responsiveness of bone in vitro by corticosteroids, PTH, PGE_2 and calcitonin. In: Talmade RV, Cohn DV, Matthews JL, eds. Hormonal control of calcium metabolism. Amsterdam: Excerpta Medica, 1981:157–162 (International Congress series no. 511).

83. Doerr P, Pirke KM. Cortisol-induced suppression of plasma testosterone in normal adult males. J Clin Endocrinol Metab 1976;43:622–628.

84. Schaison G, Durand F, Mowszowicz I. Effect of glucocorticoids on plasma testosterone in men. Acta Endocrinol (Copenh) 1978;89:126–131.

85. MacAdams MR, White RH, Chipps BE. Reduction of serum testosterone levels during chronic glucocorticoid therapy. Ann Intern Med 1986;104:648–651.

86. Vermeulen A, Verdonck L, van der Straeten M, Orie N. Capacity of the testosterone-binding globulin in human plasma and influence of specific binding of testosterone on its metabolic clearance rate. J Clin Endocrinol 1969;29:1470–1480.

87. Sakakura M, Takebe K, Nakagawa S.

▶ 223

Inhibition of luteinizing hormone secretion induced by synthetic LRH by long-term treatment with glucocorticoids in human subjects. J Clin Endocrinol Metab 1975; 40:774–779.

88. Crilly RG, Cawood M, Marshall DH, Nordin BE. Hormonal status in normal, osteoporotic and corticosteroid-treated postmenopausal women. J Royal Soc Med 1978;71:733–736.

89. Goulding A, Gold E. Effects of chronic prednisolone treatment on bone resorption and bone composition in intact and in ovariectomized rats receiving β-estradiol. Endocrinology 1988;122:482–487.

90. Sprague RG, Power MH, Mason HL, et al. Observations on the physiologic effects of cortisone and ACTH in man. Arch Intern Med 1950;85:199–258.

91. Lukert BP, Johnson, Robinson RG. Estrogen and progesterone replacement therapy reduces glucocorticoid-induced bone loss. J Bone Miner Res 1992;7:1063–1069.

92. Boe J, Skoogh BE. Is long-term treatment with inhaled steroids in adults hazardous? Eur Respir J 1992;5:1037–1039.

93. Smith MJ, Hodson ME. Effect of long-term inhaled high dose beclomethasone dipropionate on adrenal function. Thorax 1983;38:676–681.

94. Gordon ACH, McDonald CF, Thompson, SA, Frame MH, Pottage A, Crompton GK. Dose of inhaled budesonide required to produce clinical suppression of plasma cortisol. Eur J Respir Dis 1987;71:10–14.

95. Jennings BH, Andersson KE, Johansson SA. The assessment of the systemic effects of inhaled glucocorticosteroids. Eur J Clin Pharmacol 1991;41:11–16.

96. Puolijoki H, Liippo K, Herrala J, Salmi J, Tala E. Inhaled beclomethasone decreases serum osteocalcin in postmenopausal asthmatic women. Bone 1992;13:285–288.

97. Seeman E, Wagner HW, Offord KP, Kumar R, Johnson WJ, Riggs BL. Differential effects of endocrine dysfunction on the axial and appendicular skeleton. J Clin Invest 1982;69:1302–1309.

98. Lukert BP, Raisz LG. Glucocorticoid-induced osteoporosis: pathogenesis and management. Ann Intern Med 1990; 112:352–364.

99. Hodgson SF. Corticosteroid-induced osteoporosis. Endocrinol Metab Clin North Am 1990;19:95–111.

100. Villareal DT, Civitelli R, Gennari C, Avioli LV. Is there an effective treatment for glucocorticoid-induced osteoporosis? Calcif Tissue Int 1991;49:141–142.

101. Kimberly RP. Mechanisms of action, dosage schedules, and side effects of steroid therapy. Curr Opin Rheumatol 1991;3:373–379.

102. Reid IR, Schooler BA, Stewart AW. Prevention of glucocorticoid-induced osteoporosis. J Bone Miner Res 1990;5:619–623.

103. Fauci AS. Alternate-day corticosteroid therapy. Am J Med 1978;64:729–731.

104. Gluck OS, Murphy WA, Hahn TJ, Hahn B. Bone loss in adults receiving alternate day glucocorticoid therapy. Arthritis Rheum 1981;24:892–898.

105. Hahn TJ, Halstead LR, Strates B, Imbimbo B, Baran DT. Comparison of subacute effects of oxazacort and prednisone on mineral metabolism in man. Calcif Tissue Int 1980;31:109–115.

106. Devogelaer JP, Juaux JP, Dufour JP, et al. Bone-sparing action of deflazacort versus equipotent doses of prednisone: a double-blind study in males with rheumatoid arthritis. In: Christiansen C, Johansen JS, Riis BJ, eds. Osteoporosis. Copenhagen: Osteoporosis Aps, 1987:1014–1015.

107. Olgaard K, Storm T, Wowern NV, et al. Glucocorticoid-induced osteoporosis in the lumbar spine, forearm, and mandible of nephrotic patients: a double-blind study on the high-dose, long-term effects of prednisone versus deflazacort. Calcif Tissue Int 1992;50:490–497.

108. Gennari C. Differential effect of glucocorticoids on calcium absorption and bone mass. Br J Rheumatol 1993;32:11–14.

109. Medici TC, Ruegsegger P. Does alternate-day cloprednol therapy prevent bone loss? A longitudinal double-blind, controlled clinical study. Clin Pharmacol Ther 1990;48:455–466.

110. Aloia JF, Cohn SH, Ostuni JA, Cane R, Ellis K. Prevention of involutional bone

loss by exercise. Ann Intern Med 1978;39:356–358.

111. Hahn TJ, Halstead LR, Teitelbaum SL, Hahn BH. Altered mineral metabolism in glucocorticoid-induced osteopenia: effect of 25-hydroxyvitamin D administration. J Clin Invest 1979;64:655–665.

112. Braun JJ, Birkenhager-Frenkel DH, Rietveld AH, et al. Influence of 1α-(OH)D₃ administration on bone and bone mineral metabolism in patients on chronic glucocorticoid treatment: a double blind controlled study. Clin Endocrinol (Oxf) 1983;19(2):265–273.

113. Reid IR, Ibbertson HK. Calcium supplements in the prevention of steroid-induced osteoporosis. Am J Clin Nutr 1986;44(2):287–299.

114. Sambrook P, Birmingham J, Kelly P, et al. Prevention of corticosteroid osteoporosis. N Engl J Med 1993;328:1747–1752.

115. Sambrook PN, Eisman JA, Yeates MG, Pocock NA, Eberl S, Champion GD. Osteoporosis in rheumatoid arthritis: safety of low dose corticosteroids. Ann Rheum Dis 1986;45:950–953.

116. Reid IR. Steroid osteoporosis. Calcif Tissue Int 1989;45:63–67.

117. Suzuki Y, Ichikawa Y, Saito E, Homma M. Importance of increased urinary calcium excretion in the development of secondary hyperparathyroidism of patients under glucocorticoid therapy. Metabolism 1983;32:151–156.

118. Reid IR, Heap SW, King AR, Ibbertson HK. Two-year follow-up of bisphosphonate (APD) treatment in steroid osteoporosis. Lancet 1988;2:1144.

119. Ringe JD, Welzel D. Salmon calcitonin in the therapy of corticosteroid-induced osteoporosis. Eur J Clin Pharmacol 1987:33:35–39.

120. Ringe JD. Treatment of primary osteoporosis with calcium and salmon calcitonin. Dtsch Med Wochenschr 1990; 115:1176–1182.

121. Reid IR, France JT, Pybus J, Ibbertson HK. Plasma testosterone concentrations in asthmatic men treated with glucocorticoids. BMJ 1985;291:574.

122. Clarke BL, Ebeling PR, Jones JD, O'Fallon WM, Riggs BL, Fitzpatrick LA.

Increased bone turnover with aging in men is not due to testosterone deficiency. Submitted to the Endocrine Society, Las Vegas, NV 1993;1617A.

123. Greenberg C, Kukrejas C, Bowser EN, Hargis GK, Henderson WJ, Williams GA. Effects of estradiol and progesterone on calcitonin secretion. Endocrinology 1986;118:2594–2598.

124. Christiansen C, Riis BJ, Nilas L, Rodbro P, Deftos L. Uncoupling of bone formation and resorption by combines estrogen and progestogen therapy in postmenopausal osteoporosis. Lancet 1985;ii: 800–801.

125. Grecu EO, Simmons R, Baylink DJ, Haloran BP, Spencer ME. Effects of medroxyprogesterone acetate on some parameters of calcium metabolism in patients with glucocorticoid-induced osteoporosis. Bone Miner 1991;13:153–161.

126. Kleerekoper M, Mendlovic DB. Sodium fluoride therapy of postmenopausal osteoporosis. Endocr Rev 1993;14:312–323.

127. Rickers H, Deding A, Christiansen C, Rodbro P, Naestoft J. Corticosteroid-induced osteopenia and vitamin D metabolism. Effect of vitamin D₂, calcium, phosphate and sodium fluoride administration. Clin Endocrinol 1982;16:409–415.

128. Meunier PJ, Dempster DW, Edouard C, Chapuy MC, Arlot M, Charhon S. Bone histomorphometry in corticosteroid-induced osteoporosis in Cushing's syndrome. Adv Exp Med Biol 1984;171:191–200.

129. Hedlund LR, Gallagher JC. Increase incidence of hip fracture in osteoporotic women treated with sodium fluoride. J Bone Min Res 1989;4(2):223–225.

130. Morris HG, Jorgenson JR, Jenkins SA. Plasma growth hormone concentrations in corticosteroid-treated children. J Clin Invest 1968;47:427–435.

131. Gourmelen M, Girard F, Binoux M. Serum somatomedin/insulin-like growth factor (IGF) and IGF carrier levels in patients with Cushing's syndrome or receiving glucocorticoid therapy. J Clin Endocrinol Metab 1982;54:885–892.

132. Unterman TG, Phillips LS. Glucocorticoid effects on somatomedins and so-

▶ 225

matomedin inhibitors. J Clin Endocrinol Metab 1985;61:618–626.

133. Hahn TJ. Steroid and drug induced osteopenia. In: MJ Favus, ed. Primer on the metabolic bone diseases and disorders of mineral metabolism. Kelseyville, Calif: American Society for Bone and Mineral Research, 1990:158–162.

134. Pocock NA, Eismon JA, Dunstan CR, Evans RA, Thomas DH, Huq NL. Recovery from steroid-induced osteoporosis. Ann Intern Med 1982;107:319–323.

135. Lufkin EG, Wahner HW, Bergstralk EJ. Reversibility of steroid-induced osteoporosis. Am J Med 1988;85:887–888.

226 ◄

9 ▸ Calcium and Vitamin D in the Pathogenesis and Treatment of Osteoporosis

▶ ▶ ▶ Susan M. Ott

Calcium

"Calcium to prevent osteoporosis" is in the news, on television, in the magazines, and in the on-line instructions for the Medline search program that give "calcium intake and osteoporosis" as the example for how to search for key words. Performing the search reveals great diversity, from Kanis's "Calcium supplementation of the diet—not justified by the present evidence" (1) to Nordin and Heaney's "Calcium supplementation of the diet—justified by present evidence" (2). Reviewing those papers, I have come to agree with Parfitt's conclusion: ". . . calcium deficiency, once variously regarded as a non-existent condition in human beings, and as the major cause of age-related bone loss, now occupies a middle ground as one of many contributors to fracture risk, not the most important but the easiest to correct" (3).

The first part of this chapter reviews the published evidence about the mechanisms of calcium effects on the skeleton, including the requirements to match the obligatory losses, regulation of parathyroid hormone (PTH), and other biochemical effects. The remodeling barrier is discussed in relationship to any therapy that blocks bone resorption. The effect of calcium may also relate to mechanical strain and physicochemical mechanisms. The physiology of calcium absorption is reviewed, showing the influence of calcium intake, the absorbability of different preparations, and the effects of food, gastric acidity, and aging. A variety of studies give data relating to possible therapeutic effects of calcium: epidemiologic surveys, relationships between calcium intake and fracture, calcium balance data, and clinical studies of calcium intake and bone mineral density (BMD), which are cross-sectional, longitudinal, prospective, and randomized. Finally, some practical aspects of calcium therapy are considered. The second part of the chapter considers vitamin D.

The following frustrations must be kept in mind when interpreting calcium studies: (1) In calcium physiology, relationships are seldom linear. For example, as calcium intake increases, the percent absorbed by the intestine decreases, so urine excretion is not a direct function of intake. Changes in bone mass are also nonlinear; acute effects are often more pronounced than chronic ones. (2) Bone changes slowly; the remodeling system takes months to readjust to manipulation. This means studies must be long term and measurement techniques must be precise. (3) Calcium is not the most important factor in bone loss, and studies not meticulously controlled for other factors will fail to see a calcium effect. (4) Commercial interests interject bias to the research. (5) There is no good way to validate calcium intake and people are notorious for their lack of reliability in reporting what they actually eat (4). (6) Information or misinformation about nutrition in general and calcium specifically is so abundant that it influences behavior of study participants.

Mechanisms of Calcium Effects on the Skeleton

The mechanistic details of the effects of calcium on the skeleton are complex. Calcium must be ingested to avoid deficiency. Beyond that, calcium alters the bone-related hormones and possibly the local hormones induced by mechanical stress. Calcium could alter the physicochemical properties of the bone mineral.

REQUIREMENTS TO MATCH OBLIGATORY LOSSES

Many people would like to believe that they could prevent osteoporosis by increasing their calcium intake. Merely providing adequate or even excess calcium, however, is not sufficient to prevent bone loss. Because the colon, kidney, and skin cannot perfectly conserve calcium, it is a physiologic imperative that at some level the dietary calcium will be too low to meet obligatory losses. To maintain stable plasma calcium levels, calcium would then be removed from the bone. The magnitude of this required calcium intake is still uncertain.

Calcium kinetic studies have attempted to define obligatory calcium losses. The intestines both absorb and secrete calcium. In pathologic conditions the intestine can secrete large amounts of calcium, which exacerbates calcium deficiency. In normal people, the intestinal calcium loss from digestive juices and desquamated epithelial cells is about 140 mg/d, but some of this is reabsorbed (5). Dermal losses of calcium amount to about 60 mg/d (6).

Urine calcium concentration varies greatly, and not all of this variation can be explained by the calcium intake. Even when calcium absorption is measured, it explains only about 46% of the variability in urine calcium content (7). Cross-sectional calcium balance studies provide useful information (discussed later), but they do not necessarily demonstrate the magnitude of obligatory losses, especially from the kidney. Studies that show high urine calcium values may be misleading if the urine calcium is assumed to represent a renal *loss* rather than a renal *response* to increased calcium load. If there is primary bone loss, the urine calcium value increases. Dramatic examples are astronauts or immobilized patients with spinal cord injuries, whose urine calcium level exceeds 450 mg/d (8). Patients maintained on chronic parenteral nutrition also have increased urinary calcium values, especially when the nutrition is initiated (9). Infusing more calcium does not solve this problem; it may exacerbate it. The infused calcium can decrease the circulating PTH level and, therefore, the tubular resorption of calcium will decrease and urine calcium content will increase even more.

▶ 229

The kidneys are capable of preserving calcium. Patients with malabsorption have urine calcium values as low as 7 mg/d, even with serum calcium values in the normal range. Thus, there is hardly any normal "obligatory" urine calcium loss. In elderly patients, however, renal tubular function may be impaired. Excessive salt loading, protein loads, or diuretics (including caffeine) will also prevent the kidney from conserving calcium.

Calcium balance studies reported by Malm (10) in 1958 in healthy middle-aged male prisoners showed that 38 of 39 were in positive calcium balance on a calcium intake of 937 mg/d. When the intake was dropped to 460 mg/d, 3 of 26 adapted immediately and 3 did not adapt. The other 20 men had an initial period of negative balance and then slowly adapted over 188 days to neutral or slightly negative balance; only 7 of these regained the deficit caused by the initial period of calcium loss. The adaptation was at the level of increased gastrointestinal absorption and not from better urine conservation. This study demonstrates that short-term responses to a low-calcium diet differ from long-term adaptations. Although the study shows that normal adults are capable of stable calcium metabolism on a limited intake of 460 mg/d, the results cannot be extrapolated to other ages. Children require more calcium because they should be growing. Elderly persons may not be able to absorb or conserve calcium as well as middle-aged men.

Thus, the magnitude of the "obligatory" calcium losses in healthy adults is about 250 mg/d. The obligatory losses may increase with age or disease. One mechanism by which increased calcium intake may help to prevent osteoporosis is by replacing calcium that is inevitably lost through the skin, intestine, and kidney.

The major mechanism whereby calcium affects bone is probably through inhibition of PTH secretion. With dietary calcium deficiency, PTH levels increase and lead to increased bone resorption as well as increased activation frequency, with subsequent loss of bone mass. When excess calcium is ingested, PTH production is suppressed. This chronic suppression could help to stabilize bone mass.

The role of PTH itself in control of bone mass is perplexing. PTH stimulates osteoblastic activity, especially on trabecular surfaces. In some cases this effect predominates over the increased resorption, and osteosclerosis results. Patients with renal failure and secondary hyperparathyroidism often have increased BMD of the spine, but decreased cortical bone mass (11). Patients with osteoporosis treated with PTH show increases at the spine but decreases at cortical sites (12). With primary hyperparathyroidism, there is also more bone at trabecular sites such as spine and iliac crest relative to the cortical bone of the proximal femur (13). Thus, it is interesting that many of the clinical studies of calcium supplements suggest more beneficial effects on cortical bone.

Parathyroid effects on bone also are modulated by estrogen. With estrogen deficiency, the bone is more sensitive to the resorbing effects of PTH (14). This could be mediated by interleukins, especially interleukin-6, which enhance resorption. PTH can stimulate release of the interleukins, an effect that is inhibited by estrogen (15,16)(see Chapter 2). The role of calcium in this scheme is not clear, but since calcium can inhibit PTH secretion, it could partially offset the negative effects of estrogen deficiency.

Several studies have measured the effects of calcium on PTH and vitamin D, and most show an inhibition. In healthy elderly people after 6 months of 1.2 g of calcium daily, serum PTH levels fell from 41 to 33 pg/mL, and 1,25-dihydroxyvitamin D (1,25(OH)$_2$D) from 38 to 30 pg/mL (17). In another study of elderly persons 1 g calcium per day reduced PTH from 50 to 42 pg/mL (18). In clinical trials in normal postmenopausal women, calcium-treated groups showed decreased PTH (19) and 1,25(OH)$_2$D levels (20). Short-term studies of various calcium preparations showed decreased PTH levels in normal persons (21). Not all reports showed decreases in PTH after calcium (22,23). In a group of 59 normal premenopausal women, an extra 610 mg calcium daily for 3 years did not result in significant change in PTH levels (24). Since PTH measurements are variable, some of the studies that showed no changes may have had too few subjects.

Most studies have shown that increased calcium intake decreases PTH, and it appears that the converse is also true. When 9 subjects went from high calcium diet (2 g/d) to low (300 mg/d), PTH concentrations increased and remained elevated for the next 8 weeks (25).

Osteoporosis

OTHER BIOCHEMICAL EFFECTS

Whether by inhibition of PTH or by other mechanisms, calcium treatment appears to block bone resorption. Bone formation may decrease as a consequence of decreased turnover, but in some cases the improved mineralization will result in an increased bone formation. Urine hydroxyproline, an imperfect marker of bone resorption, was decreased after a calcium challenge in women with postmenopausal osteoporosis (26). Women given calcium for 8 days showed decreased urine hydroxyproline levels (27). In clinical trials of postmenopausal women, urine hydroxyproline concentration decreased (28) from about 18 to 13 μmol/mmol (29) and from about 36 to 27 mg/g creatinine (19). In perimenopausal women studied by Riis and colleagues (23), the urine hydroxyproline level decreased with estrogen but not with calcium.

▶ 231

In uncomplicated osteoporosis, osteocalcin is a marker of bone formation. In one study of elderly persons given calcium, no change was seen in osteocalcin level (18). In children given calcium supplements as part of a randomized trial, the osteocalcin level was lower in those given the calcium, 48 versus 54 μg/L (30). Osteocalcin also decreased in calcium-treated perimenopausal women in a study by Elders and coworkers (28) but not by Riis and colleagues (23).

Calcium kinetic studies in women treated with 24 oz milk daily showed decreased bone formation and resorption (31). In a cross-sectional study using calcium kinetics, the net absorbed calcium correlated negatively to bone resorption rate ($r = -0.03$) and positively to bone mineralization rate ($r = 0.29$)(32).

DISCUSSION OF REMODELING BARRIER

Adult bone undergoes constant remodeling by discrete units referred to as BMUs (for bone modeling units or basic multicellular units). Bone volume depends on the number of BMUs as well as the formation and resorption rates at each BMU. On the trabecular surfaces of bone, remodeling at the BMU begins with activation, followed by osteoclastic resorption and then bone formation. PTH is one of the factors identified in activation. Inhibition of activation results in decreased numbers of BMUs, and this alone will result in decreased overall bone formation and resorption rates. The net effect on bone volume would be positive, because each BMU usually resorbs more bone than it forms. The BMUs are all in different phases of remodeling. If all activation or resorption suddenly stopped while formation continued, the previously resorbed cavities would fill with new bone, and the bone volume would increase by about 5% to 10%, depending on the initial rate of turnover. After the cavities were filled up (this would take one formation period, or about 3 months), the bone volume would stabilize. The increase in bone volume would not exceed 5% to 10%, which can be termed a remodeling barrier. Agents that block activation or resorption cannot break this barrier. Only anabolic agents, which stimulate osteoblasts to form more bone than has been resorbed, can increase the bone volume beyond this amount.

Calcium probably acts by inhibiting PTH, which leads to decreased activation. This is only a partial inhibition and does not usually result in much new bone formation. But the rate of bone loss can be attenuated. In addition, calcium may improve mineralization of existing osteoid, especially when there was calcium deficiency (as noted from bone biopsy results, which are discussed later in this chapter). No current evidence indicates that calcium has anabolic effects on the osteoblasts.

RELATION TO MECHANICAL STRAIN

Mechanical stresses stimulate bone formation; conversely, decreased stress stimulates bone resorption. The magnitude of the bone gain or loss is modulated by systemic and local hormones, which of course interact with each other. Lanyon (33) reported a series of elegant studies in a turkey model in which the ulna was separated from its muscles and therefore unloaded. A calcium-insufficient diet caused a 15% reduction in bone area, and unloading worsened the loss to 32%. Loading partially reversed this to 25% of the initial value. This was in contrast to studies carried out in animals with a normal calcium diet, in which loading was osteogenic (34).

These findings are supported by a study in which bone density of the femur decreased in exercising and sedentary women with moderate calcium intake (−1.1% and −0.99%). With a high calcium intake, the bone density improved by 0.87% in the sedentary group and 2.9% in the exercising group. The same findings were not seen at other skeletal sites (35). Prince and colleagues (29) found that exercise plus calcium gave significantly better improvement in BMD than exercise alone. Additive effects of physical activity and calcium were not seen in the study by Smith and colleagues (36), however. One explanation may have been that the group randomly assigned to both exercise and calcium was older and more frail.

PHYSICOCHEMICAL MECHANISMS

Calcium may directly influence the bone density, probably by physicochemical mechanisms. Burnell and colleagues found evidence for calcium deficiency at the level of the bone crystal structure (37). In 25% of women with postmenopausal osteoporosis there was a higher ratio of sodium to calcium by analysis of the chemical composition of bone biopsies; the percent of mineral within the bone itself was decreased. This correlated with decreased total body calcium measurements. When the patients were treated with calcium and either calcitonin, stanozolol, or placebo, those with the skeletal calcium deficiency showed the best response, whether or not they took active medication with the calcium (38).

Physiology of Calcium Absorption

Most calcium is absorbed in the small intestine. About 4% is absorbed from the colon, between 7 and 26 hours after ingestion (39). Calcium may be absorbed via both D-dependent and independent mechanisms. The D-dependent mechanism is saturated with calcium meals containing 120 mg calcium (40). ▶ 233

Women vary in their ability to absorb calcium (41). The fractional absorption, adjusted to an intake of 0.8 g/d, ranged from .10 to .55 in normal postmenopausal women (42). Even with the same calcium load, individuals can vary about 10% from one time to another (43). Riggs and colleagues (44) compared osteoporotic women to normals and found that 17 of 35 women had lower than normal intestinal absorption of calcium. In a study by Need and coworkers (45), normal postmenopausal women were separated into calcium absorbers or nonabsorbers based on a radiocalcium absorption test. Then after 1 g calcium, the absorbers decreased hydroxyproline excretion and had a greater increase in fasting urine calcium/creatinine level. The nonabsorbers did not have a change in hydroxyproline excretion.

INFLUENCE OF CALCIUM INTAKE

The absorption of calcium is under homeostatic control, and higher intakes result in lower absorption (41). Combining data from 273 balance studies, Heaney and Recker (42) found a highly significant correlation between the logarithm of absorption fraction and the logarithm of calcium intake ($r = -0.53$). The percentage of osteoporotic women in positive calcium balance increases from 60% to 86% when intake increases from 800 to 1200 mg/d but shows no further increase at 2200 mg/d (46). The fractional calcium absorption of women treated with 24 oz milk daily decreases after one year (31). Conversely, when calcium intake is decreased from 2000 to 300 mg/d, whole body calcium retention increases by 43%, along with an increase in PTH, a transient increase in 1,25-$(OH)_2D$, and a decrease in urine calcium levels (25).

ABSORPTION OF DIFFERENT PREPARATIONS

Different Salts: Using the washout method, measured calcium absorption from milk is similar to that from the carbonate, acetate, lactate, gluconate, and citrate salts (47). The fractional absorption of calcium varies between 0.04 and 0.4 with different foods, but the solubility of the calcium salt (specifically carbonate, phosphate, and citrate) plays little role in this variability. In the solubility range of 0.1 to 10 mM, which includes most commonly used sources of calcium, there is no difference in calcium absorption (48). Calcium carbonate, lactate, and gluconate all inhibit PTH to the same extent (49). However, calcium gluconate is not as well absorbed as calcium pyrrolidone carboxlylate (50). In Australian women with postmenopausal osteoporosis, urine calcium increases and hydroxyproline decreases similarly with Calsup or Caltrate brands of calcium carbonate or with Sandocal, an effervescent lactogluconate (26). Somewhat different results were reported from New Zealand, where effervescent tablets containing carbonate and citrate (Spar-Cal and Calcium-Sandoz) had significantly higher absorption than calcium carbonate (Os-Cal) or hydroxyapatite (Ossopan) (21). A more recent study in 12 normal women also showed calcium-Sandoz had higher urine calcium excretion than Os-Cal; however, the effervescent tablet also contained 1 g NaCl per tablet (51).

Not all calcium preparations are absorbed equally, and one of the reasons is that they have different rates of dissolution. It is less expensive to manufacture calcium carbonate in a compact form that will not readily dissolve. The dissolution of 27 brands of calcium varies from under 33% to 75% (52). Those brands in the group with the best dissolution are: Calcium (Giant Food), Calcium Concentrate 600 (Hudson), Natural Calcium (Giant Food), and Os-Cal (Marion). The authors did not test chewable tablets, which have high dissolution due to mastication. That this difference in dissolution might change bioavailability was tested for two preparations with high (Caltrate 600) and low dissolution (Calcium 600, Rugby). The preparation with high dissolution had greater net calcium absorption, 32% of the dose compared to 19% (53).

I was skeptical about the importance of dissolution until one of my patients told me that she had forgotten to take her calcium tablets, which she purchased from a health food store. She put them in the pocket of her apron, and discovered them there after the apron had been through the cycles on the washer and the dryer! Another patient switched to a brand from a health food store, and, when she came in to have her BMD measured, densities were seen overlying the spine. These changed position after a couple of hours and were not seen on a scan several days later (after she changed to a chewable form of calcium) (Figure 9-1).

Citrate: Several investigators have examined the absorption of calcium citrate (Table 9-1; 47,48,54–57). The urine excretion of calcium 2 hours following a dose increases more after calcium citrate than after calcium carbonate (58,59), but this does not necessarily mean that there was more gastrointestinal

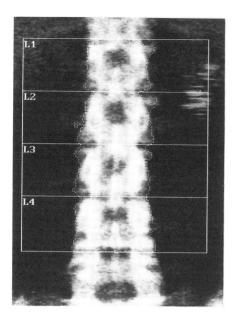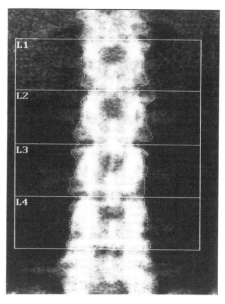

FIGURE 9-1 Dual energy x-ray absorptiometry printouts from a woman who had ingested calcium supplements from a health food store. The undigested supplements can be seen as dense spots near L-1 and L-2 (left). Several days later the procedure was repeated, and the abnormal densities were gone (right).

absorption. Urinary calcium excretion followed for 4 hours shows increased levels in subjects given citrate, which is significant at loads from 0.5 to 2.0 g (54). The fecal recovery of orally administered radiolabeled calcium suggests that citrate is absorbed better than carbonate in fasting subjects (54). A liquid form of calcium citrate and hydroxide shows even better absorption (60).

TABLE 9-1 Comparison Between Absorption of Calcium Citrate or Calcium Carbonate

| | | | Fractional Absorption | |
Author, Year	Reference	Method	Carbonate	Citrate
Heaney, 1990	48	Double isotope	.296	.242,.363*
Harvey, 1988	54	Fecal recovery of Ca isotope	.314	.402[†]
Miller, 1988	55	Double isotope	.264	.362[†]
Sheikh, 1987	47	Washout	.39	.30
Recker, 1985	56	Single isotope	.225	.243
Bo-Linn, 1984	57	Washout	.238	.289
Harvey, 1988	54	Increment in urine Ca	.091[‡]	.104[‡]

*Calcium citrate malate
[†]Significant difference
[‡]mg/mL glomerular filtration rate

Calcium and Vitamin D in the Pathogenesis and Treatment of Osteoporosis

Recker (56) demonstrated that calcium citrate is absorbed more readily than calcium carbonate in achlorhydric, fasting patients. In normal fasting subjects, however, there was no difference; the absorption of calcium citrate was 24% compared to 22% for calcium carbonate. When the achlorhydric patients ingested the calcium with an ordinary breakfast, there was no difference between citrate and carbonate.

Thus, it seems that calcium citrate may, in some situations, be absorbed more efficiently than calcium carbonate. In the only large, randomized, controlled trial comparing the effects of these two preparations (calcium carbonate and calcium citrate-maleate) there were no significant differences between the groups, although for some measurement sites the calcium citrate-maleate group tended to have better results (20).

EFFECTS OF FOODS ON CALCIUM ECONOMY

Although other nutrients may not influence calcium absorption, they may alter the excretion of calcium. The term "calcium economy," coined by Heaney (5), emphasizes the importance of both the intake and outgo of calcium.

Protein and Phosphate: Encouraged by groups who feel that we should all be strict vegetarians, the lay literature has a strong bias that protein intake is harmful to the bones. Even protein from dairy products, they claim, can worsen osteoporosis (61). Several legitimate studies have been done, which suggest that protein can alter the urine calcium. The magnitude of this change, however, is small. The different phosphate contents of proteins can add complexity, because phosphate decreases urine calcium whereas amino acids increase it. These effects are probably at the level of the kidney. Nonmeat protein causes increased urine calcium (62), but meat intake does not increase urine calcium as much as isolated amino acids (46). In nine normal subjects, 54 g protein increased the urine calcium after a few hours, without a measurable change in glomerular filtration rate (63). However, other studies have shown that protein increases both the urine calcium and the glomerular filtration rate (GFR) (64,65). In an interesting study in six normal women, a change in protein intake from 44 to 102 g resulted in a significant increase in urine calcium, which was abolished by ingesting 5.8 g bicarbonate with the protein (66). The effect on urine calcium would only be important if it led to a negative calcium balance. Studies using stool and urine collection techniques have demonstrated that protein from meat does not change the calcium balance (67). Balance studies with isotopes in 170 women showed a significant influence of nitrogen on calcium balance (68). The magnitude of the effect was small, so that a 50% increase in protein above the mean would result in a loss of 32 mg calcium per day.

Comparing vegetarians to nonvegetarians, Hunt and colleagues (69) found no difference in bone mass. The vegetarians had a significantly lower protein intake, but they also had a lower calcium intake (1316 versus 1097 mg/d, including supplements). Since vegetarians may have other life-style differences that favor bone strength, it is difficult to use these studies to evaluate protein intake. No controlled trials have been done to determine the effect of changes in protein.

Phosphate can decrease urine calcium and increase PTH secretion. Rats, but fortunately not human beings, are sensitive to phosphate and easily develop renal failure with phosphate loads. In young women, a diet with low calcium (400 mg) and high phosphate (1700 mg) resulted in elevated PTH after 4 weeks, without changes in $1,25(OH)_2D$ (70). This study did not examine the effects of the high phosphate or low calcium independently, but another study of young women who did not have a high-phosphate diet showed that calcium restriction could evoke a persistent PTH response (71). A high-phosphate diet, up to 2000 mg/d, does not interfere with intestinal absorption of calcium (72).

▶ 237

Caffeine: Caffeine also increases urine loss of calcium through an effect on the kidney. The caffeine effect can be measured and is statistically significant, but becomes clinically significant only at large intakes. Using calcium balance techniques in 170 subjects, Heaney and Recker (68) showed a significant regression of caffeine on calcium balance. A 50% increase in caffeine from a baseline of two cups daily predicted an extra 6 mg/d loss of calcium. Hasling and colleagues (73) showed that 1000 mg coffee daily increased the urine calcium level by only 64 mg.

Magnesium: Although little appears in the medical literature about the effect of magnesium on osteoporosis or on calcium absorption, the notion that beneficial effects exist seems entrenched in the lay literature, and many patients firmly believe that they cannot absorb calcium without magnesium supplements. The literature search revealed one incredible article that demonstrates how some of these misconceptions are perpetuated. A report by Abraham and Grewal (74) concluded that magnesium supplements increased bone mass. Twenty-six women, mean age 53 and on hormone replacement therapy, participated in the study. Seven chose not to take the supplements and were used as controls. The supplement contained 500 mg calcium and 200 mg magnesium, and an extra 400 mg magnesium was given. All the women were instructed to eat a high-fiber diet and to limit dairy products to two servings a day. Thus, the control group must have been taking a diet with low absorbable calcium. Follow-up time varied from 6 to 12 months. The BMD at the calcaneus remained stable in the control group but increased by 11% in the supplemented group. The authors never considered the possibility that the calcium in the supplement had an effect, but they felt that postmenopausal osteoporosis was due to magnesium deficiency. The study was sponsored by the company that manufactured the supplement (74).

A review of magnesium requirements, which collected 911 magnesium balance experiments from the literature, showed an allowance of 400 mg/d (75). In another 208 balance studies, a simple linear relationship was found between magnesium intake and output. Even with intakes as low as 100 mg/d, subjects were in neutral balance (76). Magnesium intake in women with osteoporosis does not correlate with the calcium balance (73).

Fiber: Calcium absorption is inhibited by fiber in the diet (77). In 12 normal men, given a high- or low-fiber diet with calcium of about 1 g, the balance was +72 mg on low fiber and −122 mg on high fiber (78). The inhibition of calcium by high fiber is not improved by increasing gastric acidity (79).

Other: For generations, parents have admonished their children to eat their spinach, but it did not help any bones. Although the calcium content in spinach is high, almost none gets absorbed. This was demonstrated clearly by Heaney and colleagues (80) who grew spinach in hydroponic solutions containing ^{45}Ca. Kale, on the other hand, contains readily absorbable calcium. Fiber from wheat bran and beans inhibits calcium absorption, and some of this is due to phytate content. Although soy beans have good absorption, common beans do not (81). Thus, the chemical content of food products may not predict the bioavailability of calcium. The absorption fractions of some of these foods, standardized to a 300-mg load with a light meal, are approximately: wheat bread, 0.42; kale, 0.40; bok choy, 0.39; calcium-enriched orange juice, 0.37; broccoli, 0.36; soy beans with low phytates, 0.32; milk, 0.31; yogurt, 0.30; chocolate milk, 0.28; soy beans with high phytate, 0.24; milk plus wheat bran, 0.23; common beans, 0.08; and spinach, 0.04 (81).

Lactose intolerance is a common problem, especially in elderly persons. An incidence of 60% was estimated from breath hydrogen tests (82). Fortunately, yogurt is well tolerated in these persons (83) and it has been documented to be well absorbed (84).

GASTRIC ACIDITY

Patients with achlorhydria do not absorb calcium carbonate when fasting, but the acid content of a normal diet is sufficient to restore normal absorption (56).

Calcium absorption is independent of gastric pH with milk, $CaCO_3$, or citrate (57). Thus, the acid content of a usual diet provides sufficient acid for usual calcium absorption.

OSTEOPOROSIS

Calcium absorption may be lower in women with osteoporosis. Spencer and co-workers (85) studied 3 patients with osteoporosis and found a negative calcium balance, which improved with calcium supplements, but not as much improvement as in young persons. The BMD correlates with calcium absorption in women with osteoporosis but not in normal women (86).

▶ 239

Studies Relating Calcium Intake to Fracture

EPIDEMIOLOGIC STUDIES

Paleontologic studies have concluded that the diet of our prehistoric ancestors contained about 1580 mg calcium and 34% protein. Skeletal remains from these cultures document strong bones (87).

Cross-cultural studies have failed to demonstrate any relationship between the customary dietary intake and the course of bone loss (88). Figure 9-2 shows results from Nordin's (89) review of spinal x-rays from individuals from several countries; the calcium intake was estimated. No relationship was found between calcium intake and the incidence of osteoporosis. The dietary intake was low, for example, in Japan, which also had a high incidence of osteoporosis. But in Jamaica, with a similarly low calcium intake, the incidence of osteoporosis was negligible.

A study by Matkovic and colleagues (90) examined the prevalence of hip fractures in two nonintermingling regions of Yugoslavia. In one region farming was dominant, and dietary intake of dairy products was high. In the other region dietary calcium intake was low. Hip fractures were more common in the region with the low calcium intake. The conclusion was that lifelong high-calcium intake reduced the risk of hip fractures. Although this is a plausible explanation, it is not definitive. There could have been hereditary differences between the two regions. Also, the region with the high dietary intake also had higher energy intake and that population may have been more physically active.

Although the international patterns of osteoporosis appear to cast doubt on the relationship between calcium intake and osteoporosis, they do not eliminate the possible positive role of calcium. Hereditary factors are much more

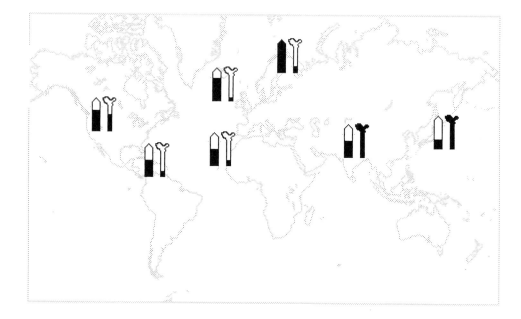

FIGURE 9-2 Calcium intake (shown by the milk cartons) and prevalence of fractures (shown by the femurs) in different countries. The maximum calcium intake was 1300 mg and the highest fracture prevalence was 40%. (*Adapted by permission from Nordin BEC. International patterns of osteoporosis. Clin Orthop 1966;45: 17–29.*)

important than dietary factors in determining bone mass. Studies on twins have suggested that about 80% of peak bone mass is determined by inherited factors, and all other life-style factors, including diet, account for the remaining 20% (91). Also, there can be serious errors in the estimation of calcium intake from the tremendously different diets of different cultures. "Hidden" sources of calcium have already been identified for some of these: soups made in China from boiling bones in vinegar have a high calcium content (92). Tortillas made from corn have a high calcium content because the stones used to grind the flour were traditionally made of limestone. In some countries chewing on chicken bones is habitual.

Fujita and Fukase (93) have identified another complexity in examining the relationship between dietary calcium, bone mass, and risk of osteoporosis. The Japanese calcium intake is only about 400 mg/d, and the bone mass in Japanese women is lower than in American women, where the average calcium intake is higher. However, despite the lower bone mass, the Japanese women have fewer than half as many hip fractures as American women. The other factors that determine fractures include the overall structure of the proximal femur, the pattern of physical activity, the quality of the bone, and the nature of falls.

Table 9-2 shows studies that have related the prevalence of fractures to calcium intake (44,82,94–105). In an early cross-sectional study of 2063 outpatients or staff members, there was no significant difference between high- and low-calcium intake and the prevalence of spine fractures. Also, no difference was noted in the calcium intake between patients with and without fracture (97). Several other cross-sectional studies have agreed with these results. On the other hand, Riggs and coworkers (44) did find that osteoporotic patients had lower calcium intake than controls.

Case-control studies have shown more variable results (see Table 9-2). In Chinese persons the relative risk in those with the lowest calcium intake was 1.9 compared to those with high intakes, but a similar study in English (101) women found a relative risk of 1.0 (102). Recently, Kanis and colleagues (100) conducted a population-based survey of hip fractures in 14 centers from 6 countries in southern Europe. They identified 2086 women with hip fractures and 3532 age-matched controls. The relative risk of hip fracture was 0.75 in women taking calcium. The risk decreased with longer duration of calcium use.

▶ 241

FRACTURE INCIDENCE STUDIES

In three longitudinal studies of fracture incidence, results are inconsistent. Holbrook and colleagues (96) found a relative risk of 0.6 for each 198 mg calcium intake. But Wickham and coworkers (95) found no change in risk in a 15-year study. The incidence of arm or wrist fractures, in a study of 9704 women followed for 2 years, showed a relative risk of 1.01 for dietary calcium intake for every 5000 mg/wk; thus, calcium intake did not help in predicting these fractures (92).

Osteoporotic patients may have a lower intake of all nutrients, not only calcium. Women with hip fractures were randomly assigned to groups, one of which received daily oral nutrition supplements containing 20 g protein for a mean of 32 days. The clinical outcome was significantly better in the supplemented group (106).

Calcium Balance as a Parameter of Bone Health

Because 99% of the calcium is within the bone, a positive calcium balance indicates an increasing bone mass. Several investigators have studied the effect of calcium intake on calcium balance. Although these studies do not necessarily show the amount of calcium needed to meet obligatory losses, they do show that there may be a relationship between the calcium intake and bone health. In other

Osteoporosis

TABLE 9-2 Studies Comparing Fractures to Calcium Intake

Author, year	Reference	Study Design	Number of Normals	Number of Fractures	Subjects	Type of Fracture	Result	Comments
Kelsey, 1992	94	lg × 2.2 y	9704	250	Community women >65 y	Arm	↔	No change in risk
Wickham, 1989	95	lg × 15 y	1356	44	Random community	Hip	↔	No change in risk
Holbrook, 1988	96	lg × 14 y	957	33	Elderly population	Hip	+	Relative risk = .6/198 mg
Smith, 1965	97	xs	2063		Outpts or staff	Spine	↔	No difference between high and low calcium intake; also no difference between fracture and nonfracture
Kleerekoper, 1989	98	xs	397	266	Postmenopausal women	Vertebra	↔	No difference in Ca intake
Riggs, 1967	44	xs	166	83	Clinic pts	Spine	+	Ca intake 617 in pts, 712 control ($P<.05$)
Wootton, 1979	99	xs	72	110	Hosp pts	Hip	↔	No difference in Ca intake
Kanis, 1992	100	case-c	2086	3532	Population	Hip	+	Relative risk 0.75 for women taking Ca
Lau, 1988	101	case-c	800	400	Chinese	Hip	+	Relative risk 1.9 lowest-highest quartile
Cooper, 1988	102	case-c	600	300	Hosp/community	Hip	↔	Relative risk 1.0 in women; in men some protection with intake >1041 mg/d
Nieves, 1992	103	case-c	168	161	Hosp pts	Hip	↔	No risk from current or teenage intake
Hurxthal, 1969	104	case-c	53	53	Clinic pts	Spine	+	Fracture cases 21% lower Ca intake
Myburgh, 1990	105	case-c	25	25	Athletes	Stress	+	Fracture cases 697 mg/d versus 832 mg/d in control
Wheeler, 1991	82	case-c	15	15	Hosp pts	Hip	↔	No difference in Ca intake

words, calcium can both supply the needed mineral as well as adjust the hormonal milieu to avoid excessive bone resorption. In a variety of subjects with serial measurements of bone mass, calcium balance correlated with the trend in bone mass measurements (107,108). This fits in with the current view of calcium economy, that retained calcium is deposited into bone and not into the soft tissues.

In classic balance studies, Heaney and colleagues (7) measured 130 perimenopausal women who consumed their usual calcium intake. This is an important aspect of the design because when the calcium intake is changed, the period of flux to readjust takes months, and studies done during this time are difficult, if not impossible, to interpret. The calcium absorption correlated significantly with calcium balance. The regression of calcium intake versus calcium balance intercepted the x-axis at 1.24 g/d. In postmenopausal women not taking estrogen, the intercept increased to 1.5 g/d. With estrogen replacement therapy the intercept ("requirement") returned to the premenopausal level (109). Hasling and coworkers (73) recently performed balance studies in 85 osteoporotic patients and showed similar results: at zero balance from regression equation the dietary intake was 1380 mg/d.

▶ 243

In 49 patients receiving calcium supplements from 8 days to 44 years, the calcium balance correlated inversely with duration of supplementation. A more positive balance was found in short-term users. This is consistent with the theory that calcium blocks bone activation frequency. The study was complicated by the fact that some patients also received vitamin D and estrogen (110).

Eighteen balance studies in 14-year-old girls showed that the main determinant of calcium balance was the dietary intake of calcium ($r = 0.67$). There was no urinary adaptation to low-calcium intake. In fact, one girl had a urine calcium level of 250 mg/d despite a dietary intake of only 270 mg/d, and one wonders if she had an abnormality in renal tubular function (111).

Studies Relating Calcium Intake to Bone Density

CROSS-SECTIONAL

A quantitative review of the literature suggested that calcium intake showed positive correlations with bone mass (112). Table 9-3 (69,97,104,113–140) lists some studies that have compared calcium intake to BMD. Of 31 studies located in the medical literature, none had negative results. About half did not show any significant relationship between calcium intake and bone mass. The rest showed either a significant correlation, or mixed results (positive by one technique and neutral by another). These studies varied greatly in design, and the correlation

Osteoporosis

TABLE 9-3 Cross-sectional Studies of Bone Mass and Calcium Intake

Author, Year	Reference	Number	Type	Bone Mineral Density Determination	Result	Comment
Bauer, 1993	113	9704	Normal women > 65 y	SPA	↔	No association with Ca, relative risk = 1.1
Yano, 1985	114	2120	Elderly Japanese	SPA arm, heel	+	Significant
Smith, 1965	97	2063	Outpatients or staff	Femur, hand	↔	No difference between high and low Ca intake
Hurxthal, 1969	104	398	Healthy men, women	Density sp	+	r = .178 for men and .260 for women
Johnell, 1984	115	395	Women age 49 y	SPA	↔	No correlation to calcium intake
Sowers, 1985	116	324	Community, 55–80 y	SPA	↔	No correlation to calcium intake
Mazess, 1991	117	300	Normals, 20–39 y	SPA, DPA sp, hip	↔	No correlation to calcium intake
Hunt, 1989	69	290	Elderly women	SPA	↔	No difference between vegetarian and nonvegetarian, no correlation with Ca intake

Reference	No.	Population	Method	Effect	Comments
Elders, 1989	118	Normal women, 46–55 y	DPA spine	+/↔	Lower BMD in lowest versus highest tertile in premenopausal women; no difference in peri or postmenopause.
Stevenson, 1989	119	Normal women, 21–68 y	DPA sp, hip	↔	No correlation to Ca intake
Sandler, 1985	120	Postmenopausal women	CT arm	↔	No correlation with current intake
Picard, 1988	121	Normal women, 40–50 y	SPA, DPA sp	+	BMD higher in group taking >1000 mg/d than <500 mg/d
Halioua, 1989	122	Normal premenopausal	SPA	+	Significant, $r = 0.36$
Cauley, 1988	123	Postmenopausal	QCT arm	+	Diet Ca $r = .17$, $P < .01$; higher BMD in women with high lifelong Ca intake
Chan, 1991	124	Children	SPA	+	Correlation .3 between BMD and Ca intake
Angus, 1988	125	Normal women	SPA, DPA sp, hip	↔	No correlation to Ca intake

Calcium and Vitamin D in the Pathogenesis and Treatment of Osteoporosis

Osteoporosis

TABLE 9-3 Cross-sectional Studies of Bone Mass and Calcium Intake (continued)

Author, Year	Reference	Number	Type	Bone Mineral Density Determination	Result	Comment
Anton, 1991	126	131	Normal, 52–92 y	DPA	+	Correlation to Ca intake $P < .03$, $r = .19$
Nilas, 1984	127	103	Early postmenopause	SPA	↔	No difference low-medium-high Ca intake
McCulloch, 1990	128	101	Normal, 20–35 y	QCT heel	↔	No correlation to Ca intake
Freudenheim, 1986	129	84	Normal women	SPA arm	↔	No correlation between usual intake and initial BMD
Wolman, 1992	130	67	Athletes	QCT sp	+	Significant relationship to Ca intake (no r reported)
Buchanan, 1988	131	63	Patients, 49–90 y	QCT sp	+/↔	$r = .24$, $P = .08$, several on medications
Desai, 1987	132	60	Normal, 30–40 y	DPA sp, hip	↔	No correlation to Ca intake

Author, year	Ref	Population	Method		Findings
Kanders, 1988	133	Normal young women	DPA, SPA	+/↔	No correlation BMD with Ca $r = .21$ at spine and .27 at radius, but those with intake >800 mg/d were higher than those <800 mg/d
Stevenson, 1988	134	Postmenopausal	TBC, QCT sp, arm	↔	No correlation to Ca intake
Block, 1989	135	Young men	QCT sp, DPA hip	+/↔	$r = .12$ QCT (NS) and .35 DPA (significant)
Lukert, 1987	136	Normal perimenopausal	SPA	+	Correlation to Ca:P ratio, $r = .29$
Sentipal, 1991	137	Girls, 8–18 y	DXA sp	+	Correlation to calcium intake $P = .04$, r not given
Kelly, 1990	138	Normal men	SPA, DPA sp, hip	+	Diet Ca versus sp $r = 49$; hip $r = .64$, arm NS
Vinther, 1953	139	Nursing home	x-ray	+	Patients with greater Ca intake had less demineralization on x-ray
Leuenberger, 1989	140	Normal women, 19–21 y	QCT spine	↔	No correlation with Ca intake ($r = -.5$)

BMD, bone mineral density; DPA, dual photon absorptiometry; DXA, dual energy x-ray absorptiometry; QCT, quantitative computed tomography; sp, spine; SPA, single photon absorptiometry; TBC, total body calcium

Calcium and Vitamin D in the Pathogenesis and Treatment of Osteoporosis

coefficients were not large, but the overall impression gained from reviewing these studies is that calcium has a weak positive effect on bone mass.

LONGITUDINAL

Longitudinal studies of bone density also have variable results, as shown in Table 9-4 (141–149). The studies with the greatest patient-years of follow-up showed no significant difference between the change in bone mass and the calcium intake.

PROSPECTIVE CLINICAL TRIALS

Prospective studies of calcium are shown in Table 9-5 (19,20,22–24,26,28–31,35,36,111,127,150–161). The results of these studies are mixed. None showed dramatic improvement in BMD, although in several studies the calcium-treated group lost less than the controls, who were not randomized.

CONTROL GROUPS IN CLINICAL TRIALS

Several randomized clinical trials of various medications for osteoporosis have provided calcium supplementation to both the treated and the placebo groups (Figure 9-3; 162–168). The lack of regard for calcium as a therapy for osteoporosis is evident in some of the reports that consider these placebo groups to be "untreated." From the viewpoint of calcium treatment, these are all uncontrolled prospective studies. Although the various treatments usually increased bone mass significantly greater than did calcium, the calcium groups generally showed either stable bone mass or a loss of about 1% a year. In comparison, a placebo group of 18 women with postmenopausal osteoporosis with a mean calcium intake of 700 mg/d showed a decrease in single photon absorptiometry of 3.3% a year (169). Another study showed a decrease in total body calcium of 1.8% yearly (170).

RANDOMIZED TRIALS OF CALCIUM TREATMENT

Table 9-5 shows details of controlled, randomized trials of calcium therapy (19,20,22,23,24,26,28,29,30,35,36,150–153). This study design is the most convincing. Figure 9-3 shows the results from those studies that reported changes in bone mass in sufficient detail to calculate the percent change per year. The plotted results show that the preponderance of data support a positive role of calcium, even though in some studies the effect is small. It appears that the effects on the spine, which has a larger proportion of cancellous bone, are less bene-

TABLE 9-4 Longitudinal Studies of Bone Mass and Calcium Intake

Author, Year	Reference	Years of Study	Numbers of Patients	Type of Patient	Bone Mineral Density Determination	Result	Comment
Slemenda, 1992	141	16	111	Male twins, 63 y	SPA	↔	Dietary Ca not related to bone loss
van Beresteijn, 1990	142, 143	8	154	Perimenopausal	SPA, DPA sp	↔	No difference between high and low at baseline or in rates after 8 y, DPA at end of study only
Milne, 1977	144	5	252	Normal men, women >62 y	Hand	↔	Bone loss unrelated to Ca intake
Riggs, 1987	145	4	106	Healthy women	SPA, DPA sp	↔	No correlation with Ca intake
Recker, 1992	146	3.4	156	College students	DPA sp	+/↔	Ca intake $r = .12$ (NS), but Ca/protein $r = .199$, $P < .02$
Slemenda, 1987	147	3	84	Normal women, 42–58 y	SPA	↔	Dietary Ca not related to bone loss
Aloia, 1983	148	up to 6	44	Normal women, 45–55 y	TBC, SPA	+/↔	No correlation with change in SPA but $r = .39$, $P = .03$ with change in TBC
Dawson-Hughes, 1987	149	0.6	76	Postmenopausal	DPA sp	+	Lowest quartile (<400 mg/d) showed loss of −3% versus gain of 1.2% in highest quartile

DPA, dual photon absorptiometry; sp, spine; SPA, single photon absorptiometry; TBC, total body calcium

▶ 249

Calcium and Vitamin D in the Pathogenesis and Treatment of Osteoporosis

TABLE 9-5 Clinical Trials of Calcium

Author, Year	Reference	Design	Calcium Number	Control Number	Subjects	Duration (y)	Dose/d	Measurement
Dawson-Hughes, 1990	20	db-bl	150	150	Postmenopausal with Ca intake > 650 mg/d	2	0.5 g	SPA, DPA sp, hip
Smith, 1989	150	db-bl	55	62	Healthy women	4	1.5 g	SPA wrist, humerus
Reid, 1993	19	db-bl	61	61	Postmenopausal, mean 10 y	2	1 g	DXA tb, sp, hip
Johnston, 1992	30	db-bl	45	45	Twin children	3	1 g	SPA, DPA sp, hip
Orwoll, 1989	22	db-bl	41	36	Healthy men	3	1 g	SPA, QCT sp
Prince, 1991	29	db-bl	39	41	Postmenopausal, low BMD	2	1 g	SPA
Smith, 1981	36	db-bl	22	29	Elderly	3	0.750 g	SPA
Riis, 1987	23	db-bl	15	13	Normal perimeno-pausal	2	2 g	SPA, DPA sp, tb, hip
Nelson, 1991	35	db-bl	18	18	Postmenopausal	1	0.8 g	QCT, DPA sp, tb, hip
Elders, 1991	28	rand	198	97	Normal, 46–55	2	1 g, 2 g	DPA sp
Baran, 1990	24	rand	20	17	Normal premeno-pausal	3	0.5 g dairy	DPA sp
Fujita, 1990	151	rand	12	21	Pmop > 70y	2	0.9 g	SPA, QCT
Recker, 1977	152	rand	22	20	Normal, postmenopausal nuns	2	1 g	SPA, hand

Author, Year	Ref	Type	N	N	Population	Duration	Calcium dose	Method
Lamke, 1978	153	rand	20	20	Postmenopausal Colles fracture	1	1 g	X-ray spect. hip
Horsman, 1977	154	semi-rand	24	18	Normal postmenopausal	2	0.8 g	Hand, SPA
Nordin, 1980	155	pros	20	41	Pmop vertebral fracture	2.5	1.2 g	Metacarpal
Ettinger, 1987	156	pros	44	25	Normal perimeno-pausal	2	1 g	SPA, QCT
Albanese, 1975	157	pros	12	17	Normal elderly	3	0.75 g	Finger
Recker, 1985	31	pros	13	9	Healthy postmenopausal	2	24 oz milk	Ca balance
Matkovic, 1990	111	pros	22	9	14 y	2	Pills or milk to 1.6 g	SPA, DPA
Nilas, 1984	127	pros	103	0	Perimenopausal	2	0.5 g	SPA
Polley, 1987	158	pros	136	52	Postmenopausal with Ca intake <1000 mg/d	0.75	1g pill or ~0.5 g diet	SPA
Almustafa, 1992	159	pros	49	0	Various osteoporosis	"1–10"	1.2–2 g	Fracture
Need, 1986	160	pros	38	0	Patients with high resorption	0.8	1 g	SPA
Lee, 1981	161	pros	20	0	Elderly women	0.5	2 oz cheese +0.35 g +vit D	Hand x-ray density

BMD, bone mineral density; db-bl, double-blind; DPA, dual photon absorptiometry; DXA, dual energy x-ray absorptiometry; pmop, postmenopausal osteoporosis; pros, prospective; QCT, quantitative computed tomography; rand, randomized; sp, spine; SPA, single photon absorptiometry; tb, total body

▶ 251

Calcium and Vitamin D in the Pathogenesis and Treatment of Osteoporosis

Osteoporosis

TABLE 9-5 Clinical Trials of Calcium (continued)

Author	Group	Upper Extremity, %/y Calcium	Upper Extremity, %/y Control	Total Body, %/y Calcium	Total Body, %/y Control	Spine, %/y Calcium	Spine, %/y Control	Hip, %/y Calcium	Hip, %/y Control	Results
Dawson-Hughes, 1990	Early menopause	−0.09	−1.00			−1.44	−1.47	−0.31	−0.44	↔
	Late menopause	−0.05	−0.36			−0.68	−1.13	0.08	−0.66	↔
	Late <400	0.25	−1.20			−0.06	−1.50	0.30	−1.10	+
Smith, 1989	Postmenopause	−1.21	−2.26							+
	All	−1.12	−1.78	−0.52	−0.91					+
Reid, 1993		7.20	6.10			0.71	0.29	−0.15	−0.38	+
Johnston, 1992		−1.00	−1.00			6.70	6.50	5.10	5.00	+
Orwoll, 1989		−0.50	−2.60			−2.30	−2.30			↔
Prince, 1991						0.87	0.85			+
Smith, 1981	Exercise	−0.10	0.76							↔
	No exercise	0.53	−1.10							+
Riis, 1987		−1.86	−3.67	−2.62	−3.98	−1.57	−0.76			+/↔
Nelson, 1991		0.95	−0.27	−2.20	−2.70	1.40	0.38	2.00	−1.10	+/↔
Elders, 1991	1 g					−0.65	−1.70			+
	2 g					−0.35				+
Baran, 1990						−0.13	−0.97			+
Fujita, 1990		3.70	−3.60			0.19	−5.30			+

Recker, 1977	−1.80	−2.80			
Lamke, 1978	3.00	1.00			
Horsman, 1977	−0.04	−1.50			
Nordin, 1980			−5.00	−4.50	
Ettinger, 1987	−0.45	−1.00			
Albanese, 1975	2.00	−2.20			
Recker, 1985					
Matkovic, 1990	7.00	5.00	4.00	4.00	
Nilas, 1984	−2.00				
Polley, 1987	0.20	−0.37			
Almustafa, 1992					
Need, 1986	−1.10				
Lee, 1981					

\+ ↕ + ↕ ↕ + + ↕ ↕ + ↕ ↕ ↕

▶ 253

Calcium and Vitamin D in the Pathogenesis and Treatment of Osteoporosis

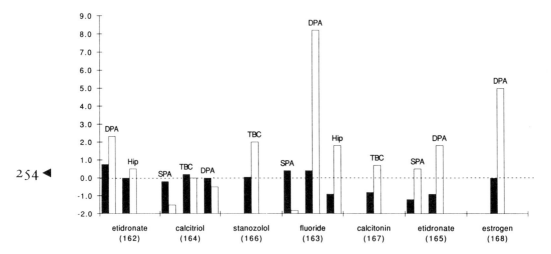

Change in bone mass, %/y

FIGURE 9-3 Change in bone mass from clinical trials in women with postmenopausal osteoporosis. The solid bars represent groups treated with calcium; those shown with open bars also received the treatments noted. Note that the abscissa is at −2%/y, which is the "historical control" of bone loss expected without calcium supplements. Numbers in parentheses indicate references. DPA, dual photon absorptiometry at the spine; Hip, dual photon absorptiometry at the hip; TBC, total body calcium; SPA, single photon absorptiometry at the radius.

ficial than at the cortical bone of the radius or metacarpals. This differential effect is the reverse of that seen in studies of infused PTH or drugs such as fluoride, etidronate, or estrogen. With these drugs, which increase PTH, there is more increase of cancellous bone than cortical.

The randomized studies do not provide much information about the dose-response relationship for calcium. One study used two doses of 1 and 2 g/d, and the higher dose showed a better response (−0.7 versus −1.3%/2 y), but it was not statistically significant (28). Dawson-Hughes and colleagues (20) chose women based on their usual calcium intake, so that one group ingested less than 400 mg/d initially, and the other group ate between 400 and 650 mg/d. They all received 500 mg calcium supplement. The subjects with the lower intakes had greater improvement in BMD, but this was not designed to test dose-response. It does show that the women with initial lower calcium intakes are more likely to respond to treatment.

Perimenopausal women may respond less well to calcium supplementation than postmenopausal women. Clearly, women are losing bone rapidly when they first go through estrogen withdrawal, and the calcium release from bone may supply an excess of extracellular calcium. Dawson-Hughes and colleagues (20) found that perimenopausal women showed no benefit from calcium

254 ◀

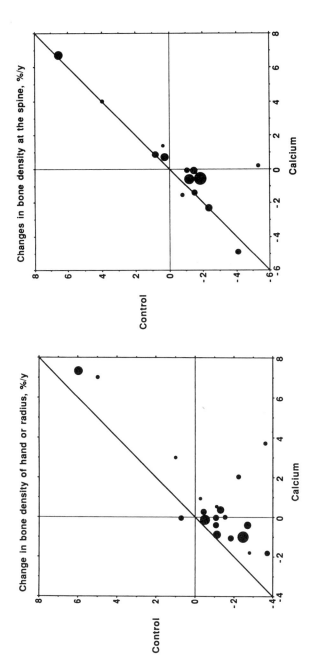

FIGURE 9-4 Results from controlled studies of calcium supplements. The areas of the points are proportional to the number of subject-years in the studies. Those studies in which calcium was better than control are under the 45 degree line of identity.

Calcium and Vitamin D in the Pathogenesis and Treatment of Osteoporosis

therapy. Likewise, Smith and coworkers (150) found better results in the post-menopausal women. Ettinger and colleagues (156), who studied perimeno-pausal women, showed no beneficial effect of calcium. Riis and coworkers (23) also studied perimenopausal women, and those treated with calcium did significantly worse than those given estrogen replacement; however, the calcium group still fared better than the untreated placebo group.

Only one randomized study has been done in children (30). This study used the twin model, thus improving the statistical power. The results showed that the twins with calcium supplementation had greater increases in bone mass at the forearm. The improvement was only seen in the prepubertal children.

ADJUNCT THERAPY

Some treatment programs being developed for osteoporosis are able to increase the bone mass. Antiresorbing drugs can increase bone volume by about 10% and fluoride can increase it dramatically. However, bone mass will not be able to show response to treatment if there is not sufficient calcium available to deposit into the newly made bone. In this situation, the goal is not to be in calcium balance but to be in calcium excess. For example, in a study of fluoride, patients given calcium supplementation did not develop the expected degree of osteomalacia (171). Little data are available about the amount of calcium needed to optimize other therapies for osteoporosis. Currently, the requirement for calcium seems so logical that most clinical trials ensure calcium intake in their patients.

BONE BIOPSIES

In a small study, 5 women with postmenopausal osteoporosis underwent bone biopsies before and after 2 years of taking 1200 mg calcium. They showed improvement in the mineralization lag time. This was due to an increased double-labeled surface; osteoid surfaces were unchanged (22).

In 3 children, dietary calcium deficiency (about 125 mg/d) with normal 25-hydroxyvitamin D (25-(OH)D) levels led to severe osteomalacia, with osteoid volumes of 4% to 9% and decreased tetracycline labeling. After treatment with calcium, repeat biopsies showed normal values (172).

Steiniche and colleagues (168) performed bone biopsies in 11 women with postmenopausal osteoporosis after treatment with 2 g calcium daily for a year. They reported a significant decrease in the osteoid surfaces (11.5% to 8.9%), and osteoid thickness (10.2 to 6.3 μm). Bone volume, eroded surfaces, and mineralizing surfaces did not change significantly, although the latter increased slightly (6.8% to 9.4%).

Other studies have not found significant changes on bone biopsies from osteoporotic women treated with calcium (165,167,173,174). Ott and Chesnut (164) performed biopsies on 32 women after 2 years of calcium treatment. The number of osteoclasts decreased from 0.9 to 0.5, and the mineralizing surface increased from 3.0% to 4.1%. No significant changes were seen in the bone or osteoid volume, bone formation rates, or trabecular thickness. Chesnut and colleagues (166) described decreased osteoid thickness without other significant changes. In comparison, biopsies from women with osteoporosis taking a placebo for one year showed that the bone volume decreased significantly. Mineralization parameters, including double-labeled surface and bone apposition rate, are stable (169).

▶ 257

SUMMARY

The preponderance of data from controlled clinical trials suggests that calcium has a beneficial effect on bone mass. The cross-sectional and prospective studies of calcium intake are more variable, and the largest studies do not show significant effects. Although at first glance these findings seem incompatible, several reasonable explanations are offered. (1) The magnitude of the calcium effect is small, especially in comparison to the large variation in bone mass, and thus is more likely to be seen in a controlled trial than in a population study. (2) Part of the mechanism of the calcium effect is probably to reduce bone resorption via a reduction in activation, so that the largest gains in BMD would occur during the first year. These changes would be easier to measure in a clinical trial. (3) Other factors are more potent than calcium. This is especially true of estrogen, which can easily overwhelm any calcium effect. (4) Calcium requirements vary. (5) Assessment of dietary intake of calcium is difficult. Furthermore, the media constantly barrage women with messages to take more calcium, and those women who are at a higher risk for osteoporosis may have unwittingly increased their intake, which will cause errors in cross-sectional studies.

In conclusion, it is logical to ensure adequate calcium intake for women who have osteoporosis or who are at risk of getting it. More data on necessary doses are still needed, but a total calcium intake of 1000 to 1500 mg/d is suggested by the current evidence.

Practical Aspects of Calcium Therapy

DIFFERENT SALTS, FOODS, ACIDITY

Calcium carbonate is the most efficient source of calcium and is the least expensive. If a supplement is prescribed, it should be one with good dissolution.

Chewable tablets are a safe bet. Because calcium is absorbed better with food, it should be given with meals. Also, calcium carbonate is an antacid, and it causes a rebound gastric acidity when given on an empty stomach.

The dairy industry and its spokesmen insist that supplements are not as good as natural sources such as dairy products. Although there is no evidence for this, the viewpoint has infiltrated literature to patients and physicians alike. Dairy products contain protein, cholesterol, and calories, which may not be welcome. Furthermore, those who think that calcium from food sources is inexpensive (175) probably do not grocery shop.

For the patients who want to get all their intake from food sources, consideration should be given to calcium-fortified food such as orange juice. Also, spinach and common beans should not be used as calcium sources. Eggs and canned fish without bones have little calcium, and cottage cheese has less than most people think (Figure 9-5). Many foods are now labeled with nutrient content, and fortunately it is easy to calculate calcium content because the printed values are given as a percent of recommended dietary allowance which is 1000 mg (176).

Before prescribing calcium, physicians should be aware of the calcium intake from the patient's diet. Too many doctors prescribe 500 mg calcium daily, assuming that all patients consume the average amount of calcium. This may be unnecessary in the woman who loves milk and insufficient in a patient who avoids all dairy products.

MODULATE DIURNAL RHYTHM?

Calcium metabolism participates in diurnal rhythms. More bone is resorbed at night. It is not clear if this is related to nighttime fasting, to recumbent posture, or to hormonal variations independent of the diet. Some have postulated that calcium taken at bedtime might alleviate the nocturnal resorption, but as yet no evidence supports this theory.

COST

Calcium supplements vary in price. The cost to the pharmacist for one month dosage at 500 mg/d ranges from $2.07 to $16.98 (177). In 1984, a survey by Consumer Reports showed the cost per 1000 mg to be $0.12 for TUMS, up to $2.33 for calcium orotate. Os-Cal cost twice as much as TUMS (178). Physicians should be aware of these costs when they suggest calcium supplements to their patients. Unfortunately, some of the lowest priced calcium carbonate is not as biologically available, so it is not wise merely to recommend the cheapest brand. Because TUMS is a chewable form with known bioavailability, it is the brand I usually recommend.

An adequate amount of calcium for optimal bone strength is 1000 to 1500 mg each day. This can be taken by a combination of diet and supplements. The best supplement is chewable calcium carbonate (for example, TUMS). Each regular TUMS contains 200 mg of calcium, and should be taken with food. Here are calcium contents of some foods:

▶ 259

Item	Serving	Calcium in mg
Milk (whole or skim)	One 8oz glass	290
American cheese	1 oz	150
Cheddar cheese	1 oz	200
Parmesan cheese,grated	1 oz	400
Swiss cheese	1 oz	250
Cottage cheese	1/4 cup	50
Ice cream	1/2 cup	110
Yogurt	1 cup	300
Broccoli	1 cup	150
Collards	1 cup	350
Kale	1 cup	200
Tofu	1"x2"x3"	100
Figs	10 figs	250
Oysters	1 cup	200
Canned pink salmon	3 oz	150
Canned sardines	8 medium	350
Orange juice with calcium (Citrus Hill)	6 oz glass	200

Some foods do not contain very much calcium, despite what you may have heard:
Fresh fish, including salmon, does not contain much calcium. (The calcium in the canned fish comes from the bones.)
Asparagus, cabbage, corn, carrots, cauliflower, lettuce, peas, or potatoes do not contain much calcium. Beans contain calcium but it doesn't get absorbed very well
Spinach has lots of calcium but it does not get absorbed at all!
Eggs do not have calcium, unless you eat the shells.

Learn to read the nutritional labels on food you buy. It's easy for calcium! The U.S. RDA for calcium is 1000mg. The labels give the percentage of this amount. So to calculate the mg of calcium, just add a zero to the number on the label. For example, if a serving contains 15% of the U.S. RDA, it has 150mg of calcium.

FIGURE 9-5 Example of information given to patients about calcium in food.

SIDE EFFECTS

The risks of side effects from a reasonable dose of calcium (1000 mg/d) are very low. Ringe (179) has estimated that the risk of nephrolithiasis is "low" in normal women. Only those patients who have already had a kidney stone and who have absorptive hypercalciuria should not take excess calcium. Many kidney stones are caused by calcium oxalate, and the oxalate component is more responsible for the stone than the calcium. Limiting the dietary calcium allows more absorption of oxalate because calcium binds oxalate in the intestine. A recent survey of 45,619 men showed that dietary calcium intake was *inversely* associated with the risk of kidney stones; the relative risk of a stone for men in the highest quintile was 0.56 compared with the lowest quintile (180).

Some patients insist that calcium makes them constipated, although in blinded trials this complication is no more frequent than with placebo (181). Others complain of gastritis, which might be caused by taking calcium carbonate between meals, thus stimulating rebound acid production.

Vitamin D

The remainder of this chapter reviews the relationship between vitamin D and osteoporosis, with particular attention to clinical studies of vitamin D therapy. The mechanisms of skeletal effects are considered, using studies in bone tissue and serum PTH and markers of bone turnover. The divergent results of the changes in vitamin D with aging or osteoporosis are reported. Therapeutic trials of vitamin D and its metabolites are critically reviewed.

Brief Review of Vitamin D Physiology

Vitamin D was misnamed years ago, before the steroid nature of the hormone was known. Cholecalciferol (vitamin D) is formed in the skin from cholesterol precursors, after exposure to ultraviolet light. It may also be ingested from animal or plant sources. The molecule is hydroxylated at the 25 position in the liver to form 25-hydroxyvitamin D and then at the 1 position in the kidney to form 1,25-dihydroxyvitamin D, the most active metabolite. The renal 1α-hydroxylase is carefully regulated, primarily by PTH, phosphate, and calcium. Growth hormone and estrogen also can modify activity of the enzyme. $1,25$-$(OH)_2D$ circulates in both free and bound forms, bound to D-binding protein. Intracellular receptors for $1,25(OH)_2D$ are found in many cells, and the receptor-hormone complex binds to nuclear DNA to increase transcription of specific genes. The hormone may also act via phospholipids independently of gene transcription. The actions of $1,25(OH)_2D$ are numerous and have been recently reviewed (182). In terms of calcium metabolism, the best known and probably most important action is to increase calcium absorption from the intestine (183). Synthetic $1,25(OH)_2D$ is called calcitriol.

Mechanisms of Skeletal Effects of Vitamin D

Despite reams of papers, the effects of 1,25(OH)$_2$D on bone are still not well defined. The direct and indirect effects may differ, and the net result is difficult to predict.

STUDIES OF BONE TISSUE

In Vitro Studies: In cultured osteoclasts, 1,25(OH)$_2$D has no effect (184). There are no 1,25(OH)$_2$D receptors in the mature osteoclasts, but there are receptors in osteoclast precursors. 1,25(OH)$_2$D probably increases differentiation to osteoclasts and may increase the proliferation of precursor cells (185). Early bone tissue culture studies established the reputation of 1,25(OH)$_2$D as a resorbing agent. The resorbing potency closely parallels the affinity for the 1,25(OH)$_2$D receptor (186).

In osteoblasts, the effects of 1,25(OH)$_2$D are complex (187). The effects on gene expression in cultured osteoblasts are related to the proliferative and differentiated state of the cells, and depend on the duration of exposure to vitamin D. The production of collagen or alkaline phosphatase could be either inhibited or enhanced by vitamin D (187). In rat calvaria, 1,25(OH)$_2$D inhibits collagen production (188,189).

Animal Studies: Rats given high doses of 1,25(OH)$_2$D develop osteoid accumulation (190) or impaired collagen synthesis (191). Mice given 1,25(OH)$_2$D show increased resorption and, at high doses, growth impairment (192). It is questionable whether 1,25(OH)$_2$D has any important role besides making calcium available, because osteomalacia in D-deficient animals (193) or D-resistant children (194) can be prevented with infusions of calcium.

After oophorectomy, studies in both rats and dogs have shown that 1,25(OH)$_2$D, given orally, can prevent bone loss (195–197). In the dogs after oophorectomy, 1,25(OH)$_2$D repaired bone structural loss, but bone formation decreased after 4 months (198).

Biopsy Data: Biopsy results from human beings given 1,25(OH)$_2$D do not generally suggest that this hormone increases bone formation. Of interest, despite the animal studies, bone resorption is not increased, although this is more difficult to demonstrate by histomorphometry.

In patients who have osteomalacia, 1,25(OH)$_2$D treatment results in normalization of the osteoid and improvement in the mineralization (199). In patients with renal osteodystrophy and secondary hyperparathyroidism,

Calcium and Vitamin D in the Pathogenesis and Treatment of Osteoporosis

1,25(OH)$_2$D reduces fibrosis, reduces the resorption surfaces, and reduces the bone formation rates toward normal (200). Thus, the results from biopsies may be influenced by the underlying pathology.

Mild cases of osteomalacia or renal osteodystrophy can be difficult to distinguish from osteoporosis, and this can explain some of the differences seen in biopsies of osteoporotic patients. In some studies the osteoid decreases (201,202). In osteoporotic patients, in whom initial biopsies were done to eliminate those with osteomalacia, treatment with vitamin D or derivatives does not result in significant changes (164,173,174,203).

1,25-dihydroxyvitamin D can decrease PTH secretion by increasing serum calcium and also by altering the set point of the parathyroid gland to calcium. In D deficiency, serum calcium decreases and this is a primary stimulus to PTH secretion. It is not surprising, therefore, that most studies have shown an inverse correlation between vitamin D and PTH (204–206), or an inhibition of PTH with vitamin D treatment (207,208). The magnitude of decrease can be substantial. Treatment of postmenopausal women with 1,25(OH)$_2$D at 4 µg/d for 4 days decreased PTH by 30% (209). PTH decreased by 44% in elderly women treated with calcium and 800 U of vitamin D daily (210). Studies that did not find a decrease in PTH were done when assays were less precise and probably did not have enough statistical power to demonstrate an effect.

These relationships may be more complicated with aging because the intestines may becomes less efficient at calcium absorption. Thus, Orwoll (211) showed that PTH increased with age at the same time 25-(OH)D decreased although 1,25(OH)$_2$D was the same.

EFFECT ON MARKERS OF BONE
TURNOVER OR BALANCE

Vitamin D treatment consistently results in increased urine calcium. This is probably the only undisputed finding in the clinical vitamin D literature (Table 9-6, 9-7, and 9-8). The urine hydroxyproline, however, shows various responses in different conditions, but in most clinical trials it is either unchanged or decreased (212). This suggests that most of the increased urine calcium is from increased absorption and not necessarily from bone resorption. The increased gastrointestinal absorption has been shown directly, using calcium isotopes, in women with osteoporosis (213) as well as normal women (214).

The effect on bone resorption may depend on calcium intake or on the dose of 1,25(OH)$_2$D. In normal men, 2 µg calcitriol daily for 7 days decreases hydroxyproline (208). Similarly, in postmenopausal women calcitriol at 4 µg/d for

4 days resulted in decreased hydroxyproline 5 days later (209). The urine hydroxyproline level was unchanged at a dose of 1 μg/d of 1α-(OH)D, but increased at a dose of 2 μg/d (215). When normal men were placed on a low-calcium diet (400 mg/d), calcitriol, 3 μg/d, led to a negative balance (216). But when the dietary calcium was 880 mg/d and calcitriol was 2 μg/d the men were in calcium balance (217). Thus, bone resorption is more likely when higher doses of vitamin D are combined with lower calcium intakes. The alkaline phosphatase level tends to decrease with vitamin D therapy (see Tables 9-6, 9-7, and 9-8).

Osteocalcin: Several studies have shown that treatment with calcitriol consistently increases serum osteocalcin levels (208,218). This increase may be greater in osteoporotic patients than in normal individuals (219). Initial levels of osteocalcin were lower in osteoporotic patients, but they increased after calcitriol treatment (220). $1,25(OH)_2D$ levels correlate with osteocalcin in osteoporotic women (221). However, there is not a concomitant increase in alkaline phosphatase (220).

▶ 263

The function of osteocalcin is still uncertain. Under some conditions in cultured osteoblasts, chronic vitamin D exposure may inhibit alkaline phosphatase and collagen production, but stimulate osteocalcin (187). In normal persons, both alkaline phosphatase and osteocalcin levels have been shown to correlate with bone formation rates. However, osteocalcin is not always a marker for bone formation. In patients with osteomalacia, the osteocalcin levels are abnormally high, even though mineralization rates are low (222). Thus, the physiologic implications of the increased osteocalcin with $1,25(OH)_2D$ are currently unclear.

Recovery from Vitamin D Deficiency

In the face of uncertainty about the physiologic role of $1,25(OH)_2D$ on bone, studies of recovery from vitamin D deficiency are interesting. When treated with vitamin D, the $1,25(OH)_2D$ levels rapidly rise to supranormal levels of 200 pg/mL and stay elevated for several months, despite normal serum calcium values. It is tempting to speculate that these high levels play some role in the recovery from osteomalacia (223,224).

Changes in D Metabolism with Aging or Osteoporosis

SKIN AND MUSCLE

Less vitamin D is produced in the skin in elderly individuals. Skin samples from persons, aged 77 to 82, produced half the previtamin D as skin from 8 to 18 year

TABLE 9-6 Clinical Trials of Vitamin D

Author, Year	Reference	Design	Number Treated	Number Control	Subjects	Years of Study	% Dropout	Dose	Calcium Dose
Chapuy, 1992	210	db-bl	1634	1636	Ambulatory women, mean 84+6 y	1.5	46	800 U/d	1.2 g
Heikinheimo, 1992	270	rand, open	341	458	Mean age, 86 y	3.5	NA	150,000 U/y IM	none
Dawson-Hughes, 1991	271	db-bl	124	125	Healthy postmenopausal	1	10	400 U/d	0.377 g
Nordin, 1985	86	rand	68	68	Healthy, 65–74 y	2	20	15,000 U/wk	none
Orwoll, 1990	207	db-bl	41	36	Healthy men	3	NA	1000 U/d	1 g in vit D group only
Nordin, 1980	155	pros	25	23	Pmop, vertebral fracture	2.2	NA	10–50,000 U/d	1.2 g in control group only
Riggs, 1976	272	pros	9	9	Pmop, vertebral fracture	1	NA	50,000 2×/wk	1.5–2.5 g

d, decreased; db-bl, double blind; ES, eroded surface; i, increased; NA, not available; nc, no change; OS, osteoid surface; pmop, postmenopausal osteoporosis; pros, prospective; rand, randomized

olds (225). Thus, especially in very elderly persons, the dietary intake of vitamin D becomes relatively more important.

Muscle weakness has been associated with aging, and this could contribute to fracture risk in elderly men and women. Patients with abnormal electromyograms have lower 1,25(OH)₂D levels than age-matched normal controls (226). A double-blind trial of calcitriol in elderly subjects, however, showed no difference in muscle strength between placebo and calcitriol groups (227).

GENERAL

Levels of 25-(OH)D: The serum levels of 25-(OH)D vary greatly around the world (228). This is largely due to differences in sun exposure and to addition of vitamin D to dairy products. Several studies from northern Europe and the United States have shown that elderly persons have lower 25-(OH)D levels than younger persons (205,211,229,230). Seasonal changes are often reported. In Belgium, 25-(OH)D levels are lower in older persons than younger ones in the summer. The low wintertime 25-(OH)D levels normalized with replacement (231). Nursing home patients in Virginia had low 25-(OH)D levels without seasonal variation (232). In one report from Japan, however, the 25-(OH)D levels were similar in elderly women (up to age 79) and premenopausal women (233).

Osteoporosis

Result	Site	Bone Mass, %/y		Fracture (% Patients)		Alkaline Phosphatase	PTH	Urine Calcium	Bone Biopsy	Osteocalcin
		D	Control	D	Control					
+	Hip	1.8	−3.1	7.5	10.9	d	d			nc
+				16.4	21.8	d				
+	Body	−0.10	−0.05							
	Spine	0.85	0.15							
+	Hand	Better								
↔	Wrist	−0.9	−1.3			nc	d	i		nc
	Spine	−2.5	−2.1							
—	Hand	Worse		Worse						
+						d	d	i	d ES, d OS	

▶ 265

In New York, elderly persons had values in the range of 8 to 43 ng/mL, which is considered the normal range (234).

Reported 25-(OH)D levels in osteoporotic patients are variable. In Italy women with compression fractures had greater levels than controls (235). Finnish patients with hip fracture had lower 25-(OH)D levels than controls (236), but in England the patients with hip fractures had similar vitamin D status to patients who underwent hip replacement (237). Another Finnish study showed that the low 25-(OH)D levels were associated with elevated PTH levels (238). There is no association between 25-(OH)D levels and bone density (229,239).

Levels of 1,25(OH)$_2$D: Studies of 1,25(OH)$_2$D in elderly patients have shown conflicting results. Because 1,25(OH)$_2$D is bound to a D-binding protein, some investigators have measured this binding protein to estimate the free level. Decreased 1,25(OH)$_2$D concentrations have been reported from the United Kingdom, where 90% of geriatric patients had subnormal values (205); Israel (240); New York (234); Japan (233); Australia, where free levels were measured (241); and Belgium, where levels were normal in summer but not in winter (231). In one US study of 86 normal individuals, 1,25(OH)$_2$D slightly increased until age 65 in women, and it decreased after age 65 in men and women (242).

However, normal 1,25(OH)$_2$D levels are found in elderly patients from Oregon (211), Virginia (232), Denmark (243), and California (244). Although

TABLE 9-7   Clinical Trials of 1α-Hydroxyvitamin D

Author, Year	Reference	Design	Number	Number Control	Subjects	Years of Study	Dose, μg/d	Calcium Dose
Orimo, 1982	275	db-bl	234	242	Osteoporosis pain or fracture	0.5	0.75	none
Orimo, 1987	276	rand, not bl	38	48	Pmop, vertebral fracture	2	1	1g in half of each group
Shiraki, 1985	277	rand, not bl	20	23	Pmop	2	.5 and 1	none
Hoikka, 1980	201	db-bl	19	18	Hip fracture	0.5	1	2.5 g
Sørensen, 1977	202	rand, placebo	15	11	Pmop, fracture	0.25	2	1g
Nordin, 1980	155	pros	21	61	Pmop, vertebral fracture	1	1–2	1.2 g in control group only
Harju, 1989	238	pros	9	11	Hip fracture	0.2	0.5	1 g in vitamin D group only
Fujita, 1990	278	placebo	9	16	Pmop	1	1	NA
Lindholm, 1977	279	pros	16	0	Various osteoporosis	0.5–1.5	.5–2	1–2 g
Krølner, 1980	280	pros	15	0	Various osteoporosis	2	0.5–1.0	no
Lund, 1985	281	pros	22	0	Various osteoporosis	1–5	1	NA

d, decreased; db-bl, double-blind; i, increased; NA, not available; nc, no change; OV, osteoid volume; pmop, postmenopausal osteoporosis; pros, prospective; rand, randomized.

the 1,25(OH)$_2$D levels and production were normal in older men who had a normal GFR, they had a higher PTH level, so the kidneys may have required more stimulation to maintain the concentrations. In a study of healthy women, PTH and 1,25(OH)$_2$D both increased with age, but the intestinal vitamin D receptors decreased (245). A resistance to 1,25(OH)$_2$D action has been suggested from data showing increasing 1,25(OH)$_2$D and PTH levels with stable calcium absorption (41).

LEVELS OF 1,25(OH)$_2$D IN WOMEN
WITH OSTEOPOROSIS

According to Riggs and Melton's (246) postulated pathophysiology of osteoporosis, 1,25(OH)$_2$D levels are low in both types of osteoporosis. In type I (postmenopausal) the bone loss from estrogen deficiency is rapid, releasing calcium into the circulation. This inhibits 1α-hydroxylase activity. In type II os-

Measure-ment	Result	Bone Mass %/y		Alkaline Phos-phatase	Hydroxy-Proline	PTH	Urine Calcium	Bone Biopsy
		Vit D	Control					
Hand density	+							
Fracture	+			nc				
SPA	+	3.6, 5.5	−6.50	d		d		
SPA, bone biopsy	↔	0.00	2.50	nc			i	d OV
SPA, bone biopsy	+	25.00		d	nc	d	i	d OV
Metacarpal, vertebral fracture	—							
Bone biopsy	+					d		d OV
SPA, QCT spine	+	9	−10					
SPA, bone biopsy	+			d			i	
DPA	+	5.50						
DPA, SPA, Bone biopsy	+							

teoporosis (senile) the aging kidneys are unable to produce a sufficient amount of $1,25(OH)_2D$, and calcium absorption is limited.

Several studies have measured the levels of this sterol in women with osteoporosis, compared to similarly aged women without fractures. The results are not consistent (Figure 9-6) (219,221,247–256), but the largest studies have found no significant differences.

Studying patients immediately after surgery may be misleading; $1,25(OH)_2D$ levels did not increase after vitamin D treatment in patients with either hip replacement or hip fracture, but after 6 months this response was normal in both groups (237).

These findings can also be complicated by patients who have osteomalacia, which may mimic osteoporosis. In a subset of Finnish women who had experienced a hip fracture, very high $1,25(OH)_2D$ concentrations were seen that were not explained by PTH (238). These patients could have been in a recovery phase of D deficiency, in which $1,25(OH)_2D$ levels are high for months. Also,

TABLE 9-8 Clinical Trials of Calcitriol

Author, Year	Refer-ence	Design	N	N Control	Subjects	Years	% Drop-out	Dose, μg/d	Calcium Dose	Measurement
Tilyard, 1992	282	rand,open	314	308	Pmop, vert fx	3	30	0.5	1g in control group only	Fracture
Falch, 1987	283	rand, sg-bl	47	39	Pmop, Colles fracture	3	11	0.5	none	DPA arm, fracture
Ott, 1989	164	db-bl	43	43	Pmop, vert fx	2	16	0.53	1g or less	DPA, TBC, SPA, Bx, fracture
Jensen, 1982, 1985	284, 285	db-bl	29	29	Normal, 70 y	1	26	0.37	0.5 g	SPA, fracture
Gallagher, 1990	173	db-bl	25	25	Pmop, vert fx	2	20	0.62	1g or less	DPA, SPA, TBBMC, Bx, fracture
Christiansen, 1981	286	db-bl	21	23	Perimenopausal	1	9	0.25	0.5g	SPA
Aloia, 1988	174	db-bl	17	17	Pmop, vert fx	2	20	0.8	1g or less	TBC, SPA, DPA, Bx, fracture
Gallagher, 1982	287	db-bl	10	8	Pmop, vert fx	0.5	10	0.5	none	Ca balance, Bx, SPA
Gallagher, 1989	288	db-bl	29	33	Pmop, vert fx	1	NA	0.55	none reported	Fx
Caniggia, 1988, 1990	289, 290	pros	270	0	Pmop, vert fx, impaired Ca transport	1 to 8	NA	1	none	SPA, TBBMC in subset
Need, 1986	160	pros	37	38	Pmop with malabsorption	0.8	NA	0.25	1g	SPA
Caniggia, 1984	291	db-bl	7	7	Pmop	1	21	0.5	none	SPA, Bx
Fujita, 1990	278	db-bl vs 1α(OH)D	401	195	Outpatients, half with fracture	0.58	NA	0.5	none	Hand density

Result	Upper Extremity %/y		Total Body %/y		Spine %/y		Fracture (% patients)		Alkaline Phosphatase	OH-proline	PTH	Urine Calcium	Bone Biopsy	Osteocalcin
	D	Control	D	Control	D	Control	D	Control						
+	−1.00	−1.40					5	20				i		
↕							31	20						
↕	−1.50	−0.20	0.00	0.20	−0.50	0.00	26	16	nc	nc	d	i	nc	
−	−1.70	0.60							d					
+	−1.03	−0.53	0.10	−0.93	0.97	−1.96	44	41	nc	d		i	nc	
−	−2.10	−1.90							nc			i		
+	1.26	−1.63	0.96	−0.73	0.18	−4.30	25	33	d	d	nc	i	nc	nc
+	−1.50								nc	d	nc	i	d ES	
+							29	53						
↕			1.20	nd					nc	nc		i		i
+	−0.55	−1.10										i		
↕									nc	d		i	i BV	

BV, bone volume; Bx, bone biopsy; d, decreased; db-bl, double-blind; DPA, dual photon absorptiometry; ES, eroded surface; i, increased; nc, no change; pmop, post-menopausal osteoporosis; pros, prospective; rand, randomized; SPA, single photon absorptiometry; TBBMC, total body bone mineral content; TBC, total body calcium; vert fx, vertebral fracture

Calcium and Vitamin D in the Pathogenesis and Treatment of Osteoporosis

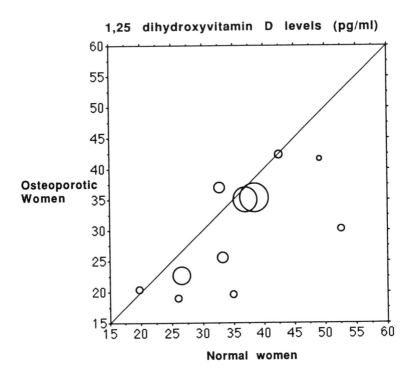

1,25 dihydroxyvitamin D levels (pg/ml)

Osteoporotic Women

Normal women

FIGURE 9-6 Studies of 1,25(OH)₂D levels in osteoporotic and normal women. The areas of the points are proportional to the numbers of subjects in the studies. Those studies in which normal women had higher vitamin D levels are below the 45 degree line of identity.

there could have been subclinical malabsorption. English women with hip fractures generally had 1,25(OH)₂D levels that were similar to elderly controls, but a subset with histologic evidence of decreased mineralization had increased levels (255).

The substrate status could also affect the results. In women with post-menopausal osteoporosis, treatment with 25-(OH)D increases both calcium absorption and 1,25(OH)₂D levels (250,257).

ESTROGEN AND 1,25(OH)₂D

The total circulating 1,25(OH)₂D increases after estrogen therapy in postmenopausal women, but there is disagreement about the free levels, because estrogen can increase the D-binding proteins. Cheema and coworkers (258) reported increased free levels, whereas Bouillon and colleagues (259) calculated normal free levels. Whether or not the free levels increased, there was more biologic effect. Gallagher and colleagues (260) found that estrogen increased circulating 1,25(OH)₂D; this was associated with increased calcium absorption.

Although estrogen does have measurable effects on the 1α-hydroxylase activity, natural menopause itself does not appear to result in abnormal $1,25(OH)_2D$ metabolism. Cross-sectional studies comparing early postmenopausal women to premenopausal women have shown normal $1,25(OH)_2D$ levels (261) or decreased total levels but normal free concentrations (262).

Falch (263) found no difference in circulating 25-(OH)D, $1,25(OH)_2D$ or D-binding protein in women followed longitudinally from 2 to 4 years prior to menopause until 4 to 6 years after the natural menopause. During this time bone loss was rapid. Therefore, the bone loss was apparently not caused by vitamin D metabolism. Similar results were reported by Hartwell and colleagues (261) in a longitudinal study of 10 women who went through natural menopause with no change in $1,25(OH)_2D$ or D-binding protein levels.

▶ 271

RESPONSIVENESS OF 1α-HYDROXYLASE

Parathyroid hormone stimulates 1α-hydroxylase, and several studies have examined the activity of this enzyme in elderly or osteoporotic patients. This can be tested directly, with PTH infusions, or indirectly with a low-calcium diet. With the low-calcium diet, similar responses are seen in premenopausal and postmenopausal women (258,262). Slovik and colleagues (256) found that direct infusion of PTH caused increases in $1,25(OH)_2D$ in normal women but not in women with osteoporosis. Sørensen and coworkers (254), however, reported that PTH caused a similar increase in $1,25(OH)_2D$ in osteoporotic patients and controls. Some of this discrepancy could be due to different ages or severity of osteoporosis. Investigators at the Mayo Clinic found a similar increase in $1,25(OH)_2D$ levels in normals and in patients with vertebral fractures. In patients with hip fractures, however, the baseline $1,25(OH)_2D$ levels were lower than normal and they responded less well to PTH (252).

KIDNEY FAILURE AND $1,25(OH)_2D$

Different degrees of renal function could explain some of the variable reports of $1,25(OH)_2D$ levels in elderly women (264). Because these women often have serum creatinine values within the "normal" range, the degree of renal insufficiency is overlooked, especially in thin, osteoporotic women. The creatinine clearance may be as low as 25 mL/min with serum creatinine value of 1.2 mg/dL. Renal failure can cause reduced levels of $1,25(OH)_2D$ because the final hydroxylation occurs in the renal tubules. Tsai and coworkers (252) reported a linear relationship between GFR and the ability of PTH to increase $1,25(OH)_2D$. In men living in a Veterans Administration nursing home, the

Calcium and Vitamin D in the Pathogenesis and Treatment of Osteoporosis

fracture incidence was related to increased blood urea nitrogen and decreased 1,25(OH)$_2$D levels (265).

Phosphate excretion is also diminished with renal insufficiency, which further reduces 1,25(OH)$_2$D production. Portale and colleagues (266) showed that dietary phosphate restriction could increase 1,25(OH)$_2$D production in mild renal insufficiency.

Goodman and Coburn (267) have reviewed the use of 1,25(OH)$_2$D in cases with recognized early renal failure. Renal osteodystrophy is almost always present by the time patients require dialysis. Often the parathyroid gland has already undergone so much hypertrophy that medical management is not possible. Therefore, nephrologists have attempted to treat patients with moderate renal failure to prevent the hyperparathyroidism. Some of the early reports of using calcitriol were worrisome because the renal function seemed to deteriorate. Later studies, in which both serum calcium and phosphate were carefully monitored, did not show any worsening of renal function beyond that seen in control subjects. Treatment with calcitriol controls development of hyperparathyroidism significantly better than placebo treatment.

CALCIUM ABSORPTION

Low levels of vitamin D in elderly or osteoporotic women are associated with decreases in calcium absorption from the gut. Calcium malabsorption in osteoporotic patients with low 25-(OH)D levels can be corrected by administering vitamin D (268). However, even with D replacement, calcium absorption may remain suboptimal in some patients. For example, in one study the calcium absorption increased from .36 to .57 in normal women given vitamin D, but in women with fractures absorption was .41 before treatment and only .44 afterward (269). Calcium absorption is correlated with 1,25(OH)$_2$D in both normal and osteoporotic women, but the regression intercept is lower in the women with osteoporosis, suggesting a partial gut resistance (247).

Orally administered 1,25(OH)$_2$D can probably increase calcium absorption by acting on the intestine directly, before it is itself absorbed. If oral 1,25(OH)$_2$D or 25-(OH)D were given to achieve similar 1,25(OH)$_2$D serum levels, the oral 1,25(OH)$_2$D would increase calcium absorption to a greater extent (269).

RELATIONSHIP BETWEEN D AND BONE DENSITY

Few studies have compared the 25-(OH)D levels to BMD. There was no correlation between 25-(OH)D and BMD in 122 normal women after adjusting for age (229). In another study, the 25-(OH)D level was low in 49 of 539 subjects, and they had a lower BMD (206). In 22 normal women followed longitudinally through menopause, a negative correlation was found between vitamin D intake and bone mass at the distal but not the proximal radius (204). In 16 elderly women followed for 4 years, the 25-(OH)D levels correlated to the change in BMD, $r=0.6$ (136).

RELATIONSHIP BETWEEN 1,25(OH)$_2$D
AND BONE DENSITY

In 22 normal women followed longitudinally through menopause there was a trend for 1,25(OH)$_2$D to correlate negatively with bone loss (204). However, in a cross-sectional study of 103 patients with osteoporosis, 1,25(OH)$_2$D did not correlate with BMD (221).

▶ 273

Studies of Vitamin D Supplements

Table 9-6 gives details of clinical trials of vitamin D (86,155,207,210,270–273). Recent studies from Europe have shown improvement in fracture rates in elderly persons treated with simple vitamin D replacement. A double-blind trial was conducted in 3270 French women, with a mean age of 84 years. After 18 months, the number of hip fractures was 43% lower and nonvertebral fractures 32% lower in the women treated with 800 units vitamin D and 1.2 g calcium. PTH decreased and BMD increased by 2.7%, whereas in the placebo group the BMD decreased by 4.6% (210). In another study, elderly persons, mean age 86, were randomly treated with a yearly injection of large doses of vitamin D (150,000 units). Fractures were seen in 22% of the untreated group and 16% of the treated group after 3.5 years (270). These studies emphasize the fact that many elderly patients may have subclinical vitamin D deficiency due to inadequate sun exposure and decreased conversion of 25-(OH)D even when skin is exposed. These studies were performed in countries that do not add vitamin D to milk or dairy products, so it is uncertain if the benefits would be so definite in the United States, but even in this fortified land many elderly people have low 25-D levels.

   Large weekly doses of vitamin D, however, may not be beneficial. Nordin (155) showed that women given 50,000 units twice weekly for an average of 2.2 years had more fractures than placebo- or calcium-treated patients; BMD decreased by 48 units, compared to a decrease of 26 units with placebo and no change with calcium.

   Studies of 24,25(OH)$_2$D in normal perimenopausal women (273) or osteoporotic subjects (274) have shown no beneficial effect.

Calcium and Vitamin D in the Pathogenesis and Treatment of Osteoporosis

Calcitriol and Other Analogs in Treatment of Osteoporosis

THERAPEUTIC TRIALS OF 1α-HYDROXYVITAMIN D

1α-Hydroxyvitamin D [1α-(OH)D] is a synthetic vitamin D sterol that is metabolized in the liver to $1,25(OH)_2D$. The dose is generally about twice that of calcitriol. Unlike calcitriol, there is no direct stimulation of the intestine as the drug is being absorbed. Also, any process that affects liver metabolism could alter the pharmacology of 1α-(OH)D. This metabolite has been studied in Europe and Japan, but not in the United States. Details of studies in Table 7 (155,201,202,238,275–281) document some of the varied results.

THERAPEUTIC TRIALS OF CALCITRIOL

Details of reported trials of calcitriol are in Table 8 (160,164,173,174,278, 282–291), and the results of controlled trials that presented bone mass data are shown on Figure 9-7. The results do not suggest a mandate for this therapy in the treatment of osteoporosis. At the radius, all but one controlled study showed a loss of bone mass in the calcitriol groups. At the spine, the bone mass did not increase significantly in the calcitriol groups, but in some studies the calcitriol groups lost less bone than the placebo groups. A large uncontrolled study from Italy reported gains in BMD at the wrist, but this study enrolled only women who had documented low calcium absorption, and the dietary calcium was only about 500 mg/d (289–291).

Three of the studies were conducted in the United States, using an identical protocol (165,173,174). Postmenopausal women with vertebral compression fractures were randomly assigned to calcitriol or placebo groups. Initially all subjects were placed on calcium intake of 1000 mg/d, using supplements if necessary. They also received a multiple vitamin containing 400 units vitamin D. The aim of the study was to give high doses of calcitriol, reducing the calcium intake if necessary. The study medication was increased every one or 2 weeks, and calcium in blood and urine was monitored. If hypercalciuria or hypercalcemia developed, the calcium intake was decreased to 500 mg/d. If hypercalciuria persisted, then the dose of the study medication was decreased. The study lasted 2 years, and bone mass was measured at the radius, spine, and total body. Bone biopsies were also performed at the beginning and end of the study.

These studies came to different conclusions. Aloia and colleagues (174) and Gallagher and coworkers (173) found significantly better change in bone mass in the calcitriol groups compared to placebo groups. *Women treated with calcitriol did not significantly gain bone mass,* but those treated with placebo had lost

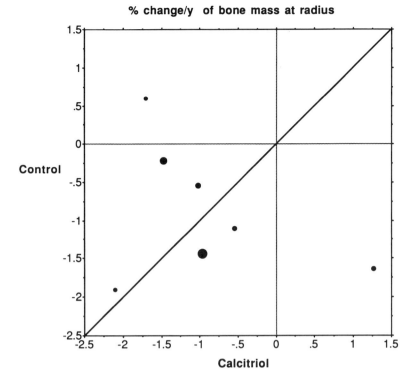

% change/y of bone mass at radius

Control

Calcitriol

▶ 275

FIGURE 9-7 Results of controlled studies of calcitriol in women with postmeno-pausal osteoporosis. The areas of the points are proportional to the number of subject-years in the studies. Those studies in which calcitriol group was better than control group are under the 45 degree line of identity.

bone mass, and this accounted for the difference between groups. The calcitriol-treated patients reported by Ott and Chesnut (164) also did not gain bone mass. The placebo controls, however, did not lose significant amounts of bone mass, and so there was no difference between calcitriol and placebo groups.

Various explanations have been offered to explain the differences in these studies. The one most frequently used and the most illogical is that the dose was not high enough in Ott's study. The mean dose for Aloia was 0.80 µg/d; and for Ott 0.53 µg/day. The doses were variable, and at 24 months the dose was 0.62 µg/day in Gallagher's study and only 0.43 µg/d in Ott's study. The differences arose because the investigators had different levels of concern about the urine calcium content. In all three studies, the urine calcium level rose dramatically, so even in the low-dose study, there was clearly a physiologic effect. A dose-dependent effect, however, should be seen in the treated groups. Figure 9-8 shows the *lack of a dose-dependent effect* of calcitriol in these trials. The main differences were in the placebo groups, whose women happened to lose more than those in the studies using the higher dose.

Calcium and Vitamin D in the Pathogenesis and Treatment of Osteoporosis

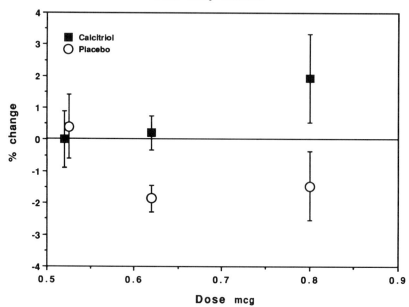

Total body calcium

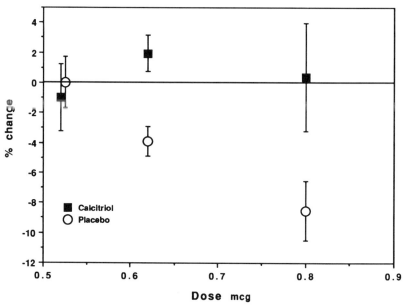

Lumbar spine

FIGURE 9-8 Lack of dose-response in US studies of calcitriol in women with post-menopausal osteoporosis. The bone density did not increase significantly in any of the three studies. The placebo groups happened to lose more bone in the studies that used the higher doses. The error bars represent one standard error.

276 ◀

Osteoporosis

Although these studies do not demonstrate a dose dependency, neither do they rule out this possibility. The studies were not designed to examine this; a randomization of doses would be necessary. When we further analyzed our data according to the mean dose tolerated by the patients, a significant correlation was found between dose and the change in bone mass. However, this is difficult to interpret, because patients who took the highest doses were those who had the lowest urinary calcium response. One plausible explanation is that some of the patients were initially more calcium deficient and were better able to tolerate the higher doses. These calcium-deficient patients would have more ability to increase their bone mass when calcium became available.

A more likely explanation for different results in the three American ▶ 277 studies is that the populations studied were different. The ages were similar, and all met the same exclusion criteria. The average creatinine values were not different. The mean number of fractures in the Seattle group was lower than that in other sites. However, when we analyzed our data using only those patients with severe fractures, the results were the same as with the entire group. There was no relationship between initial severity of vertebral fractures and the change in BMD after 2 years. The Seattle subjects may have been healthier in ways that were not measured. Walking and other activity was strongly encouraged for all patients in our study and that may have played a role.

Studies from Scandinavia have also shown no effect of calcitriol (see Table 9-8). There might be some hereditary differences in calcitriol response. Many of the Seattle patients were of Scandinavian heritage. Studies in Italy have been more positive, but these trials have not been controlled or randomized (289). The positive results from Japan are not surprising given the very low dietary intake of calcium (around 300 mg/day) (278). This would both enhance the efficacy of a drug that increased calcium absorption and lessen any side effects.

The most recently reported study from New Zealand (282) concluded that calcitriol treatment reduced the rate of vertebral fractures. This was a large study with 618 patients enrolled. There was a 30% dropout rate during the 3 years of study. The patients were randomly assigned (study not blind) to calcitriol, 0.5 µg/d or calcium, 1 g/d. During the first year there were new fractures in 6.7% of the calcium group and 5.3% of the calcitriol group. By the end of 3 years, 20% of the calcium group had suffered a fracture, compared to only 5% in the calcitriol group ($P < .001$). This study, like many other studies of osteoporosis, also reported the fracture rates in terms of vertebral bodies with new fractures, but that is more difficult to interpret because vertebral fractures are not independent events and after one new fracture a patient may be more likely to sustain another, possibly due to mechanical strains on the remaining vertebra. Unfortunately, bone mass was not measured in this study.

The pattern of fractures in the US and European studies was not as favorable as the New Zealand study (see Table 9-8). In these studies, from 25% to 44% of the calcitriol-treated patients had new fractures, but none had adequate power to detect differences from control. In the face of the confusing data available, it is difficult to make conclusions about the effect of calcitriol on fracture rate.

SIDE EFFECTS

Calcitriol is not a benign drug. Virtually every study has shown dramatic increases in the urine calcium levels. Ultrasound examinations of patients after 2 years of careful monitoring have shown no evidence of nephrocalcinosis in the American studies, but the doses were reduced whenever the urine calcium level exceeded 350 mg/d. Long-term use could potentially be damaging to the kidney (292). A report of children who had received calcitriol and phosphate for 0.3 to 11 years for X-linked vitamin D-resistant rickets showed nephrocalcinosis in 19 of 24 cases. All had normal serum creatinine values (293).

The early studies of calcitriol or 1α-(OH)D are replete with examples of serious hypercalcemia, some requiring hospitalization. Some of the hypercalcemia was associated with rapidly decreasing GFR, which was reversible when hypercalcemia was corrected (292). In all the American studies, dosages had to be reduced to below 0.5 μg/d in some of the patients.

In Japan, where the average calcium intake of osteoporotic women in the studies was very low (278), and in Italy, where the calcium intake was about 500 mg/d and only those with poor intestinal calcium absorption were included (289, 290), the incidence of hypercalcemia was lower. In Italy, hypercalciuria of about 300 mg/d was tolerated for several years without reported adverse effects.

Summary

In such a contentious field, where nearly every study is matched by one with different results, it is difficult to summarize or make clear conclusions. The only statement likely to gain consensus is that further research into the mechanism of vitamin D action on bone tissue is needed. Because recommendations are rather expected in a clinical review, I will hazard the following: vitamin D deficiency should be prevented, and in elderly individuals this means oral replacement with vitamin D supplements. Probably the usual amount found in multiple vitamins (400 U/d) will be sufficient in those without malabsorption. Calcitriol should not be recommended for patients with idiopathic postmenopausal osteoporosis because it does not usually improve bone mass and because it has an unacceptable risk-benefit ratio. Hypercalcemia and hypercalciuria are frequently reported. However, calcitriol could potentially be beneficial in patients who have mild intestinal malabsorption. In cases of moderate renal failure with evidence of parathyroid stimulation, calcitriol can prevent the development of "tertiary" hyperparathyroidism. These patients must be monitored carefully, with attention paid to the calcium intake.

References

1. Kanis JA, Passmore R. Calcium supplementation of the diet—I. Br Med J 1989;298:137–140.

2. Nordin BEC, Heaney RP. Calcium supplementation of the diet: justified by present evidence. Br Med J 1990;300:1056–1060.

3. Parfitt AM. Dietary risk factors for age-related bone loss and fractures. Lancet 1983;2:1181–1185.

4. Cummings SR, Block G, McHenry K, Baron RB. Evaluation of two food frequency methods of measuring dietary calcium intake. Am J Epidemiol 1987;126:796–802.

5. Heaney RP. Calcium in the prevention and treatment of osteoporosis. J Intern Med 1992;231:169–180.

6. Charles P, Jensen FT, Mosekilde L, Hansen HH. Calcium metabolism evaluated by ^{47}Ca kinetics: estimation of dermal calcium loss. Clin Sci 1983;65:415–422.

7. Heaney RP, Recker RR, Saville PD. Calcium balance and calcium requirements in middle-aged women. Am J Clin Nutr 1977;30:1603–1611.

8. Tavassoli M. Medical problems of space flight. Am J Med 1986;81:850–854.

9. Lipkin EW, Ott SM, Chesnut CH, Chait A. Mineral loss in the parenteral nutrition patient. Am J Clin Nutr 1988;47:515–523.

10. Malm OJ. Calcium requirement and adaptation in adult men. Scand J Clin Lab Invest 1958;10:1–289.

11. Shane E, delaCruz L, Ott SM. Photon absorptiometry and bone histomorphometry show preferential loss of cortical bone in renal patients. J Bone Miner Res 1988;3(suppl 1):595.

12. Neer M, Slovik DM, Daly M, Potts T Jr, Nussbaum SR. Treatment of postmenopausal osteoporosis with daily parathyroid hormone plus calcitriol. Osteoporosis Int 1993;3:204–205.

13. Silverberg SJ, Shane E, delaCruz L, et al. Skeletal disease in primary hyperparathyroidism. J Bone Miner Res 1989;4:283–291.

14. Cosman F, Shen V, Xie F, Seibel M, Ratcliffe A, Lindsay R. Estrogen protection against bone resorbing effects of parathyroid hormone infusion. Assessment by use of biochemical markers. Ann Intern Med 1993;118:337–343.

15. Jilka RL, Hangoc G, Girasole G, et al. Increased osteoclast development after estrogen loss: mediation by interleukin-6. Science 1992;257:88–91.

16. Ishimi Y, Miyarua C, Jin CH, et al. IL-6 is produced by osteoblasts and induces bone resorption. J Immunol 1990;145:3297–3303.

17. Kochersberger G, Westlund R, Lyles KW. The metabolic effects of calcium supplementation in the elderly. J Am Geriatr Soc 1991;39:192–196.

18. Kochersberger G, Bales C, Lobaugh B, Lyles KW. Calcium supplementation lowers serum parathyroid hormone levels in elderly subjects. J Gerontol 1990;45:M159–M162.

19. Reid IR, Ames RW, Evans MC, Gamble GD, Sharpe SJ. Effect of calcium-supplementation on bone loss in postmenopausal women. N Engl J Med 1993;328:460–464.

20. Dawson-Hughes B, Dallal GE, Krall EA, Sadowski L, Sahyoun N, Tannenbaum S. A controlled trial of the effect of calcium

supplementation on bone density in post menopausal women. N Engl J Med 1990; 323:878–883.

21. Reid IR, Hannan SF, Schooler BA, Ibbertson HK. The acute biochemical effects of four proprietary calcium preparations. Aust N Z J Med 1986;16:193–197.

22. Orwoll ES, McClung MR, Oviatt SK, Recker RR, Weigel RM. Histomorphometric effects of calcium or calcium plus 25-hydroxyvitamin D$_3$ therapy in senile osteoporosis. J Bone Miner Res 1989;4:81–88.

23. Riis B, Thomsen K, Christiansen C. Does calcium supplementation prevent postmenopausal bone loss? N Engl J Med 1987;316:173–177.

24. Baran D, Sorensen A, Grimes J, et al. Dietary modification with dairy products for preventing vertebral bone loss in premenopausal women: A three-year prospective study. J Clin Endocrinol Metab 1989;70:264–270.

25. Dawson-Hughes B, Stern DT, Shipp CC, Rasmussen HM. Effect of lowering dietary calcium intake on fractional whole body calcium retention. J Clin Endocrinol Metab 1988;67:62–68.

26. Need AG, Horowitz M, Morris HA, Nordin BEC. Effects of three different calcium preparations on urinary calcium and hydroxyproline excretion in postmenopausal osteoporotic women. Eur J Clin Nutr 1991;45:357–361.

27. Horowitz M, Need AG, Philcox JC, Nordin BEC. Effect of calcium supplementation on urinary hydroxyproline in osteoporotic postmenopausal women. Am J Clin Nutr 1984;39:857–859.

28. Elders PJM, Netelenbos JC, Lips P, et al. Calcium supplementation reduces vertebral bone loss in perimenopausal women: A controlled trial in 248 women between 46 and 55 years of age. J Clin Endocrinol Metab 1991;73:533–540.

29. Prince RL, Smith M, Dick IM, et al. Prevention of postmenopausal osteoporosis: a comparative study of exercise, calcium supplementation, and hormone-replacement therapy. N Engl J Med 1991;325:1189–1195.

30. Johnston CC Jr, Miller JZ, Slemenda CW, et al. Calcium supplementation and increases in bone mineral density in children. N Engl J Med 1992;327:82–87.

31. Recker RR, Heaney RP. The effect of milk supplements on calcium metabolism, bone metabolism and calcium balance. Am J Clin Nutr 1985;41:254–263.

32. Hasling C, Charles P, Jensen FT, Mosekilde L. Calcium metabolism in postmenopausal osteoporosis: the influence of dietary calcium and net absorbed calcium. J Bone Miner Res 1990;5:939–946.

33. Lanyon LE. Strain-related bone modeling and remodeling. Top Geriatr Rehab 1989;4:13–24.

34. Lanyon LE, Rubin CT, Baust G. Modulation of bone loss during calcium insufficiency by controlled dynamic loading. Calcif Tissue Int 1986;38:209–216.

35. Nelson ME, Fisher EC, Dilmanian FA, Dallal GE, Evans WJ. A 1-y walking program and increased dietary calcium in postmenopausal women: effects on bone. Am J Clin Nutr 1991;53:1304–1311.

36. Smith EL Jr, Reddan W, Smith PE. Physical activity and calcium modalities for bone mineral increase in aged women. Med Sci Sports Exerc 1981;13:60–64.

37. Burnell JM, Baylink DJ, Chesnut CH III, Mathews MW, Teubner EJ. Bone matrix and mineral abnormalities in postmenopausal osteoporosis. Metabolism 1982;31:1113–1120.

38. Burnell JM, Baylink DJ, Chesnut CH III, Teubner EJ. The role of skeletal calcium deficiency in postmenopausal osteoporosis. Calcif Tissue Int 1986;38:187–192.

39. Barger-Lux MJ, Heaney RP, Recker RR. Time course of calcium absorption in humans: evidence for a colonic component. Calcif Tissue Int 1989;44:308–311.

40. Sheikh MS, Ramirez A, Emmett M, Santa Ana C, Schiller LR, Fordtran JS. Role of vitamin D-dependent and vitamin D-independent mechanisms in absorption of food calcium. J Clin Invest 1988;81:126–132.

41. Eastell R, Yergey AL, Vieira NE, Cedel SL, Kumar R, Riggs BL. Interrelationship among vitamin D metabolism,

true calcium absorption, parathyroid function, and age in women: evidence of an age-related intestinal resistance of 1,25-dihydroxyvitamin D action. J Bone Miner Res 1991;6:125–132.

42. Heaney RP, Recker RR. Distribution of calcium absorption in middle-aged women. Am J Clin Nutr 1986;43:299–305.

43. Heaney RP, Recker RR, Hinders SM. Variability of calcium absorption. Am J Clin Nutr 1988;47:262–264.

44. Riggs BL, Kelly PJ, Kinney VR, Scholz DA, Bianco AJ Jr. Calcium deficiency and osteoporosis. J Bone Joint Surg 1967;49–A:915–924.

45. Need AG, Horowitz M, Philcox JC, Nordin BEC. Biochemical effects of a calcium supplement in osteoporotic postmenopausal women with normal absorption and malabsorption of calcium. Miner Electrolyte Metab 1987;13:112–116.

46. Spencer H. Osteoporosis: goals of therapy. Hosp Pract 1982;131–148.

47. Sheikh MS, Santa Ana CA, Nicar MJ, Schiller LR, Fordtran JS. Gastrointestinal absorption of calcium from milk and calcium salts. N Engl J Med 1987;317:532–536.

48. Heaney RP, Recker RR, Weaver CM. Absorbability of calcium sources: the limited role of solubility. Calcif Tissue Int 1990;46:300–304.

49. Goddard M, Young G, Marcus R. Short-term effects of calcium carbonate, lactate, and gluconate on the calcium-parathyroid axis in normal elderly men and women. Am J Clin Nutr 1986;44:653–658.

50. Marchandise X, Pagniez D, Ythier H, Gilquin B, Duquesnoy B, Wemeau JL. Influence of accompanying anion on intestinal radiocalcium absorption. Calcif Tissue Int 1987;40:8–11.

51. Johnson RN. A study of five calcium supplements: estimation of calcium absorption and sodium content. Eur J Clin Nutr 1991;45:117–119.

52. Brennan MJ, Duncan WE, Wartofsky L, Butler VM, Wray HL. In vitro dissolution of calcium carbonate preparations. Calcif Tissue Int 1991;49:308–312.

53. Sheikh MS, Fordtran JS. Calcium bioavailability from two calcium carbonate preparations. N Engl J Med 1990;323:921.

54. Harvey JA, Zobitz MM, Pak CYC. Dose dependency of calcium absorption: a comparison of calcium carbonate and calcium citrate. J Bone Miner Res 1988;3:253–258.

55. Miller JZ, Smith DL, Flora L, Slemenda C, Jiang X, Johnston CC Jr. Calcium absorption from calcium carbonate and a new form of calcium (CCM) in healthy male and female adolescents. Am J Clin Nutr 1988;48:1291–1294.

56. Recker RR. Calcium absorption and achlorhydria. N Engl J Med 1985;313:70–73.

57. Bo-Linn GW, Davis GR, Buddrus DJ, Morawski SG, Santa Ana C, Fordtran JS. An evaluation of the importance of gastric acid secretion in the absorption of dietary calcium. J Clin Invest 1984;73:640–647.

58. Pak CYC, Avioli LV. Factors affecting absorbability of calcium from calcium salts and food. Calcif Tissue Int 1988;43:55–60.

59. Nicar MJ, Pak CYC. Calcium bioavailability from calcium carbonate and calcium citrate. J Clin Endocrinol Metab 1985;61:391–393.

60. Pak CYC, Harvey JA, Hsu MC. Enhanced calcium bioavailability from a solubilized form of calcium citrate. J Clin Endocrinol Metab 1987;65:801–805.

61. Lappe FM. Diet for a small planet. New York: Ballantine Books, 1991.

62. Margen S, Chu J-Y, Kaufmann NA, Calloway DH. Studies in calcium metabolism. I. The calciuretic effect of dietary protein. Am J Clin Nutr 1974;27:584–589.

63. Allen LH, Bartlett RS, Block GD. Reduction of renal calcium reabsorption in man by consumption of dietary protein. J Nutr 1979;109:1345–1350.

64. Kim Y, Linkswiler HM. Effect of level of protein intake on calcium metabolism and on parathyroid and renal function in the adult human male. J Nutr 1979;109:1399–1404.

65. Chu J-Y, Margen S, Costa FM. Studies in calcium metabolism: II. Effects of low calcium and variable protein intake on human calcium metabolism. Am J Clin Nutr 1975;28:1028–1035.

▶281

66. Lutz J. Calcium balance and acid-base status of women as affected by increased protein intake and by sodium bicarbonate ingestion. Am J Clin Nutr 1984;39:281–288.

67. Spencer H, Kramer L, Osis D, Norris C. Effect of a high protein (meat) intake on calcium metabolism in man. Am J Clin Nutr 1978;31:2167–2180.

68. Heaney RP, Recker RR. Effects of nitrogen, phosphorus, and caffeine on calcium balance in woman. J Lab Clin Med 1982;99:46–55.

69. Hunt IF, Murphy NJ, Henderson C, et al. Bone mineral content in postmenopausal women: comparison of omnivores and vegetarians. Am J Clin Nutr 1989; 50:517–523.

70. Calvo MS, Kumar R, Heath H III. Persistently elevated parathyroid hormone secretion and action in young women after four weeks of ingesting high phosphorus, low calcium diets. J Clin Endocrinol Metab 1990;70:1334–1340.

71. Barger-Lux JM, Heaney RP. Effects of calcium restriction on metabolic characteristics of premenopausal women. J Clin Endocrinol Metab 1993;76:103–107.

72. Spencer H, Kramer L, Osis D. Factors contributing to calcium loss in aging. Am J Clin Nutr 1982;36:776–787.

73. Hasling C, Søndergaard K, Charles P, Mosekilde L. Calcium metabolism in postmenopausal osteoporotic women is determined by dietary calcium and coffee intake. J Nutr 1992;122:1119–1126. Abstract.

74. Abraham GE, Grewal H. A total dietary program emphasizing magnesium instead of calcium: effect on the mineral density of calcaneous bone in postmenopausal women on hormonal therapy. J Reprod Med 1990;35:503–507.

75. Seelig MS. The requirement of magnesium by the normal adult. Am J Clin Nutr 1964;14:342–390.

76. Marshall DH, Nordin BEC, Speed R. Calcium, phosphorus and magnesium requirement. Proc Nutr Soc 1976;35:163–172.

77. James WPT, Branch WJ, Southgate DAT. Calcium binding by dietary fibre. Lancet 1978;i:638–639.

78. Kelsay JL, Behall KM, Prather ES. Effect of fiber from fruits and vegetables on metabolic responses of human subjects. Am J Clin Nutr 1979;32:1876–1880.

79. Knox TA, Kassarjian Z, Dawson-Hughes B, et al. Calcium absorption in elderly subjects on high- and low-fiber diets: effect of gastric acidity. Am J Clin Nutr 1991;53:1480–1486.

80. Heaney RP, Weaver CM, Recker RR. Calcium absorbability from spinach. Am J Clin Nutr 1988;47:707–709.

81. Heaney RP, Weaver CM. Plant constituents and food calcium absorbability. J Bone Miner Res 1992;7:136. Abstract.

82. Wheadon M, Goulding A, Barbezat GO, Campbell AJ. Lactose malabsorption and calcium intake as risk factors for osteoporosis in elderly New Zealand women. N Z Med J 1991;104:417–419.

83. Kolars JC, Levitt MD, Aouji M, Savaiano DA. Yoghurt—an autodigesting source of lactose. N Engl J Med 1984;310:1–3.

84. Smith TM, Kolars JC, Savaiano DA, Levitt MD. Absorption of calcium from milk and yogurt. Am J Clin Nutr 1985;42:1197–1200.

85. Spencer H, Menczel J, Lewin I, Samachson J. Absorption of calcium in osteoporosis. Am J Med 1964;37:223–233.

86. Nordin BEC, Baker MR, Horsman A, Peacock M. A prospective trial of the effect of vitamin D supplementation on metacarpal bone loss in elderly women. Am J Clin Nutr 1985;42:470–474.

87. Eaton SB, Konner M. Paleolithic nutrition: a consideration of its nature and current implications. N Engl J Med 1985;312:283–288.

88. Garn SM. The course of bone gain and the phases of bone loss. Orthop Clin North Am 1972;3:503–519.

89. Nordin BEC. International patterns of osteoporosis. Clin Orthop 1966;45:17–29.

90. Matkovic V, Kostial K, Simonovic I, Buzina R, Brodarec A, Nordin BEC. Bone status and fracture rates in two regions of Yugoslavia. Am J Clin Nutr 1979;32:540–549.

91. Christian JC, Yu PL, Slemenda CW, Johnston CC. Heritability of bone mass: A longitudinal study in aging male twins. Am J Hum Genet 1989;3:429–433.

92. Rosanoff A, Calloway DH. Calcium

source in Indochinese immigrants. N Engl J Med 1982;306:239–240.

93. Fujita T, Fukase M. Comparison of osteoporosis and calcium intake between Japan and the United States. Proc Soc Exp Biol Med 1992;200:149–152.

94. Kelsey JL, Browner WS, Seeley DG, Nevitt MC, Cummings SR. Risk factors for fractures of the distal forearm and proximal humerus. Am J Epidemiol 1992;135:477–489.

95. Wickham CAC, Walsh K, Cooper C, et al. Dietary calcium, physical activity, and risk of hip fracture: a prospective study. Br Med J 1989;11:299:889–892.

96. Holbrook TL, Barrett-Connor E, Wingard DL. Dietary calcium and risk of hip fracture: 14-year prospective population study. Lancet 1988;ii:1046–1049.

97. Smith RW Jr, Frame B. Concurrent axial and appendicular osteoporosis: its relation to calcium consumption. N Engl J Med 1965;273:73–78.

98. Kleerekoper M, Peterson E, Nelson D, et al. Identification of women at risk for developing postmenopausal osteoporosis with vertebral fractures: role of history and single photon absorptiometry. Bone Miner 1989;7:171–186.

99. Wootton R, Brereton PJ, Clark MB, et al. Fractured neck of femur in the elderly: an attempt to identify patients at risk. Clin Sci 1979;57:93–101.

100. Kanis JA, Johnell O, Gullberg B, et al. Evidence for efficacy of drugs affecting bone metabolism in preventing hip fracture. Br Med J 1992;305:1124–1128.

101. Lau E, Barker DJP, Cooper C. Physical activity and calcium intake in fracture of the proximal femur in Hong Kong. Br Med J 1988;297:1441–1443.

102. Cooper C, Barker DJP, Wickham C. Physical activity, muscle strength, and calcium intake in fracture of the proximal femur in Britain. Br Med J 1988;297:1443–1446.

103. Nieves JW, Grisso JA, Kelsey JL. A case-control study of hip fracture: evaluation of selected dietary variables and teenage physical activity. Osteoporosis Int 1992;1:122–127.

104. Hurxthal LM, Vose GP. The relationship of dietary calcium intake to radiographic bone density in normal and osteoporotic persons. Calcif Tissue Res 1969;4:245–256.

105. Myburgh KH, Hutchins J, Fataar AB, Hough SF, Noakes TD. Low bone density is an etiologic factor for stress fractures in athletes. Ann Intern Med 1990;113:754–759.

106. Delmi M, Rapin CH, Bengoa JM, Delmas PD, Vasey H, Bonjour JP. Dietary supplementation in elderly patients with fractured neck of the femur. Lancet 1990;335:1013–1016.

107. Hesp R, Deacon AC, Hulme P, Reeve J. Trends in trabecular and cortical bone in the radius compared with whole body calcium balance in osteoporosis. Clin Sci 1984;66:109–112.

108. Horsman A, Marshall DH, Nordin BEC, Crilly RG, Simpson M. The relation between bone loss and calcium balance in women. Clin Sci 1980;59:137–142.

109. Heaney RP, Recker RR, Saville PD. Menopausal changes in calcium balance performance. J Lab Clin Med 1978;92:953–956.

110. Stamp T, Katakity M, Goldstein AJ, Jenkins MV, Kelsey CR, Rose GA. Metabolic balance studies of mineral supplementation in osteoporosis. Clin Sci 1991;81:799–802.

111. Matkovic V, Fontana D, Tominac C, Goel P, Chesnut CH III. Factors that influence peak bone mass formation: a study of calcium balance and the inheritance of bone mass in adolescent females. Am J Clin Nutr 1990;52:878–888.

112. Cumming RG. Calcium intake and bone mass: a quantitative review of the evidence. Calcif Tissue Int 1990;47:194–201.

113. Bauer DC, Browner WS, Cauley JA, et al. Factors associated with appendicular bone mass in older women. Ann Intern Med 1993;118:657–665.

114. Yano K, Heilbrun LK, Wasnich RD, Hankin JH, Vogel JM. The relationship between diet and bone mineral content of multiple skeletal sites in elderly Japanese-American men and women living in Hawaii. Am J Clin Nutr 1985;42:877–888.

115. Johnell O, Nilsson BE. Life-style and bone mineral mass in perimenopausal women. Calcif Tissue Int 1984;36:354–356.

116. Sowers MR, Wallace RB, Lemke JH. Correlates of mid-radius bone density among postmenopausal women: a community study. Am J Clin Nutr 1985;41:1045–1053.

117. Mazess RB, Barden HS. Bone density in premenopausal women: effects of age, dietary intake, physical activity, smoking, and birth-control pills. Am J Clin Nutr 1991;53:132–142.

118. Elders PJM, Netelenbos JC, Lips P, et al. Perimenopausal bone mass and risk factors. Bone Miner 1989;7:289–299.

119. Stevenson JC, Lees B, Devenport M, Cust MP, Ganger KF. Determinants of bone density in normal women: risk factors for future osteoporosis? Br Med J 1989; 298:924–928.

120. Sandler RB, Slemenda CW, LaPorte RE, et al. Postmenopausal bone density and milk consumption in childhood and adolescence. Am J Clin Nutr 1985;42:270–274.

121. Picard D, Ste-Marie LG, Coutu D, et al. Premenopausal bone mineral content relates to height, weight and calcium intake during early adulthood. Bone Miner 1988; 4:299–309.

122. Halioua L, Anderson JJB. Lifetime calcium intake and physical activity habits: independent and combined effects on the radial bone of healthy premenopausal Caucasian women. Am J Clin Nutr 1989;49: 534–541.

123. Cauley JA, Gutai JP, Kuller LH, et al. Endogenous estrogen levels and calcium intakes in postmenopausal women. JAMA 1988;260:3150–3155.

124. Chan GM. Dietary calcium and bone mineral status of children and adolescents. Am J Dis Child 1991;145:631–634.

125. Angus RM, Sambrook PN, Pocock NA, Eisman JA. Dietary intake and bone mineral density. Bone Miner 1988;4:265–277.

126. Andon MB, Smith KT, Bracker M, Sartoris D, Saltman P, Strause L. Spinal bone density and calcium intake in healthy postmenopausal women. Am J Clin Nutr 1991;54:927–929.

127. Nilas L, Christiansen C, Rødbro P. Calcium supplementation and postmeno-pausal bone loss. Br Med J 1984;289:1103–1106.

128. McCulloch RG, Bailey DA, Houston CS, Dodd BL. Effects of physical activity, dietary calcium intake and selected lifestyle factors on bone density in young women. Can Med Assoc J 1990;142:221–227.

129. Freudenheim JL, Johnson NE, Smith EL. Relationships between usual nutrient intake and bone-mineral content of women 35–65 years of age: longitudinal and cross-sectional analysis. Am J Clin Nutr 1986;44:863–876.

130. Wolman RL, Clark P, McNally E, Harris MG, Reeve J. Dietary calcium as a statistical determinant of spinal trabecular bone density in amenorrhoeic and oestrogen-replete athletes. Bone Miner 1992;17:415–423.

131. Buchanan JR, Myers CA, Greer RB. Determinants of atraumatic vertebral fracture rates in menopausal women: biologic *v* mechanical factors. Metabolism 1988;37:400–404.

132. Desai SS, Baran DT, Grimes J, Gionet M, Milne M. Relationship of diet, axial, and appendicular bone mass in normal premenopausal women. Am J Med Sci 1987;293:218–220.

133. Kanders B, Dempster DW, Lindsay R. Interaction of calcium nutrition and physical activity on bone mass in young women. J Bone Miner Res 1988;3:145–149.

134. Stevenson JC, Whitehead MI, Padwick M, et al. Dietary intake of calcium and postmenopausal bone loss. Br Med J 1988;297:15–17.

135. Block JE, Friedlander AL, Brooks GA, Steiger P, Stubbs HA, Genant HK. Determinants of bone density among athletes engaged in weight-bearing and non–weight-bearing activity. J Appl Physiol 1989;67:1100–1105.

136. Lukert BP, Carey M, McCarty B, et al. Influence of nutritional factors on calcium-regulating hormones and bone loss. Calcif Tissue Int 1987;40:119–125.

137. Sentipal JM, Wardlaw GM, Mahan J, Matkovic V. Influence of calcium intake and growth indexes on vertebral bone min-

284 ◄

eral density in young females. Am J Clin Nutr 1991;54:425–428.

138. Kelly PJ, Pocock NA, Sambrook PN, Eisman JA. Dietary calcium, sex hormones, and bone mineral density in men. Br Med J 1990;300:1361–1364.

139. Vinther-Paulsen N. Calcium and phosphorus intake in senile osteoporosis. Geriatrics 1953;8:76–79.

140. Leuenberger PK, Buchanan JR, Myers CA, Lloyd T, Demers LM. Determination of peak trabecular bone density: interplay of dietary fiber, carbohydrate, and androgens. Am J Clin Nutr 1989; 50:955–961.

141. Slemenda CW, Christian JC, Reed T, Reister TK, Williams CJ, Johnston CC Jr. Long-term bone loss in men: effects of genetic and environmental factors. Ann Intern Med 1992;117:286–291.

142. van Beresteijn ECH, van't Hof MA, de Waard H, Raymakers JA, Duursma SA. Relation of axial bone mass to habitual calcium intake and to cortical bone loss in healthy early postmenopausal women. Bone 1990;11:7–13.

143. van Beresteijn ECH, van't Hof MA, Schaafsma G, de Waard H, Duursma SA. Habitual dietary calcium intake and cortical bone loss in perimenopausal women: a longitudinal study. Calcif Tissue Int 1990;47:338–344.

144. Milne JS, Lonergan ME. A five-year follow-up study of bone mass in older people. Ann Hum Biol 1977;4:243–252.

145. Riggs BL, Wahner HW, Melton LJ III, Richelson LS, Judd HL, O'Fallon WM. Dietary calcium intake and rates of bone loss in women. J Clin Invest 1987;80:979–982.

146. Recker RR, Davies KM, Hinders SM, Heaney RP, Stegman MR, Kimmel DB. Bone gain in young adult women. JAMA 1992;268:2403–2408.

147. Slemenda C, Hui SL, Longcope C, Johnston CC. Sex steroids and bone mass. A study of changes about the time of menopause. J Clin Invest 1987;80:1261–1269.

148. Aloia JF, Vaswani AN, Yeh JK, Ross P, Ellis K, Cohn SH. Determinants of bone mass in postmenopausal women. Arch Intern Med 1983;143:1700–1704.

149. Dawson-Hughes B, Jacques P, Shipp C. Dietary calcium intake and bone loss from the spine in healthy postmenopausal women. Am J Clin Nutr 1987;46: 685–687.

150. Smith EL, Gilligan C, Smith PE, Sempos CT. Calcium supplementation and bone loss in middle-aged women. Am J Clin Nutr 1989;50:833–842.

151. Fujita T, Fukase M, Miyamoto H, Matsumoto T, Ohue T. Increase of bone mineral density by calcium supplement with oyster shell electrolysate. Bone Miner 1990;11:85–91.

152. Recker RR, Saville PD, Heaney RP. Effect of estrogens and calcium carbonate on bone loss in postmenopausal women. Ann Intern Med 1977;87:649–655.

153. Lamke B, Sjöberg H-E, Sylvén M. Bone mineral content in women with Colles' fracture: effect of calcium supplementation. Acta Orthop Scand 1978;49:143–146.

154. Horsman A, Gallagher JC, Simpson M, Nordin BEC. Prospective trial of oestrogen and calcium in postmenopausal women. Br Med J 1977;2:789–792.

155. Nordin BEC, Horsman A, Crilly RG, Marshall DH, Simpson M. Treatment of spinal osteoporosis in postmenopausal women. Br Med J 1980;451–454.

156. Ettinger B, Genant HK, Cann CE. Postmenopausal bone loss is prevented by treatment with low-dosage estrogen with calcium. Ann Intern Med 1987;106:40–45.

157. Albanese AA, Edelson AH, Lorenze EJ Jr, Woodhull ML, Wein EH. Problems of bone health in elderly. N Y State J Med 1975;75:326–336.

158. Polley KJ, Nordin BEC, Baghurst PA, Walker CJ, Chatterton BE. Effect of calcium supplementation on forearm bone mineral content in postmenopausal women: a prospective, sequential controlled trial. J Nutr 1987;117:1929–1935.

159. Almustafa M, Doyle FH, Gutteridge DH, et al. Effects of treatments by calcium and sex hormones on vertebral fracturing in osteoporosis. Q J Med 1992;83:283–294.

160. Need AG, Chatterton BE, Walker CJ, Steurer TA, Horowitz M, Nordin BEC. Comparison of calcium, calcitriol,

ovarian hormones and nandrolone in the treatment of osteoporosis. Maturitas 1986; 8:275–280.

161. Lee CJ, Lawler GS, Johnson GH. Effects of supplementation of the diets with calcium and calcium-rich foods on bone density of elderly females with osteoporosis. Am J Clin Nutr 1981;34:819–823.

162. Watts NB, Harris ST, Genant HK, et al. Intermittent cyclical etidronate treatment of postmenopausal osteoporosis. N Engl J Med 1990;323:73–79.

163. Riggs BL, Hodgson SF, O'Fallon WM, et al. Effect of fluoride treatment on the fracture rate in postmenopausal women with osteoporosis. N Engl J Med 1990; 322:802–809.

164. Ott SM, Chesnut CH III. Calcitriol treatment is not effective in postmenopausal osteoporosis. Ann Intern Med 1989; 110:267–274.

165. Storm T, Thamsborg G, Steiniche T, Genant HK, Sorensen OH. Effect of intermittent cyclical etidronate therapy on bone mass and fracture rate in women with postmenopausal osteoporosis. N Engl J Med 1990;322:1265–1271.

166. Chesnut CH III, Ivey JL, Gruber HE, et al. Stanozolol in postmenopausal osteoporosis: therapeutic efficacy and possible mechanisms of action. Metabolism 1983;32:571–580.

167. Gruber HE, Ivey JL, Baylink DJ, et al. Long-term calcitonin therapy in postmenopausal osteoporosis. Metabolism 1984;33:295–303.

168. Steiniche T, Hasling C, Charles P, Eriksen EF, Mosekilde L, Melsen F. A randomized study on the effects of estrogen/ gestagen or high dose oral calcium on trabecular bone remodeling in postmenopausal osteoporosis. Bone 1989;10:313–320.

169. Elias C, Heaney RP, Recker RR. Placebo therapy for postmenopausal osteoporosis. Calcif Tissue Int 1985;37:6–13.

170. Chesnut CH III, Nelp WB, Baylink DJ, Denney JD. Effect of methandrostenolone on postmenopausal bone wasting as assessed by changes in total bone mineral mass. Metabolism 1977;26: 267–277.

171. Jowsey J, Riggs BL, Kelly PJ, Hoffman DL. Effect of combined therapy with sodium fluoride, vitamin D and calcium in osteoporosis. Am J Med 1972;53:43–49.

172. Marie PJ, Pettifor JM, Ross FP, Glorieux FH. Histological osteomalacia due to dietary calcium deficiency in children. N Engl J Med 1982;307:584–588.

173. Gallagher JC, Goldgar D. Treatment of postmenopausal osteoporosis with high doses of synthetic calcitriol. Ann Intern Med 1990;113:649–655.

174. Aloia J, Vaswani A, Yeh J, Ellis K, Cohn S. Calcitriol in the treatment of postmenopausal osteoporosis. In: Cohn DV, Martin TJ, Meunier PJ, eds. Calcium regulation and bone metabolism: basic and clinical aspects. Vol 9. New York: Elsevier Science Publishers, 1987:113–118.

175. Kolata G. How important is dietary calcium in preventing osteoporosis? Science 1986;233:519–520.

176. Code of Federal Regulations. Title 21. Part 104. 20. April 1993.

177. Calcium supplements. Med Lett Drugs Ther 1989;31:101–104.

178. Osteoporosis. Consumer Rep 1984; 576–580.

179. Ringe JD. The risk of nephrolithiasis with oral calcium supplementation. Calcif Tissue Int 1991;48:69–73.

180. Curhan GC, Willett WC, Rimm EB, Stampfer MJ. A prospective study of dietary calcium and other nutrients and the risk of symptomatic kidney stones. N Engl J Med 1993;328:833–838.

181. O'Connell MA, Lindberg JS, Peller TP, Cushner HM, Copley JB. Gastrointestinal tolerance of oral calcium supplements. Clin Pharm 1989;8:425–427.

182. Slatopolsky E. Update on vitamin D: 1990. Kidney Int 1990;(suppl 29):S1–S62.

183. Kumar R. Vitamin D and calcium transport. Kidney Int 1991;40:1177–1189.

184. Kahn AJ, Partridge NC. New concepts in bone remodeling: an expanding role for the osteoblast. Am J Otolaryngol 1987;8:258–264.

185. Merke J, Klaus G, Hugel U, Waldherr R, Ritz E. No 1,25-dihydroxyvitamin D_3 receptors on osteoclasts of calcium-deficient chicken despite demonstrable re-

ceptors on circulating monocytes. J Clin Invest 1986;77:312–314.

186. Stern PH, Trummel CL, Schnoes HK, DeLuca HF. Bone resorbing activity of vitamin D metabolites and congeners in vitro: influence of hydroxyl substituents in the A ring. Endocrinology 1975;97:1552–1558.

187. Owen TA, Aronow MS, Barone LM, Bettencourt B, Stein GS, Lian JB. Pleiotropic effects of vitamin D on osteoblast gene expression are related to the proliferative and differentiated state of the bone cell phenotype: dependency upon basal levels of gene expression, duration of exposure, and bone matrix competency in normal rat osteoblast cultures. Endocrinology 1991;128:1496–1504.

188. Canalis E, Lian JB. 1,25-dihydroxyvitamin D_3 effects on collagen and DNA synthesis in periosteum and periosteum-free calvaria. Bone 1985;6:457–460.

189. Raisz LG, Maina DM, Gworek SC, Dietrich JW, Canalis EM. Hormonal control of bone collagen synthesis in vitro: inhibitory effect of 1-hydroxylated vitamin D metabolites. Endocrinology 1978;102:731.

190. Boyce RW, Weisbrode SE. Histogenesis of hyperosteoidosis in $1,25(OH)_2D_3$-treated rats fed high levels of dietary calcium. Bone 1985;6:105–112.

191. Hock JM, Kream BE, Raisz LG. Autoradiographic study of the effect of 1,25-dihydroxyvitamin D_3 on bone matrix synthesis in vitamin D replete rats. Calcif Tissue Int 1982;34:347–351.

192. Marie PJ, Hott M, Garba M-T. Contrasting effects of 1,25-dihydroxyvitamin D_3 on bone matrix and mineral appositional rates in the mouse. Metabolism 1985;34:777–783.

193. Underwood JL, DeLuca HF. Vitamin D is not directly necessary for bone growth and mineralization. Am J Physiol 1984;9:E493–E498.

194. Balsan S, Garabedian M, Larchet M, et al. Long-term nocturnal calcium infusions can cure rickets and promote normal mineralization in hereditary resistance to 1,25-dihydroxyvitamin D. J Clin Invest 1986;77:1661–1667.

195. Erben RG, Weiser H, Sinowatz F, Rambeck WA, Zucker H. Vitamin D metabolites prevent vertebral osteopenia in ovariectomized rats. Calcif Tissue Int 1992;50:228–236.

196. Faugere M-C, Okamoto S, DeLuca HF, Malluche HH. Calcitriol corrects bone loss induced by oophorectomy in rats. Am J Physiol 1986;250:E35–E38.

197. Drezner MK, Nesbitt T. Role of calcitriol in prevention of osteoporosis. Part I. Metabolism 1990;39:18–23.

198. Malluche HH, Faugere M-C, Friedler RM, Fanti P. 1,25-dihydroxyvitamin D_3 corrects bone loss but suppresses bone remodeling in ovariohysterectomized beagle dogs. Endocrinology 1988;122:1998–2006.

199. Bordier P, Pechet MM, Hesse R, Marie P, Rasmussen H. Response of adult patients with osteomalacia to treatment with crystalline 1α-hydroxy vitamin D_3. N Engl J Med 1974;291:866–871.

200. Sherrard DJ, Coburn JW, Brickman AS, Singer FR, Maloney N. Skeletal response to treatment with 1,25-dihydroxyvitamin D in renal failure. Contrib Nephrol 1980;18:92–97.

201. Hoikka V, Alhava EM, Aro A, Karjalainen P, Rehnberg V. Treatment of osteoporosis with 1-alpha-hydroxycholecalciferol and calcium. Acta Med Scand 1980;207:221–224.

202. Sørensen OH, Anderson RB, Christiensen MS, et al. Treatment of senile osteoporosis with 1α-hydroxyvitamin D_3. Clin Endocrinol 1977;7:169S–175S.

203. Caniggia A, Delling G, Nuti R, Lorè F, Vattimo A. Clinical, biochemical and histological results of a double-blind trial with 1,25-hydroxyvitamin D_3, estradiol and placebo in post-menopausal osteoporosis. Acta Vitaminol Enzymol 1984;6:117–130.

204. Lukert B, Higgins J, Stoskopf M. Menopausal bone loss is partially regulated by dietary intake of vitamin D. Calcif Tissue Int 1992;51:173–179.

205. Dandona P, Menon RK, Shenoy R, Houlder S, Thomas M, Mallinson WJW. Low 1,25-dihydroxyvitamin D, secondary hyperparathyroidism, and normal osteocal-

cin in elderly subjects. J Clin Endocrinol Metab 1986;63:459.

206. Villareal DT, Civitelli R, Chines A, Avioli LV. Subclinical vitamin D deficiency in postmenopausal women with low vertebral bone mass. J Clin Endocrinol Metab 1991;72:628–634.

207. Orwoll ES, Oviatt SK, McClung MR, Deftos LJ, Sexton G. The rate of bone mineral loss in normal men and the effects of calcium and cholecalciferol supplementation. Ann Intern Med 1990;112:29–34.

208. Bollerslev J, Gram J, Nielsen HK, et al. Effect of a short course of 1,25-dihydroxyvitamin D₃ on biochemical markers of bone remodeling in adult male volunteers. Bone 1991;12:339–343.

209. Geusens P, Vanderschueren D, Verstraeten A, Dequeker J, Devos P, Bouillon R. Short-term course of 1,25(OH)₂D₃ stimulates osteoblasts but not osteoclasts in osteoporosis and osteoarthritis. Calcif Tissue Int 1991;49:168–173.

210. Chapuy MC, Arlot ME, Duboeuf F, et al. Vitamin D₃ and calcium to prevent hip fractures in elderly women. N Engl J Med 1992;327:1637–1642.

211. Orwoll ES, Meier DE. Alterations in calcium, vitamin D, and parathyroid hormone physiology in normal men with aging: relationship to the development of senile osteopenia. J Clin Endocrinol Metab 1986;63:1262.

212. Tjellesen L, Christiansen C, Rødbro P. Effect of 1,25-dihydroxyvitamin D₃ on biochemical indices of bone turnover in postmenopausal women. Acta Med Scand 1984;215:411–415.

213. Riggs BL, Nelson KI. Effect of long term treatment with calcitriol on calcium absorption and mineral metabolism in postmenopausal osteoporosis. J Clin Endocrinol Metab 1985;61:457–461.

214. Adams ND, Gray RW, Lemann J Jr, Cheung HS. Effects of calcitriol administration on calcium metabolism in healthy men. Kidney Int 1982;21:90–97.

215. Marshall DH, Nordin BEC. The effect of 1α-hydroxyvitamin D₃ with and without oestrogens on calcium balance in post-menopausal women. Clin Endocrinol 1977;7:159S–168S.

216. Maierhofer WJ, Gray RW, Cheung HS, Lemann J Jr. Bone resorption stimulated by elevated serum 1,25-(OH)₂-vitamin D concentrations in healthy men. Kidney Int 1983;24:555–560.

217. Maierhofer WJ, Lemann J Jr, Gray RW, Cheung HS. Dietary calcium and serum 1,25-(OH)₂-vitamin D concentrations as determinants of calcium balance in healthy men. Kidney Int 1984;26:752–759.

218. Zerwekh JE, Sakhaee K, Pak CYC. Short-term 1,25-dihydroxyvitamin D₃ administration raises serum osteocalcin in patients with postmenopausal osteoporosis. J Clin Endocrinol Metab 1985;60:615.

219. Duda RJ Jr, Kumar R, Nelson KI, Zinsmeister AR, Mann KG, Riggs BL. 1,25-dihydroxyvitamin D stimulation test for osteoblast function in normal and osteoporotic postmenopausal women. J Clin Invest 1987;79:1249–1253.

220. Cannigia A, Nuti R, Galli M, Loré F, Turchetti V, Righi GA. Effects of a long-term treatment with 1,25-dihydroxyvitamin D₃ on osteocalcin in postmenopausal osteoporosis. Calcif Tissue Int 1986;38:328–332.

221. Hartwell D, Riis BJ, Christiansen C. Comparison of vitamin D metabolism in early healthy and late osteoporotic postmenopausal women. Calcif Tissue Int 1990;47:332–337.

222. Demiaux B, Arlot ME, Chapuy MC, Meunier PJ, Delmas PD. Serum osteocalcin is increased in patients with osteomalacia: Correlations with biochemical and histomorphometric findings. J Clin Endocrinol Metab 1992;74:1146–1151.

223. Papapoulos SE, Clemens TL, Fraher LJ, Gleed J, O'Riordan JLH. Metabolites of vitamin D in human vitamin-D deficiency: effect of vitamin D₃ or 1,25-dihydroxycholecalciferol. Lancet 1980;612–615.

224. Stanbury SW, Taylor CM, Lumb GA, et al. Formation of vitamin D metabolites following correction of human vitamin D deficiency. Miner Electrolyte Metab 1981;5:212–227.

225. MacLaughlin J, Holick MF. Aging decreases the capacity of human skin to produce vitamin D₃. J Clin Invest 1985;76:1536–1538.

226. Heyburn PJ, Peacock M, Casson IF, Crilly RG, Taylor GA. Vitamin D metabolites in post-menopausal women and their relationship to the myopathic electromyogram. Eur J Clin Invest 1983;13:41–44.

227. Grady D, Halloran B, Cummings S, et al. 1,25-dihydroxyvitamin D_3 and muscle strength in the elderly: a randomized controlled trial. J Clin Endocrinol Metab 1991;73:1111–1117.

228. McKenna MJ. Differences in vitamin D status between countries in young adults and the elderly. Am J Med 1992; 93:69–77.

229. Tsai K-S, Wahner HW, Offord KP, Melton LJ III, Kumar R, Riggs BL. Effect of aging on vitamin D stores and bone density in women. Calcif Tissue Int 1987; 40:241–243.

230. Aksnes L, Rodland O, Odegaard OR, Bakke KJ, Aarskog D. Serum levels of vitamin D metabolites in the elderly. Acta Endocrinol (Copenh) 1989;121:27–33.

231. Bouillon RA, Auwerx JH, Lissens WD, Pelemans WK. Vitamin D status in the elderly: seasonal substrate deficiency causes 1,25-dihydroxycholecalciferol deficiency. Am J Clin Nutr 1987;45:755–763.

232. McMurtry CT, Young SE, Downs RW, Adler RA. Mild vitamin D deficiency and secondary hyperparathyroidism in nursing home patients receiving adequate dietary vitamin D. J Am Geriatr Soc 1992;40:343–347.

233. Fujisawa Y, Kida K, Matsuda H. Role of change in vitamin D metabolism with age in calcium and phosphorus metabolism in normal human subjects. J Clin Endocrinol Metab 1984;59:719–726.

234. Clemens TL, Zhou X-Y, Myles M, Endres D, Lindsay R. Serum vitamin D_2 and vitamin D_3 metabolite concentrations and absorption of vitamin D_2 in elderly subjects. J Clin Endocrinol Metab 1986; 63:656.

235. Loré F, Di Cairano G, Periti P, Caniggia A. Effect of the administration of 1,25-dihydroxyvitamin D_3 on serum levels of 25-hydroxyvitamin D in postmenopausal osteoporosis. Calcif Tissue Int 1982;34:539–541.

236. Punnonen R, Salmi J, Tuimala R, Jarvinen M, Pystynen P. Vitamin D deficiency in women with femoral neck fracture. Maturitas 1986;8:291–295.

237. Hordon LD, Peacock M. Vitamin D metabolism in women with femoral neck fracture. Bone Miner 1987;2:413–426.

238. Harju E, Punnonen R, Tuimala R, Salmi J, Paronen I. Vitamin D and calcitonin treatment in patients with femoral neck fracture: a prospective controlled clinical study J Int Med Res 1989;17:226–242.

239. Weisman Y, Salama R, Harell A, Edelstein S. Serum 24,25-dihydroxyvitamin D and 25-hydroxyvitamin D concentrations in femoral neck fracture. Br Med J 1978;2:1196–1197.

240. Sagiv P, Lidor C, Hallel T, Edestein S. Decrease in bone level of 1,25-dihydroxyvitamin D in women over 45 years old. Calcif Tissue Int 1992;51: 24–26.

241. Prince R, Dick I, Boyd F, Kent N, Garcia-Webb P. The effects of dietary calcium deprivation on serum calcitriol levels in premenopausal and postmenopausal women. Metabolism 1988;37:727–731.

242. Epstein S, Bryce G, Hinman JW, et al. The influence of age on bone mineral regulating hormones. Bone 1986,7:421–425.

243. Hartwell D, Rødbro P, Jensen SB, Thomsen K, Christiansen C. Vitamin D metabolites—relation to age, menopause and endometriosis. Scand J Clin Lab Invest 1990;50:115–121.

244. Halloran BP, Portale AA, Lonergan ET, Morris RC Jr. Production and metabolic clearance of 1,25-dihydroxyvitamin D in men: effect of advancing age. J Clin Endocrinol Metab 1990;70:318–323.

245. Ebeling PR, Sandgren ME, DiMagno EP, Lane AW, DeLuca HF, Riggs BL. Evidence of an age-related decrease in intestinal responsiveness to vitamin D: relationship between serum 1,25-dihydroxyvitamin D_3 and intestinal vitamin D receptor concentrations in normal women. J Clin Endocrinol Metab 1992;75:176–182.

246. Riggs BL, Melton LJ. Evidence for two distinct syndromes of involutional osteoporosis. Am J Med 1983;75:899–901.

247. Morris HA, Need AG, Horowitz M, O'Loughlin PD, Nordin BEC. Calcium absorption in normal and osteoporotic postmenopausal women. Calcif Tissue Int 1991;49:240–243.

248. Aloia JF, Cohn SH, Vaswani A, Yeh JK, Yuen K, Ellis K. Risk factors for postmenopausal osteoporosis. Am J Med 1985;78:95–100.

249. Gallagher JC, Riggs BL, Eisman J, Hamstra A, Arnaud SB, DeLuca HF. Intestinal calcium absorption and serum vitamin D metabolites in normal subjects and osteoporotic patients. J Clin Invest 1979;64: 729–736.

250. Francis RM, Peacock M, Taylor GA, Storer JH, Nordin BEC. Calcium malabsorption in elderly women with vertebral fractures: evidence for resistance to the action of vitamin D metabolites on the bowel. Clin Sci 1984;66:103–107.

251. Stevenson JC, Allen PR, Abeyasekera G, Hill PA. Osteoporosis with hip fracture: changes in calcium regulating hormones. Eur J Clin Invest 1986;16:357–360.

252. Tsai K-S, Heath H III, Kumar R, Riggs BL. Impaired vitamin D metabolism with aging in women: possible role in pathogenesis of senile osteoporosis. J Clin Invest 1984;73:1668–1672.

253. Riggs BL, Hamstra A, DeLuca HF. Assessment of 25 hydroxyvitamin D 1 hydroxylase reserve in postmenopausal osteoporosis by administration of parathyroid extract. J Clin Endocrinol Metab 1981;53:833–835.

254. Sørensen OH, Lumholtz B, Lund B, et al. Acute effects of parathyroid hormone on vitamin D metabolism in patients with the bone loss of aging. J Clin Endocrinol Metab 1982;54:1258–1261.

255. Hordon LD, Peacock M. Osteomalacia and osteoporosis in femoral neck fracture. Bone Miner 1990;11:247–259.

256. Slovik DM, Adams JS, Neer RM, Holick MF, Potts JT Jr. Deficient production of 1,25-dihydroxyvitamin D in elderly osteoporotic patients. N Engl J Med 1981; 305:372–374.

257. Zerwekh JE, Sakhaee K, Glass K, Pak CYC. Long term 25-hydroxyvitamin D3 therapy in postmenopausal osteoporosis: demonstration of responsive and nonresponsive subgroups. J Clin Endocrinol Metab 1983;56:410–413.

258. Cheema C, Grant BF, Marcus R. Effects of estrogen on circulating "free" and total 1,25-dihydroxyvitamin D and on the parathyroid-vitamin D axis in postmenopausal women. J Clin Invest 1989;83: 537–542.

259. Bouillon R, Van Assche FA, Van Baelen H, Heyns W, De Moor P. Influence of vitamin D-binding protein on the serum concentration of 1,25-dihydroxyvitamin D3: significance of the free 1,25-dihydroxyvitamin D3 concentration. J Clin Invest 1981;67:589–596.

260. Gallagher JC, Riggs BL, DeLuca HF. Effect of estrogen on calcium absorption and serum vitamin D metabolites in postmenopausal osteoporosis. J Clin Endocrinol Metab 1980;51:1359–1364.

261. Hartwell D, Riis BJ, Christiansen C. Changes in vitamin D metabolism during natural and medical menopause. J Clin Endocrinol Metab 1990;71:127–132.

262. Prince RL, Dick I, Garcia-Webb P, Retallack RW. The effects of the menopause on calcitriol and parathyroid hormone: responses to a low dietary calcium stress test. J Clin Endocrinol Metab 1990;70:1119–1123.

263. Falch JA, Oftebro H, Haug E. Early postmenopausal bone loss is not associated with a decrease in circulating levels of 25-hydroxyvitamin D, 1,25-dihydroxyvitamin D, or vitamin D-binding protein. J Clin Endocrinol Metab 1987;64:836–839.

264. Buchanan JR, Myers CA, Greer RB III. Effect of declining renal function on bone density in aging women. Calcif Tissue Int 1988;43:1–6.

265. Rudman D, Rudman IW, Mattson DE, Nagraj HS, Caindec N, Jackson DL. Fractures in the men of a Veterans Administration nursing home: relation to 1,25-dihydroxyvitamin D. J Am Coll Nutr 1989;8:324–334.

266. Portale AA, Halloran BP, Murphy MM, Morris RC. Oral intake of phosphorus can determine the serum concentration of 1,25-dihydroxyvitamin D by determin-

ing its production rate in humans. J Clin Invest 1986;77:7–12.

267. Goodman WG, Coburn JW. The use of 1,25-dihydroxyvitamin D_3 in early renal failure. Annu Rev Med 1992;43:227–237.

268. Francis RM, Peacock M. Storer JH, Davies AEJ, Brown WB, Nordin BEC. Calcium malabsorption in the elderly: the effect of treatment with oral 25-hydroxyvitamin D_3. Eur J Clin Invest 1983;13:391–396.

269. Francis RM, Peacock M. Local action of oral, 1,25-dihydroxycholecalciferol on calcium absorption in osteoporosis. Am J Clin Nutr 1987;46:315–318.

270. Heikinheimo RJ, Inkovaara JA, Harju EJ, et al. Annual injection of vitamin D and fractures of aged bones. Calcif Tissue Int 1992;51:105–110.

271. Dawson-Hughes B, Dallal GE, Krall EA, Harris S, Sokoll LJ, Falconer G. Effect of vitamin D supplementation on wintertime and overall bone loss in healthy postmenopausal women. Ann Intern Med 1991;115:505–512.

272. Riggs BL, Jowsey J, Kelly PJ, Hoffman DL, Arnaud CD. Effects of oral therapy with calcium and vitamin D in primary osteoporosis. J Clin Endocrinol Metab 1976;42:1139–1144.

273. Riis BJ, Thomsen K, Christiansen C. Does 24R,25(OH)$_2$-vitamin D_3 prevent postmenopausal bone loss? Calcif Tissue Int 1986;39:128–132.

274. Reeve J, Tellez M, Green JR, et al. Long-term treatment of osteoporosis with 24,25-dihydroxycholecalciferol. Acta Endocrinol 1982;101:636–640.

275. Orimo H, Inoue T, Fujita T, Itami Y. Clinical experience with 1α-OH-D_3: senile osteoporosis. In: Norman AW, ed. Vitamin D: chemical, biochemical and clinical endocrinology of calcium metabolism. Berlin: Walter de Gruyter, 1982:1239–1243.

276. Orimo H, Shiraki M, Hayashi T, Nakamura T. Reduced occurrence of vertebral crush fractures in senile osteoporosis treated with 1α(OH)-vitamin D_3. Bone Miner 1987;3:47–52.

277. Shiraki M, Orimo H, Ito H, et al. Long-term treatment of postmeno-

pausal osteoporosis with active vitamin D_3, 1-alpha-hydroxycholecalciferol (1α-OHD$_3$) and 1,24 dihydroxycholecalciferol (1,24(OH)$_2$D$_3$). Endocrinol Jpn 1985;32:305–315.

278. Fujita T. Studies in osteoporosis in Japan. Metabolism 1990;39:39–42.

279. Lindholm TS, Sevastikoglou JA, Lindgren U. Long-term treatment of osteoporotic patients with 1α-OH-D_3 and calcium. In: Norman AW, ed. Vitamin D: biochemical, chemical and clinical aspects related to calcium metabolism. Berlin: Walter de Gruyter, 1977:635–637.

280. Krølner B, Nielsen SP, Lund B, Lund BJ, Sørensen OH, Jacobsen S. Lumbar spine bone mineral content in postmenopausal osteoporosis. Calcif Tissue Int 1980;31:77A.

281. Lund B, Hjorth L, Kjaer I, et al. Treatment of osteoporosis of ageing with 1α-hydroxycholecalciferol. Lancet 1975;1168–1171.

282. Tilyard MW, Spears GFS, Thomson J, Dovey S. Treatment of postmenopausal osteoporosis with calcitriol or calcium. N Engl J Med 1992;326:357–362.

283. Falch JA, Odegaard OR, Finnanger AM, Matheson I. Postmenopausal osteoporosis: no effect of three years treatment with 1,25-dihydroxycholecalciferol. Acta Med Scand 1987;221:199–204.

284. Jensen GF, Christiansen C, Transbøl I. Treatment of post menopausal osteoporosis. A controlled therapeutic trial comparing oestrogen/gestagen, 1,25-dihydroxyvitamin D_3 and calcium. Clin Endocrinol 1982;16:515–524.

285. Jensen GF, Meinecke B, Boesen J, Transbøl I. Does 1,25(OH)$_2$D$_3$ accelerate spinal bone loss? A controlled therapeutic trial in 70-year-old women. Clin Orthop 1985;192:215–221.

286. Christiansen C, Christensen MS, Rødbro P, Hagen C, Transbøl I. Effect of 1,25-dihydroxy-vitamin D_3 in itself or combined with hormone treatment in preventing postmenopausal osteoporosis. Eur J Clin Invest 1981;11:305–309.

287. Gallagher JC, Jerpbak CM, Jee WSS, Johnson KA, DeLuca HF, Riggs BL. 1,25-dihydroxyvitamin D_3: short- and

long-term effects on bone and calcium metabolism in patients with postmenopausal osteoporosis. Proc Natl Acad Sci USA 1982;79:3325–3329.

288. Gallagher JC, Riggs BL, Recker RR, Goldgar D. The effect of calcitriol on patients with postmenopausal osteoporosis with special reference to fracture frequency. Proc Soc Exp Biol Med 1989; 191:287–292.

289. Caniggia A. Long-term calcitriol treatment in post-menopausal osteoporosis: Follow-up of two hundred patients. In: Norman AW, ed. Vitamin D: molecular, cellular and clinical endocrinology. Berlin: Walter de Gruyter, 1988:807–816.

290. Caniggia A, Nuti R, Lore F, Martini G, Turchetti V, Righi G. Long-term treatment with calcitriol in postmenopausal osteoporosis. Metabolism 1990;39:43–49.

291. Cannigia A, Nuti R, Loré F, Vattimo A. The hormonal form of vitamin D in the pathophysiology and therapy of postmenopausal osteoporosis. J Endocrinol Invest 1984;7:373–378.

292. Lund B, Sørensen OH, Lund BJ. 1α-hydroxycholecalciferol and renal function. Lancet 1978;2:731.

293. Verge CF, Lam A, Simpson JM, Cowell CT, Howard NJ, Silink M. Effects of therapy in X-linked hypophosphatemic rickets. N Engl J Med 1991;325:1843–1848.

10 ▸ The Relationship of Estrogen to Bone Health

▶ ▶ ▶ Robert Marcus

The profound impact of menopausal estrogen withdrawal on skeletal integrity has been appreciated since the seminal contributions of Albright and Reifenstein (1) more than 40 years ago. Over the last 15 years, careful and properly controlled clinical trials clearly show that estrogen replacement therapy (ERT) maintains bone mass throughout the skeleton of menopausal women. In addition, epidemiologic studies indicate substantial protection against osteoporotic fracture for menopausal women who receive long-term treatment. This chapter discusses the relationship of women's endocrine reproductive status to skeletal health, including the consequences of interrupting menstrual function during young adult life, the changes in skeletal homeostasis at the time of natural menopause, the skeletal effects of ERT, and several practical aspects of estrogen administration. Nonskeletal aspects of hormone replacement have received intense scrutiny in recent years and are summarized only briefly in this chapter.

Estrogen Withdrawal in Young Women

Even temporary cessation of menstrual function may lead to bone loss. Treatment of endometriosis with a gonadotropin-releasing hormone analog profoundly lowers circulating estrogen concentrations and is accompanied by increased bone turnover and loss of bone, particularly from trabecular sites (2–5). Following treatment, resumption of normal gonadal function restores bone density in virtually all cases. Full recovery of bone mass depends on treatment duration. To date, most treatment protocols have not exceeded 6 months, the length of two remodeling cycles. With sustained or repeated courses of therapy, concern about permanent bone loss must be raised.

Klibanski and colleagues (6) and others (7,8) have called attention to deficits in bone mass in women with amenorrhea due to prolactin-secreting pituitary tumors. These deficits appear to depend solely on the reduction in circulating estrogen, since hyperprolactinemia in the absence of hypogonadism is not associated with a decreased bone mass (9).

Numerous reports document the presence of bone mineral deficits in young women athletes whose rigorous exercise has resulted in loss of menses (10–12). These women exhibit hypogondatropic hypogonadism and show significant reductions in bone mineral density (BMD) despite impressive levels of skeletal loading. As opposed to the straightforward pathophysiology described above for gonadotropin analogs, inadequate nutritional status also contributes to bone loss in the amenorrheic athletes. The observed deficits are of sufficient magnitude to create a substantial risk of injury and fracture (11,13). Moreover, the abnormalities in nutrient intake and menstrual function are often of sufficient duration to jeopardize full recovery of bone mass (14).

Young women who are rendered precipitously hypogonadal by oophorectomy are particularly vulnerable to severe bone loss. Cann and colleagues (15) observed an average trabecular bone loss of 12.4% 2 years after oophorectomy of premenopausal women. This striking decrease is influenced by patient age. Little difference in bone mass has been observed between 50-year-old women who have experienced a natural menopause and those who have recently undergone oophorectomy (16).

Young women with idiopathic primary ovarian failure have spinal trabecular bone mass averaging about 50% of age-predicted values (17). A more common example of premature ovarian failure is the young woman with breast cancer who has become hypogonadal following chemotherapy and cannot take replacement estrogen. No completely satisfactory therapy is currently available for such patients, although bisphosphonates and calcitonin may conserve bone mass. Some evidence points to a favorable skeletal effect of tamoxifen in these patients (18–20). However, much of the skeletal protective effect of this drug reflects experience in older women who are well beyond the age of natural menopause. Tamoxifen is a competitive inhibitor of estrogen action. It acts as an agonist when no estrogen is present but is an effective antagonist in women with endogenous estrogen production. The impact of tamoxifen on bone health would therefore be of particular concern for healthy young women who may be considered candidates to receive hormonal prophylaxis against breast cancer.

The skeletal consequences of altered menstrual function short of amenorrhea are less well understood. Pryor and colleagues (21) presented evidence for loss of spinal trabecular bone at an annual rate as great as 4% among healthy young women who experience as few as one or two anovulatory or short-luteal phase cycles per year. This report aroused a great deal of controversy but has not yet been either confirmed or refuted.

Menopausal Changes in Calcium Balance and Bone Remodeling

In an extensive study of calcium balance performance, Heaney and coworkers (22) demonstrated a modest stable daily calcium loss of about 20 mg in normal premenopausal women. As women entered menopause, the degree of negative calcium balance increased to about 38 mg, reflecting decreased efficiency of intestinal calcium absorption and increased urinary calcium excretion. Although such a loss may appear trivial, extrapolated over a decade it would amount to about 13% of an original bone calcium mass of 1000 g. Using radiotracer kinetic methods to study bone remodeling, the authors found virtually identical rates of mineral accretion and resorption in premenopausal women and postmenopausal women who were taking estrogen (23). Untreated menopausal women showed higher values for accretion and an even larger increase in resorption, indicative of a generalized rise in bone remodeling activity. These changes clearly reflect the loss of endogenous estrogen and are obviated by hormone replacement.

▶ 295

The following sequence gives a plausible model for the menopausal changes in calcium balance performance: (1) reduction in circulating estrogen promotes secretion by osteoblasts of interleukin-6 and other osteoclast-recruiting cytokines (see Chapter 2); (2) osteoclast recruitment initiates an increased level of bone resorption, which, in turn, increases plasma ionized calcium activity, suppresses parathyroid hormone (PTH) secretion, and increases the load of calcium filtered by the kidney; (3) suppressed PTH concentrations decrease renal calcium conservation; in addition, (4) suppressed PTH decreases renal production of 1,25-dihydroxyvitamin D (1,25(OH)$_2$D) thereby decreasing the efficiency of intestinal calcium absorption. When estrogen is replenished, bone remodeling is suppressed, 1,25(OH)$_2$D levels rise (24,25) intestinal calcium absorption improves (22,24), and calcium balance is restored (22).

Descriptions of menopausal changes in bone mass vary with skeletal location and measurement technique. Although a few studies have reported no menopausal change in the rate of bone loss (25,26), the concept of accelerated menopausal bone loss in the absence of estrogen replacement has become axiomatic and receives support from a wide variety of studies (27-37). Gallagher and colleagues (35) observed threefold greater decreases in total body calcium in the 25 years after menopause than in a similar time frame before menopause. The largest change was within 5 years of last menses, during which time the annual loss was 10-fold greater than the premenopausal rate. Similarly, Harris and Dawson-Hughes (37) measured an annual spinal bone loss, adjusted for body size and dietary calcium intake, of 2.2% within 2 years, and about 1% beyond the sixth postmenopausal year.

Uncertainty persists about when accelerated bone loss actually begins. Slemenda and colleagues (33) examined the relationships between bone loss and sex steroids in a large group of perimenopausal and early postmenopausal women who were studied sequentially for 3 years. The term "perimenopausal" indicated women who were close to average age of menopause, and who still had menstrual periods, albeit at irregular intervals. The women were divided into two groups, "early" and "late," based on plasma gonadotropin concentrations. Subjects with follicle-stimulating hormone (FSH) levels greater than 40 mIU/mL were designated "late," and subjects with normal FSH levels were recorded as "early." No loss of bone from the radius was detected during the early perimenopausal phase, but an annual decrease in bone mass of 1% was observed in both the late peri- and postmenopausal women. These results were correlated with circulating estradiol concentrations (100 pg/mL for "early" and 48 pg/mL for "late") and were mirrored in the levels of osteocalcin, a marker of bone turnover.

In general agreement with these results is a recent study by Recker and coworkers (34), who followed bone mineral status of 75 perimenopausal women who still experienced menstrual periods and had plasma FSH concentrations less than 25 mIU/mL. When bone mass at multiple sites was regressed over time, not a single slope differed from zero. The average plasma estradiol concentration for this study group, 108 pg/mL, corresponds to the "early" perimenopausal group of Slemenda and coworkers (33), with whom the bone measurements are also in good agreement. It is not possible to determine from the paper of Recker and colleagues (34) how many of the subjects entered the "late' perimenopausal phase during this study.

Regardless of timing, considerable individual variation is observed in absolute rates of bone loss. In the study of Harris and Dawson-Hughes (37), values for annual change in spinal BMD ranged from −6% to +4%, and at the femoral neck ranged from −8% to +6%. Some, but certainly not all, of this variation may be attributed to measurement imprecision. Several laboratories have attempted to develop clinical or biochemical algorithms to predict which women are at risk for "rapid" bone loss (38). Although a number of formulae have been proposed, predication of treatment on this type of information has not been shown to be advantageous.

Several years following last menses, annual rates of bone loss decrease, remaining stable over subsequent decades at approximately 1% at most skeletal sites (35–37,39). Body weight appears to influence this loss, with heavier subjects relatively protected (40). Some evidence also supports a protective role for higher endogenous levels of estrone, which is the most abundant circulating estrogen in postmenopausal women (41). By contrast, Manolagas and colleagues (42) reported no significant differences in circulating androgens or estrogens in oophorectomized women with either fast or slow rates of bone loss. In view of the powerful skeletal effects of exogenous estrogen, it is somewhat surprising for endogenous estrogen not also to be protective. However, even in the cross-sectional study of Cauley and coworkers (41), which demonstrated a significant relationship between bone mass and circulating estrone, women in the highest estrone quartile had concentrations below 100 pg/mL, which, given its relatively low estrogenic potency, are certainly below the 60 to 70 pg/mL of 17β-estradiol shown to be necessary to suppress bone remodeling.

Specific Aspects of Estrogen-Dependent Trabecular Bone Loss

Remodeling constitutes the pathway through which bone is lost or gained from the adult skeleton. Because remodeling occurs exclusively on bone surfaces, it is not surprising that changes in trabecular bone, with its enormous surface area/mass ratio, are particularly dramatic following estrogen withdrawal. Trabecular bone can be lost either through generalized trabecular thinning or through drop-out of entire trabecular elements. Dropout occurs when exuberant resorption results in trabecular perforation, offering no scaffold for new bone formation to take place. Parfitt (43) introduced the concept that "killer osteoclasts" erode deeper cavities than normal in response to estrogen deficiency, resulting in trabecular perforation and loss of trabecular connectivity. Since connectivity is a critical determinant of bone strength, the implications of this model for fracture risk are profound. Direct proof of the killer osteoclast model has not yet been provided, but, if validated, this concept would describe a unique skeletal response not seen in other settings of disordered bone remodeling.

Skeletal Effects of Estrogen Replacement

The ability of appropriate doses of estrogen, administered in a timely fashion, to conserve bone mass in menopausal women can no longer be doubted. In 1976, Lindsay and colleagues (44) reported results from a group of oophorectomized women randomly assigned to receive estrogen (mestranol, average dose 24 μg/d) or placebo. The placebo group progressively lost bone (measured at the metacarpal), but increased bone mineral was observed in the treatment group, a finding that persisted over 10 years of follow-up (45; Figure 10-1). Treatment was also associated with improved indices of vertebral deformity. In a controlled clinical trial, Recker and colleagues (46) compared the effects of placebo, conjugated equine estrogens (0.625 mg with methyltestosterone 5 mg for 21 days

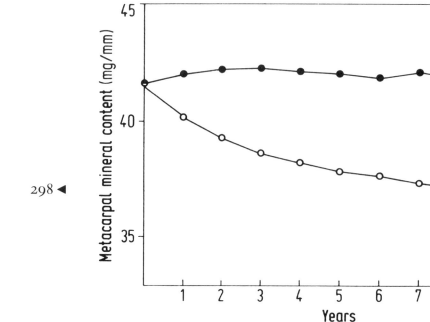

FIGURE 10-1 Effect of estrogen on metacarpal mineral content in oophorecto-mized women. Black circles represent women treated continuously with estrogen; open circles represent women treated with placebo. (*Reproduced by permission from Lindsay R, Hart DM, Forrest C, Baird C. Prevention of spinal osteoporosis in oophorectomised women. Lancet 1980;ii:1151–1153.*)

each month), and calcium carbonate (1000 mg/d) in 60 postmenopausal women. Although significant loss of forearm bone mass was observed (by single photon absorptiometry) in the control and calcium groups, regressions against time were not significant for the estrogen group. Although protocol details vary from one study to the next, similar protective effects on bone mass have been consistently demonstrated by other groups (47–51).

Physiologic Basis of Skeletal Conservation

The molecular events by which estrogen protects bone are not fully understood. A parsimonious interpretation of the available data shows the major actions of estrogen to occur at two sites: bone, where estrogen directly suppresses resorp-tion, and kidney, where the hormone alters renal phosphorus handling and pro-motes the activation of vitamin D.

Recent evidence from the laboratory of Manolagas and Jilka (see Chapter 2) suggests that release of interleukin-6 and other cytokines by osteoblasts plays a critical role in osteoclast recruitment and initiation of remodeling. Further evidence points to a powerful modulatory action of estrogen on this system. Administration of estrogen to postmenopausal women leads to a number of characteristic biochemical changes that reflect this action. Reductions in urinary excretion of calcium and hydroxyproline mirror the direct inhibition of bone resorption (52–54), and, as a coupled response, are accompanied by reduced circulating levels of osteocalcin, a marker of bone formation (54).

Estrogen administration also reduces the plasma concentrations of calcium and inorganic phosphorus (53–55). Whereas lower calcium levels are due primarily to decreased bone resorption, increased renal phosphorus clearance contributes to the reduced concentrations of inorganic phosphorus. Estrogen increases plasma levels of the active vitamin D metabolite, $1,25(OH)_2D$, or calcitriol (24,25). This increase represents a rise in the "free," or unbound fraction of the hormone, as well as in the total plasma concentration (25), and normalizes intestinal calcium absorption efficiency (24). The mechanisms by which calcitriol levels increase are not precisely understood, but appear to be related either to reductions in plasma phosphorus concentration, or to a direct stimulatory effect of estrogen on the renal 1α-hydroxylase system (55).

▶ 299

Effects of Estrogen on Fracture

Because of the great number of subjects and duration of study required to document a protective effect against fractures, primary support for such an effect comes from epidemiologic literature rather than from clinical trials. Case-control epidemiologic studies confirm a lower risk of hip, forearm, and vertebral fracture for women who have taken estrogen (56–62) and suggest the magnitude of such protection to be about 60%. Full realization of this benefit requires sustained hormone administration, probably for at least 5 years (57).

Estrogen is generally assumed to protect against fracture by conserving bone mass. Although this assumption is certainly consistent with the evidence, other possible mechanisms may also contribute to observed reductions in fracture risk. Participants in epidemiologic studies did not randomly decide to take estrogen, and pretreatment characteristics of these women might themselves underlie a lower fracture risk. For example, a woman's decision to take estrogen may be influenced by her approach to numerous life-style options, such as regular exercise, dietary moderation, and use of alcohol or tobacco, all of which may independently alter fracture risk.

A minimum of 90% of hip fractures occur as the immediate consequence of a fall (63). Because muscle mass and leg strength predict the risk for falling (64–66), preservation of muscle is likely to make an important contribution to skeletal health. In this regard, a protective effect of long-term estrogen replacement on muscle mass and strength has been suggested and requires further investigation.

Choice of Drug and Dose Requirement

In the United States, most women treated with estrogen over the past four decades have received one oral preparation, conjugated equine estrogens (Premarin®) at a single dose, 0.625 mg/d, without the use of cyclic progestins. The fracture epidemiology thus depends heavily on this particular regimen. Until recently, experience with other forms of estrogen has centered in Europe and the United Kingdom. Most, if not all, estrogens prescribed for menopausal women provide skeletal benefit. Besides conjugated estrogens, these include 17β-estradiol, ethinyl estradiol, mestranol, and others.

Hormone doses sufficient to elevate the plasma 17β-estradiol concentration to about 70 pg/mL suppress bone remodeling and protect bone mass at the spine. For oral therapy, 0.625 mg conjugated equine estrogens daily, 1 mg 17β-estradiol, or their equivalent, generally suffice to protect spinal bone mass (67). For transdermal estrogen, the 50-μg patch is effective. Even at these doses, though, some patients may lose bone. Horsman and colleagues (68) found doses of 17β-estradiol above 25 μg/d to promote bone gain, whereas doses below 15 μg did not prevent loss. Different skeletal regions may require unique concentrations of estrogen. For example, although 0.625 mg estrone sulfate per day confers protection at the spine, higher doses may be necessary to protect the proximal femur (69).

Assessment of dosage adequacy generally requires monitoring changes in annual bone density measurements. As surrogate end points, sequential changes in biochemical markers of bone turnover, such as the urinary calcium/creatinine ratio or the plasma osteocalcin concentration, may be followed. Although there are limitations to using biochemical markers to predict changes in bone mass, these indices respond more quickly than bone density, so medication adjustments can be made in a timely fashion. For example, if the pretreatment fasting calcium/creatinine ratio is 0.12, and a repeat determination 2 months after starting conjugated equine estrogens at 0.625 mg/day is 0.10, it would appear that this dose of hormone did not effectively suppress bone turnover, and an increase to 0.9 mg/d might be warranted. This strategy, while attractive, is not without its constraints. The ability of markers to predict changes in bone mass or structure is uncertain. Of even greater concern would be the potential effect of higher estrogen doses on cardiovascular, endometrial, and breast risk profiles (see below). Consequently, I prefer to reserve the use of bone turnover markers as a basis to adjust medication only for patients with severe established osteoporosis, or with BMDs greater than 2 standard deviations below age-predicted mean values.

Route of Administration

The route of estrogen delivery appears not to be critical for the skeleton, because transdermal estradiol influences calcium retention, bone turnover, and bone mass in a similar manner to oral hormone (51). Although some estrogen-fortified creams have been successfully used in Europe, nonuniformity of absorption limits their reliability.

Differences have been observed in the response of circulating growth hormone and insulin-like growth factor I (IGF-I) to estrogen depending on route of administration. Oral therapy increases circulating concentrations of growth hormone and decreases blood levels of IGF-I, whereas transdermal estrogen increases IGF-I levels without changing those of growth hormone (70). The importance of this discrepancy is not clear at present, but since human osteoblasts possess receptors for, and respond to, both growth hormone and IGF-I (71–74), a clinically relevant consequence of this difference cannot be excluded.

The Timing of Estrogen Replacement

Concern over possible irreversible bone loss if estrogen is witheld until all menstrual periods cease has led some physicians to consider initiation of therapy before menopause. Because two longitudinal studies have failed to demonstrate accelerated bone loss in perimenopausal women whose FSH levels remain low, intervention in the early perimenopausal years is unlikely to confer measurable benefit. Insufficient data preclude making a definitive judgment about women who still have menstrual periods but whose FSH levels have increased. Replacement estrogen has not been shown to provide effective contraception. If a physician wishes to prescribe estrogen replacement for a woman who is not clearly menopausal, an oral contraceptive pill may be a superior choice.

The curvilinear nature of menopausal bone loss underlies a commonly held notion that nothing is to be gained by starting estrogen therapy once the accelerated bone loss of early menopause has subsided. No evidence actually supports this view, and fairly strong evidence argues against it. The first clinical trials to demonstrate the efficacy of estrogen were conducted with patients representing a broad age range, many of whom were in their 60s when hormone therapy was started. Lindsay and Tohme (75) evaluated the effects of oral estrogen in osteoporotic postmenopausal women who were on average more than 14 years beyond menopause. Treatment for 2 years increased vertebral bone mass and showed a trend toward increase at the proximal femur as well. A calcium-treated control group lost bone from both sites. Similarly, Lufkin and colleagues (76) compared the effects of 100-μg transdermal estrogen patches to those of placebo in 75 women, aged 47 to 75 years, with established vertebral osteoporosis. Women in the hormone group maintained or increased BMD at multiple sites, and this was associated with a reduction in vertebral fracture incidence. Thus, skeletal benefit can be achieved even when initiation of estrogen is delayed by more than a decade. There is insufficient information specifically regarding fracture outcomes in women who start estrogen at an advanced age.

Cessation of Estrogen Therapy

Although ERT is conceived as a long-term strategy for both cardiovascular and skeletal benefits, women generally do not stay on therapy for very long. In a follow-up assessment of British women who started hormone replacement in 1975, Jones and coworkers (77) found more than half had discontinued treatment within 5 years. North American pharmaceutical industry surveys suggest no more than 40% of women who are prescribed estrogen actually remain on treatment beyond one year. To some degree this may reflect an intent to prescribe short-term estrogen for control of vasomotor instability rather than as a long-term health maintenance strategy.

Uncertainty persists regarding the consequences of stopping estrogen. Lindsay and colleagues (78) observed an accelerated rate of bone loss in women who abruptly terminated ERT. In a more complex study, Christiansen and coworkers (79) randomly assigned women to estrogen or placebo for 24 months, after which the estrogen group switched to placebo or continued estrogen. The secondary placebo group lost bone over the next 12 months at the same rate observed in subjects who had taken placebo from the beginning. Thus, the authors found bone loss after termination of estrogen, but not at the accelerated rate reported by Lindsay and coworkers (78).

Use of Combination Therapy

At customary replacement doses, estrogen conserves bone through its antiresorptive effect. Because bone remodeling is a coupled phenomenon, suppressing bone resorption by any intervention will ultimately slow down formation. Such therapy is therefore unlikely to yield important increases in bone mass. Nonetheless, a rationale can be found to use estrogen in combination with agents known to stimulate bone formation. One approach has been described by Christiansen and Riis (80), who treated women with a combination of estrogen and norethisterone acetate, an androgenic progestin. Combined therapy resulted in significant increases in BMD exceeding those achieved with either agent alone. Another potential combined use of estrogen would be a treatment involving a remodeling activator, such as PTH or growth hormone. In this setting, administration of estrogen might constrain the increased level of resorption while still permitting an effective anabolic stimulus to occur. On the other hand, there is currently no established rationale for combining estrogen with other antiresorptive agents, such as bisphosphonates or calcitonin. Considerably more work is required in this area before the place of combination therapy can be established.

▶ 303

Nonskeletal Aspects of Estrogen Therapy

An informed decision to take menopausal ERT must be based on the composite effects of treatment on many aspects of health and not simply on skeletal risk. Chief among these are the effects of estrogen on mortality and morbidity related to cardiovascular, breast, and uterine disease. Ischemic heart disease is the leading cause of hospitalization and death for American women over 55 years of age. A large body of literature has emerged during the past 15 years pointing toward a substantial protective effect of prolonged ERT against cardiovascular death and morbidity (81–85). Although this conclusion is based primarily on epidemiologic studies, the effect has been consistent among several countries and across several types of analysis. The protective effect appears to be a 40% to 50% reduction in risk.

The mechanism(s) through which estrogen achieves cardiovascular protection are not well understood, although plausible models are consistent with the published evidence. In women, high-density lipoprotein (HDL) cholesterol is a highly significant predictor of ischemic heart disease risk, and estrogen increases the circulating level of this lipoprotein constituent. Similarly, estrogen reduces the levels of low-density lipoprotein (LDL) cholesterol. Changes in lipoproteins account for only a portion of estrogen's cardioprotective action, and alternative mechanisms require investigation. For example, some evidence has shown estrogen decreases the tendency to coronary artery spasm via direct actions on vascular smooth muscle.

On the opposite side of the equation is the recognized contribution of chronic unopposed estrogen use to an increase in uterine cancer risk. Although this added risk is certainly real, it can be minimized by the judicious use of cyclic progestins (86). Of more concern is a potential role for long-term estrogen use to increase the risk of breast cancer. This possibility has been examined many times over the last four decades, and the literature has generally been reassuring. However, only recently has long-term therapy (more than 10 years) been suggested for cardiovascular or skeletal protection, and most earlier reports are simply not relevant to this strategy. A few recent studies sustain the concern that as much as a 20% increase in breast cancer risk may be associated with long-term estrogen use (87–89). Short of carrying out a prospective clinical trial, this question is unlikely to be resolved with any greater precision.

Death rates from ischemic heart disease far outweigh those due to hip fracture, breast cancer, or any other disorder of elderly women. Considering an entire population, a decision to prescribe long-term estrogen should decrease overall morbidity and mortality (83). Of course, this would be of no consolation to the woman who developed breast cancer. Thus, at an individual level the decision to take estrogen must be based on an assessment of individual risks. A woman with minimal cardiovascular risk (eg, thin, athletic, nonsmoker, good HDL cholesterol) is less likely to achieve cardiovascular benefit from estrogen. If her bone mineral status were at the median for age, her skeletal risk would also be small. If one or more first-degree relatives had breast cancer, her individual risk from estrogen might outweigh the prospective benefits. On the other hand, a woman with increased cardiovascular or skeletal risk who does not have a familial contraindication to ERT is likely to benefit from estrogen. These examples are not meant to provide a treatment algorithm, but to indicate the types of considerations to be discussed with each woman before a rational decision can be reached.

References

1. Albright F, Reifenstein EC Jr. Metabolic bone disease: osteoporosis. In: Albright F, Reifenstein, EC, eds. The parathyroid glands and metabolic bone disase. Baltimore: Williams & Wilkins, 1948;145–204.

2. Steingold KA, Cedars M, Lu JKH, Randle D, Judd HL, Meldrum DR. Treatment of endometriosis with a long-acting gonadotropin-releasing hormone agonist. Obstet Gynecol 1989;69:403–411.

3. Dawood YM, Lewis V, Ramos J. Cortical and trabecular bone mineral content in women with endometriosis: effect of gonadotropin-releasing hormone agonist and danazol. Fertil Steril 1989;52:21–26.

4. Scharla SH, Minne HW, Waibel-Treber S, et al. Bone mass reduction after estrogen deprivation by long-acting gonadotropin-releasing hormone agonists and its relation to pretreatment serum concentrations of 1,25-dihydroxyvitamin D_3. J Clin Endocrinol Metab 1990;70:1055–1061.

5. Surrey ES, Judd HL. Reduction of vasomotor symptoms and bone mineral density loss with combined norethindrone and long acting gonadotropin-releasing hormone agonist therapy of symptomatic en-

dometriosis: a prospective randomized trial. J Clin Endocrinol Metab 1992;75:558–563.

6. Klibanski A, Neer RM, Beitins IZ, Ridgway EC, Zervas NT, McArthur JW. Decreased bone density in hyperprolactinemic women. N Engl J Med 1980;303:1511–1514.

7. Schlechte JA, Sherman B, Martin R. Bone density in amenorrheic women with and without hyperprolactinemia. J Clin Endocrinol Metab 1983;56:1120–1123.

8. Cann CE, Martin MC, Genant HK, Jaffe RB. Decreased spinal mineral content in amenorrheic women. JAMA 1984;251:626–629.

9. Nyström E, Leman J, Lundberg P-A, et al. Bone mineral content in normally menstruating women with hyperprolactinemia. Hormone Res 1988;29:214–217.

10. Drinkwater BL, Milson K, Chesnut CH III, et al. Bone mineral content of amenorrheic and eumenorrheic athletes. N Engl J Med 1984;311:277–281.

11. Marcus R, Cann C, Madvig P, et al. Menstrual function and bone mass in elite women distance runners. Endocrine and metabolic features. Ann Intern Med 1985;102:158–163.

12. Nelson ME, Fisher EC, Castos PD. Diet and bone status in amenorrheic runners. Am J Clin Nutr 1986;43:910–916.

13. Myburgh KH, Hutchins J, Fataar AB, Hough SF, Noakes TD. Low bone density is an etiologic factor for stress fractures in athletes. Ann Intern Med 1990, 113:754–759.

14. Lindberg JS, Powell MR, Hunt MM. Increased vertebral bone mineral in response to reduced exercise in amenorrheic runners. West J Med 1987;146:39–42.

15. Cann CE, Genant HK, Ettinger B, Gordon GS. Spinal mineral loss in oophorectomized women. Determination by quantitative computed tomography. JAMA 1980;244:2056–2059.

16. Ohta H, Masuzawa T, Ikeda T, Suda Y, Makita K, Nozawa S. Which is more osteoporosis-inducing, menopause or oophorectomy? Bone Miner 1992;19:273–285.

17. Louis O, Devroey P, Kalender W, Osteaux M. Bone loss in young hypoestrogenic women due to primary ovarian failure: spinal quantitative computed tomography. Fertil Steril 1989;52:227–231.

18. Gotfredsen A, Christiansen C, Palshof T. The effect of tamoxifen on bone mineral content in premenopausal women with breast cancer. Cancer 1984;53:853–857.

19. Love R, Mazess R, Tormey D, Barden H, Newcomb P, Jordan V. Bone mineral density in women with breast cancer treated with adjuvant tamoxifen for at least two years. Breast Cancer Res Treat 1988;12:297–301.

20. Turken S, Siris E, Seldin D, Flaster E, Hyman G, Lindsay R. Effects of tamoxifen on spinal bone density in women with breast cancer. J Natl Cancer Inst 1989;81:1086–1088.

21. Pryor JC, Vigna YM, Schechter MT, Burgess AE. Spinal bone loss and ovulatory disturbances. N Engl J Med 1990;323:1221–1227.

22. Heaney RP, Recker RR, Saville PD. Menopausal changes in calcium balance performance. J Lab Clin Med 1978;92:953–963.

23. Heaney RP, Recker RR, Saville PD. Menopausal changes in bone remodeling. J Lab Clin Med 1978;92:964–970.

24. Gallagher JC, Riggs BL, DeLuca HF. Effect of estrogen on calcium absorption and serum vitamin D metabolites in postmenopausal osteoporosis. J Clin Endocrinol Metab 1980;51:1359–1364.

25. Cheema C, Grant BF, Marcus R. Effects of estrogen on circulating "free" and total 1,25-dihydroxyvitamin D and on the parathyroid-vitamin D axis in postmenopausal women. J Clin Invest 1989;83:537–542.

25. Madsen M. Vertebral and peripheral bone mineral content by photon absorptiometry. Invest Radiol 1977;12:185–188.

26. Riggs BL, Wahner HW, Dann WL, Mazess RB, Offord KP. Differential changes in bone mineral density of the appendicular and axial skeleton with aging. J Clin Invest 1981;67:328–335.

27. Cann CE, Genant HK, Kolb FO, Ettinger B. Quantitative computed tomography for prediction of vertebral fracture risk. Bone 1985;6:1–7.

28. Firooznia H, Golimbu C, Rafii M, Schwartz MS, Alterman ER. Quantitative computed tomography assessment of spinal trabecular bone. I. Age-related regression in normal men and women. J Comput Tomogr 1984;8:91–97.

29. Krølner B, Pors Nielsen S. Bone mineral content of the lumbar spine in normal and osteoporotic women: cross-sectional and longitudinal studies. Clin Sci 1982;62:329–336.

30. Aloia JF, Vaswani A, Ellis K, Yuen K, Cohn SH. A model for involutional bone loss. J Lab Clin Med 1985;106:630–637.

31. Ribot C, Tremollieres F, Pouilles JM, Louvet JP, Guiraud R. Influence of the menopause and aging on spinal density in French women. Bone Miner 1988;5:89–97.

32. Block JE, Smith R, Glueer C-G, Steiger P, Ettinger B, Genant HK. Models of spinal trabecular bone loss as determined by quantitative computed tomography. J Bone Miner Res 1989;4:249–257.

33. Slemenda C, Hui SL, Longcope C, Johnston CC Jr. Sex steroids and bone mass. A study of changes about the time of menopause. J Clin Invest 1987;80:1261–1269.

34. Recker RR, Lappe JM, Davies M, Kimmel DB. Change in bone mass immediately before menopause. J Bone Miner Res 1992;7:857–862.

35. Gallagher JC, Goldgar D, Moy A. Total bone calcium in normal women: effect of age and menopausal status. J Bone Miner Res 1987;2:491–496.

36. Aloia JF, Vaswani A, Ross P, Cohn SH. Aging bone loss from the femur, spine, radius, and total skeleton. Metabolism 1990;39:1144–1150.

37. Harris S, Dawson-Hughes B. Rates of change in bone mineral density of the spine, heel, femoral neck and radius in healthy postmenopausal women. Bone Miner 1992;17:87–95.

38. Christiansen C, Riis BJ, Rodbro P. Screening procedure for women at risk of developing postmenopausal osteoporosis. Osteoporosis Int 1990;1:35–40.

39. Nordin BEC, Need AG, Bridges A, Horowitz M. Relative contribution of years since menopause, age, and weight to vertebral density in postmenopausal women. J Clin Endocrinol Metab 1992;74:20–23.

40. Harris S, Dallal GE, Dawson-Hughes B. Influence of body weight on rates of change in bone density of the spine, hip, and radius in postmenopausal women. Calcif Tissue Int 1992;5:19–23.

41. Cauley JA, Gutai JP, Sandler RB, LaPorte RE, Kuller LH, Sashin D. The relationship of endogenous estrogen to bone density and bone area in normal postmenopausal women. Am J Epidemiol 1986;124:752–761.

42. Manolagas SC, Anderson DC, Lindsay R. Adrenal steroids and the development of osteoporosis in oophorectomized women. Lancet 1979;ii:597–600.

43. Parfitt AM. Bone remodeling: relationship to the amount and structure of bone, and the pathogenesis and prevention of fractures. In: Riggs BL, Melton LJ III, eds. Osteoporosis: Etiology, diagnosis, and management. New York: Raven Press, 1988:72–73.

44. Lindsay R, Hart DM, Aitken JM, MacDonald EB, Anderson JB, Clarke AC. Long-term prevention of postmenopausal osteoporosis by oestrogen. Evidence for an increased bone mass after delayed onset of oestrogen treatment. Lancet 1976;i:1038–1040.

45. Lindsay R, Hart DM, Forrest C, Baird C. Prevention of spinal osteoporosis in oophorectomised women. Lancet 1980;ii:1151–1153.

46. Recker RR, Saville PD, Heaney RP. Effect of estrogens and calcium carbonate on bone loss in postmenopausal women. Ann Intern Med 1977;87:649–655.

47. Horsman A, Gallagher JC, Simpson M, Nordin BEC. Prospective trial of oestrogen and calcium in postmenopausal women. Br Med J 1977;2:789–792.

48. Nachtigall LE, Naghtigall RH, Nachtigall RD, Beckmann EM. Estrogen replacement therapy I: a 10-year prospec-

tive study in the relationship to osteoporosis. Obstet Gynecol 1979;53:277–281.

49. Riis B, Thomsen K, Christiansen C. Does calcium supplementation prevent postmenopausal bone loss? A double-blind, controlled clinical study. N Engl J Med 1987;316:173–177.

50. Civitelli R, Agnusdei D, Nardi P, Zacchei F, Avioli LV, Gennari C. Effects of one year treatment with estrogens on bone mass, intestinal calcium absorption, and 25-hydroxyvitamin D–1α-hydroxylase reserve in postmenopausal osteoporosis. Calcif Tissue Int 1988;42:77–86.

51. Stevenson JC, Cust MP, Gangar KF, Hillard TC, Lees B, Whitehead MI. Effects of transdermal versus oral hormone replacement therapy on bone density in spine and proximal femur in postmenopausal women. Lancet 1990;ii:265–269.

52. Young MM, Jasani C, Smith DA, Nordin BEC. Some effects of ethinyl oestradiol on calcium and phosphorus metabolism in osteoporosis. Clin Sci 1968;34:411–417.

53. Gallagher JC, Nordin BEC. Effects of oestrogen and progestogen therapy on calcium metabolism in post-menopausal women. In: Estrogens in the postmenopause. Basel: Frontiers Hormone Research, Karger, 1975:150–176.

54. Stock JL, Coderre JA, Mallette LE. Effects of a short course of estrogen on mineral metabolism in postmenopausal women. J Clin Endocrinol Metab 1985;61:595–600.

55. Packer E. Holloway L, Newhall K, Kanwar G, Butterfield G, Marcus R. Effects of estrogen on daylong circulating calcium, phosphorus, 1,25-dihydroxyvitamin D, and parathyroid hormone in postmenopausal women. J Bone Miner Res 1990;5:877–884.

56. Hutchinson TA, Polansky SM, Feinstein AR. Post-menopausal oestrogens protect against fractures of hip and distal radius. A case-control study. Lancet 1979;ii:705–709.

57. Weiss NS, Ure CL, Ballard JH, Williams AR, Daling JR. Decreased risk of fractures of the hip and lower forearm with postmenopausal use of estrogen. N Engl J Med 1980;303:1195–1198.

58. Paganini-Hill A, Ross RK, Gerkins VR, Henderson BE, Arthur M, Mack TM. Menopausal estrogen therapy and hip fractures. Ann Intern Med 1981;95:28–31.

59. Johnson RE, Specht EE. The risk of hip fracture in postmenopausal females with and without estrogen drug exposure. Am J Public Health 1981;71:138–144.

60. Kreiger N, Kelsey JL, Holford TR. An epidemiological study of hip fracture in postmenopausal women. Am J Epidemiol 1982;116:141–148.

61. Ettinger B, Genant HK, Cann CE. Long-term estrogen therapy prevents bone loss and fracture. Ann Intern Med 1985;102:319–324.

62. Kiel DP, Felson DT, Anderson JJ, et al. Hip fracture and the use of estrogens in postmenopausal women: the Framingham study. N Engl J Med 1987;317:1169–1174.

63. Cummings SR, Black DM, Nevitt MC, et al., and the Study of Osteoporotic Fractures Research Group. Appendicular bone density and age predict hip fracture in women. JAMA 1990;263:665–668.

64. Whipple RH, Wolfson LI, Amerman PM. The relationship of knee and ankle weakness to falls in nursing home residents: an isokinetic study. J Am Geriatr Soc 1987;35:13–20.

65. Prudham D, Grimby Evans J. Factors associated with falls in the elderly: a community study. Age Ageing 1981;10:141–146.

66. Farmer ME, Harris T, Madans JH, Wallace RB, Cornoni-Huntley J, White LR. Anthropometric indicators and hip fracture. The NHANES I epidemiologic follow-up study. J Am Geriatr Soc 1989;37:9–16.

67. Lindsay R, Hart DM, Clark DM. The minimum effective dose of estrogen for prevention of postmenopausal bone loss. Obstet Gynecol 1984;63:759–763.

68. Horsman A, Jones M, Francis R, Nordin C. The effect of estrogen dose on postmenopausal bone loss. N Engl J Med 1983;309:1405–1407.

69. Gallagher JC, Baylink D. Effect of estrone sulfate on bone mineral density of the femoral neck and spine. Annual Meeting of the American Society of Bone and Mineral Research, 1990. Abstract #802.

70. Ho KHY, Weissberger AJ. Impact of short-term estrogen administration on growth hormone secretion and action: distinct route-dependent effects on connective and bone tissue metabolism. J Bone Miner Res 1992;7:821–827.

71. Stracke H, Schultz A, Moeller D, Rossol S, Schatz H. Effect of growth hormone on osteoblasts and demonstration of somatomedin-C/IGF-1 in bone organ culture. Acta Endocrinol (Copenh) 1984;107: 16–24.

72. Chenu C, Valentin-Opran A, Chavassieux P, et al. Insulin like growth factor I hormonal regulation by growth hormone and by $1,25(OH)_2D_3$ and activity on human osteoblast-like cells in short-term cultures. Bone 1990;11:81–86.

73. Barnard R, Ng KW, Martin TJ, Waters MJ. Growth hormone (GH) receptors in clonal osteoblast-like cells mediate a mitogenic response to GH. Endocrinology 1991;128:1459–1464.

74. Ernst M, Froesch ER. Growth hormone dependent stimulation of osteoblast-like cells in serum-free cultures via local synthesis of insulin-like growth factor I. Biochem Biophys Res Commun 1988;151: 142–147.

75. Lindsay R, Tohme JF. Estrogen treatment of patients with established postmenopausal osteoporosis. Obstet Gynecol 1991;76:290–295.

76. Lufkin EG, Washner HW, O'Fallon WM, et al. Treatment of postmenopausal osteoporosis with transdermal estrogen. Ann Intern Med 1992;117:1–9.

77. Jones MM, Francis RM, Nordin BEC. Five-year follow-up of oestrogen therapy in 94 women. Maturitas 1982;4: 123–130.

78. Lindsay R, Hart DM, MacLean A, Clarke AC, Kraszewski A, Garwood J. Bone response to termination of estrogen treatment. Lancet 1978;i:1325–1327.

79. Christiansen C, Christensen MS, Transbøl I. Bone mass in postmenopausal women after withdrawal of oestrogen/gestagen replacement therapy. Lancet 1991;i:459–461.

80. Christiansen C, Riis BJ. 17β-estradiol and continuous norethisterone: a unique treatment for established osteoporosis in elderly women. J Clin Endocrinol Metab 1990;71:836–841.

81. Ross RK, Paganini-Hill A, Mack TM, Arthur M, Henderson BE. Menopausal oestrogen therapy and protection from ischaemic heart disease. Lancet 1981;i:858–860.

82. Bush TL, Barrett-Connor E, Cowan LD, et al. Cardiovascular mortality and noncontraceptive use of estrogen in women: results from the Lipid Research Clinics Program follow-up study. Circulation 1987;75:1102–1109.

83. Criqui MH, Suarez L, Barrett-Connor E, McPhillips J, Wingard DL, Garland C. Postmenopausal estrogen use and mortality. Results from a prospective study in a defined, homogeneous community. Am J Epidemiol 1988;128:606–614.

84. Stampfer MJ, Colditz GA, Willett WC, et al. Postmenopausal estrogen therapy and cardiovascular disease. Ten year follow-up from the nurses health study. N Engl J Med 1991;325:756–762.

85. Sullivan JM, Vander Zwaag R, Lemp GF, et al. Postmenopausal estrogen use and coronary atherosclerosis. Ann Intern Med 1988;108:358–363.

86. Voigt LF, Weiss NS, Chu J, Daling JR, McKnight B, van Belle G. Progestagen supplementation of exogenous oestrogens and risk of endometrial cancer. Lancet 1991;338:274–277.

87. Brinton LA, Hoover R, Fraumeni JF. Menopausal oestrogens and breast cancer risk: an expanded case-control study. Br J Cancer 1986;54:825–832.

88. Colditz GA, Stampfer MJ, Willett WC, Hennekens CH, Rosner B, Speizer FE. Prospective study of estrogen replacement therapy and risk of breast cancer in postmenopausal women. JAMA 1990;264: 2648–2653.

89. Steinberg KK, Thacker SB, Smith SJ, et al. A meta-analysis of the effect of estrogen replacement therapy on the risk of breast cancer. JAMA 1991;265:1985–1990.

11 ▸ Bisphosphonates for the Treatment of Osteoporosis

▶ ▶ ▶ Lawrence E. Mallette

This chapter summarizes the published studies of bisphosphonates for the treatment or prevention of osteoporosis and puts this information in perspective by considering the mechanisms by which osteoporosis arises and might theoretically be prevented or reversed. The reader is referred to other reviews of bisphosphonates for additional discussion (1–5).

Bisphosphonates are analogs of pyrophosphate in which the central oxygen atom is replaced by carbon. The resulting bond is stable to the action of phosphatases, and the carbon atom permits addition of a side chain that alters the spectrum of biologic activities. Bisphosphonates, like pyrophosphate, are chelators of divalent cations. In the testtube they adsorb to the surface of hydroxyapatite crystals and stabilize the crystals, slowing further crystal growth and retarding crystal dissolution. In vivo, bisphosphonates can slow bone mineralization and inhibit bone resorption. The ratio of these activities is determined by the side chain. The inhibition of bone resorption is mediated mainly by adsorbed drug, the osteoclast being thought to release the bisphosphonate in high local concentrations as it begins to resorb bone. Addition of a charged side chain such as an amino group seems to increase the bisphosphonate's ability to inhibit the osteoclast and lessen its relative inhibition of mineralization.

Table 11-1 summarizes the nomenclature of the bisphosphonates discussed in this chapter. The generic drug name is used rather than the chemical name or abbreviation.

Osteoporosis results from years of slow bone loss after a metabolic abnormality or deficiency has placed the bone remodeling sequence into negative balance. To understand how bisphosphonates might be applied to prevent or cure osteoporosis, bone remodeling must be understood (6), because the effectiveness of bisphosphonates derives from their ability to alter the remodeling process.

TABLE 11-1 Nomenclature of Bisphosphonates

Abbreviation	Chemical Name	Generic Name
AHBuBP	4-amino-1-hydroxybutylidene-1,1-bisphosphonate	alendronate
AHPrBP (APD)	3-amino-1-hydroxypropylidene-1,1-bisphosphonate	pamidronate
HEBP (EHDP)	1-hydroxyethylidene-1,1-bisphosphonate	etidronate
none	(4-chlorophenylthio)methylene-bisphosphonate	tiludronate
Cl_2MDP	dichloromethane diphosphonate	clodronate

Mechanisms of Bone Loss: Genesis of Osteoporosis

A loss of bone mass can occur only at sites where bone tissue is remodeled. Remodeling occurs on the surface of the bone trabeculae and the endosteal surface of the bone cortex. Cellular activity at these sites removes old bone and synthesizes new bone in its place.

The trabecular bone remodeling cycle, the sequential resorption of bone by osteoclasts and mononuclear cells (6) and its rebuilding by osteoblasts, is normally in neutral balance in young adults (Figure 11-1A and 1B), with allowances for local variations in balance in response to changes in load bearing of the particular bone elements. Osteoporosis develops when the bone remodeling cycle is placed into negative balance, either by a decrease in the amount of bone synthesized per cycle (Figure 11-1C) or an increased depth of resorption (Figure 11-1D).

Certain conditions can accelerate the rate of bone remodeling—that is, increase the number of remodeling sites by increasing the frequency of activation of osteoclasts. This acceleration will decrease bone mass because there will be an increased number of resorption lacunae from which bone has been removed and is not yet replaced, an increased "remodeling space" (Figure 11-2A). Once a new steady state is reached, however, no further loss occurs as long as each remodeling site is in neutral balance, with the amount of bone removed and replaced being equal (Figure 11-2B). If remodeling is in negative balance, however, bone loss will occur more rapidly if more sites are involved in remodeling (Figure 11-2C or 11-2D).

The endosteal surface of the cortex normally is in slight negative balance throughout much of adult life, but a positive balance at the subperiosteal surface normally maintains cortical thickness. An excess of parathyroid hormone (PTH) is thought to increase the depth of resorption especially in the endosteal remodeling envelope (7) and thereby accelerate thinning of the bone cortex.

The bone cortex is also remodeled by cells in "cutting cones," which carve their way through the substance of the cortex, removing and replacing

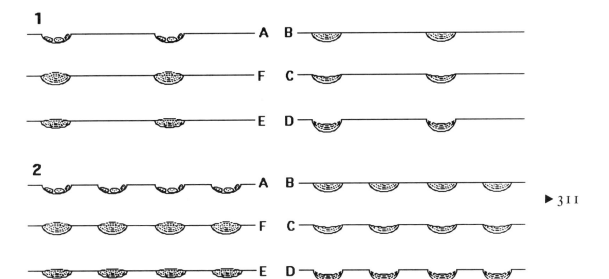

FIGURES 11-1 AND 11-2 Bone remodeling occurs at millions of sites on the trabecular or endosteal surface. Bone remodeling in the normal adult is in balance, with the amount replaced equaling the amount removed (1*A* and 1*B*). For osteoporosis to develop, less bone must be replaced in a lacuna of normal depth (1*C*), or a normal amount of bone must be placed in an abnormally deep cavity (1*D*). To cure osteoporosis, a normal amount of bone must be placed in a shallower than normal cavity (1*E*), or more bone must be placed into lacunaes of normal depth (1*F*). If bone remodeling is speeded up, the number of lacunaes in various stages of remodeling increases, that is, the remodeling space increases (2*A* versus 1*A*). This may decrease total cancellous bone mass by about 5%. With more sites being remodeled, a given degree of negative or positive balance will cause bone mass to change more rapidly (compare 2*B* through 2*F* with 1*B* through 1*F*).

bone and giving rise to the Haversian canals of the cortex. This form of cortical remodeling is not thought to contribute to the development of osteoporosis.

A loss of cancellous bone resulting from a negative balance of trabecular remodeling will predispose to fractures of the vertebrae and other bones with a high reliance on trabecular structure. A thinner cortex predisposes to fractures of tubular bones, including the femoral neck.

When a negative bone balance has developed, the trabecular plate (or cortex) first grows thinner. When the trabecula has become thin enough, an exceptionally deep resorption lacuna or two lacunae, occurring simultaneously on both sides of the plate, may penetrate through the plate. Osteoblasts that would be expected to lay down bone at this site will have lost their base on which to initiate bone formation. With subsequent rounds of resorption, the fenestration will enlarge. The eventual loss of the entire structural element will reduce the total architectural strength far more than would a uniform thinning of the plate.

▶ 311

Bisphosphonates for the Treatment of Osteoporosis

Fenestration and loss of trabecular plates will occur earlier in diseases where the depth of the resorption cavity has increased. Also, after significant thinning of the trabecular plate has occurred, an accelerated remodeling rate itself may begin to contribute to negative balance, by increasing the likelihood that osteoclasts will be excavating simultaneously on both sides of a trabecula to cause fenestration. Note, however, that fenestration will occur only after previous cycles in negative balance have thinned the trabecula sufficiently.

Since the resorption lacuna will often mark the thinnest part of the trabecular plate, the lacunar base may be the site of maximum stress and the likely point for fracture initiation, especially when the trabecular plate is thin. If so, then a decrease in the number of resorption lacunae might increase architectural stability and at least temporarily reduce the number of fractures. Eventually, however, reducing the rate of remodeling will increase the average age of the skeletal unit, which might reduce overall tensile strength. The relative quantitative importance of these two counterbalancing effects has not been established.

Although working by different mechanisms, a large number of factors can result in a negative remodeling balance. Loss of estrogen after the menopause is cited most often. Bone remodeling accelerates at the menopause, as the frequency of activation of new remodeling sites increases (6,8). Estrogen replacement will reduce the activation frequency (9) and the remodeling space. The higher activation frequency may occur in part because the effects of PTH on bone are no longer blunted by estrogen.

More importantly, estrogen deficiency places the remodeling sequence into negative balance. It does not seem to increase the depth of the resorption cavity, but it does decrease the total amount of bone synthesized by the osteoblast, either by slowing its synthetic rate slightly or shortening its life span, or both (10). In bone biopsies this is manifested as a decreased thickness of the histologically identifiable newly formed bone packets (termed a decreased mean wall thickness; see Figure 11-1C). In addition to these effects of estrogen inferred from bone biopsy studies, estrogen has been demonstrated convincingly in animal experiments to stimulate osteoblast function (11). Patients with idiopathic osteoporosis have an accentuation of the tendency toward reduced mean wall thickness (10), but it is not known whether an idiosyncratic hypersensitivity to estrogen withdrawal or unidentified intercurrent factors are responsible. Studies in vitro have shown that nicotine and alcohol also inhibit the synthetic ability of osteoblast, which may explain how they predispose to osteoporosis (12–14). Other as yet unidentified factors probably have a similar effect.

Estrogen deficiency may potentiate PTH-mediated resorption from endosteal sites and so contribute to a negative balance there (15). The clinical effect of this potentiation is to thin the bone cortex and increase the risk of femoral neck fracture. Estrogen therapy can prevent this endosteal loss (15). Suppression of endogenous PTH secretion by an increased dietary calcium intake might be predicted to have its greatest effect on the endosteal envelope. In fact, calcium supplements in postmenopausal women seem to slow the rate of loss of cortical bone more effectively than they retard spinal bone loss (16,17). Increased dietary calcium can be shown to decrease vertebral bone loss only if the basal diet is quite deficient in calcium (17).

Theoretical Basis for Increasing Bone Mass

Osteoporosis might be curable if a way could be found to reverse the negative balance of the bone remodeling sequence, placing it into positive balance, and yet maintain bone remodeling long term (Figure 11-1E and 11-1F). Bone might then be accreted on the surface of the remaining elements to increase their mass and strength. Trabecular elements that had been lost might not be rebuilt, so that baseline structural strength might not be regained fully, but the improvement in overall strength might still reduce the number of fractures. The fact that generalized skeletal sclerosis can develop sporadically in adults (18,19) demonstrates that the task of increasing bone mass is biologically possible. It may simply be a matter of finding the right combination of agents or growth factors.

A positive balance might be achieved either by stimulating the osteoblast to lay down more bone in a resorption lacuna of normal depth (see Figure 11-1F) or by decreasing the depth of the lacuna without decreasing the amount of bone synthesized at the remodeling site (see Figure 11-1E). Agents potentially capable of stimulating the osteoblast include fluoride, PTH, vitamin D congeners, and various growth factors. They are not discussed further in this chapter.

Agents that inhibit the osteoclast could potentially be used to increase bone mass, if they could be used in a fashion that did not prevent bone remodeling. The initial step in the bone remodeling cycle is the recruitment of osteoclasts to initiate bone resorption. Decreasing the number of active osteoclasts will lead to an increase in bone mass that occurs over a few weeks as the remodeling space fills in (Figure 11-2A changes to Figure 11-1A) (20). This does not, however, constitute the desired long-term continuous increase in bone mass. An agent potent enough to prevent all osteoclast activity will halt bone remodeling, so that bone mass can no longer change after the remodeling space has filled in. Then each unit of the skeleton will age, which might allow an accumulation of microdamage and an eventual decrease in overall tensile strength (21). A method must be found to diminish net resorption at each site without arresting bone remodeling.

Several classes of antiosteoclast agents are recognized. The calcitonins and other antiresorptive agents are discussed elsewhere. The bisphosphonates are perhaps the least expensive class of antiosteoclast agents with the lowest profile of adverse effects. Although their gastrointestinal absorption is below 10% and variable, they can be given orally in sufficient dosage to produce systemic effects on the skeleton. They generally cause no recognizable systemic symptoms or other adverse effects, aside from gastrointestinal irritation in a few patients.

The unanswered question concerning the bisphosphonates is how best to take advantage of their antiresorptive activity without arresting bone remodeling. One approach is based on the activation-depression-free period-repeat (ADFR) concept of Frost (22,23). Initially an agent is given to activate a large number of remodeling sites (activation). Possible activating agents include phosphate to increase endogenous PTH, synthetic PTH given by injection (24–27), triiodothyronine (28), or calcitriol (29). The goal is to recruit a large cohort of new remodeling units that will continue their activity in synchrony. The next step is to give a pulse of an osteoclast inhibitor before these osteoclasts have completed their excavations, depressing or eliminating their activity (depression). The shallower than normal resorption cavities theoretically should become the site of a normal round of bone formation, with osteoblasts depositing the usual amount of bone (see Figure 11-1E). A period of time free of pharmacotherapy is given to allow completion of the remodeling cycle (free period). The sequence is then repeated (repeat). Normal bone remodeling presumably continues at new sites that are initiated between the pulses of antiresorptive agent.

An alternate approach that evolved from the ADFR concept is intermittent therapy, omitting the activating agent and giving the pulse of antiosteoclast agent intermittently to inhibit activity at resorption sites that have recently appeared.

A third approach is to give a very low dose of bisphosphonate continuously, hoping to diminish the total resorptive activity of each osteoclast during its life span, without preventing the recruitment of osteoclasts to new remodeling sites.

Possible Inaccuracies in the Theory

Several potential problems might prevent antiresorptive agents from operating to increase bone mass or strength. First, the osteoclast may not simply dig a pit at the resorption site, but may be mobile, as suggested by time lapse photography of osteoclasts layered onto and resorbing devitalized bone or dentin. The resulting lacuna in three dimensions would then resemble a trench, with irregular outlines, rather than a simple pit. If the length of the trench were markedly greater than its width or depth, premature termination of osteoclast activity would shorten the trench, but not decrease its depth over most of its course (Figure 11-3). If the number of osteoblasts recruited were then a function of the surface area of the trench, very little positive balance would be achieved. We can hope, however, that the apparent mobility on devitalized bone surfaces is an artifact and that the osteoclast's tendency toward mobility is restrained in vivo, perhaps by the neighboring bone lining cells. Studies are needed of the areal shape of lacunae in normal bone.

Second, the osteoclast may not be responsible for the entire resorption cavity. Eriksen's morphometric data suggest that the normal osteoclast resorbs an average of 20 µm of bone over an average of 9 days and that the process is completed by mononuclear cells that resorb about 40 µm of bone over 34 days (6). The mechanism by which the mononuclear cells resorb bone and whether they are inhibited by antiosteoclast agents, including bisphosphonates, is not known. It is not known whether application of an agent that eliminated the osteoclasts early would prevent the appearance or diminish the activity of these mononuclear cells. It is also not known how important mononuclear cell function is to the eventual structural soundness of the new bone packet. A mononuclear type of cell is responsible for placing the cement line (actually a layer) that is found at the base of new packets of bone. If preparation of the surface for the new bone packet were interfered with by the antiosteoclast agent, the new bone might not be well anchored or properly structured.

When resorptive activity of the osteoclast is inhibited pharmacologically and it fails to complete its resorption lacuna, is it possible that abnormal bone is

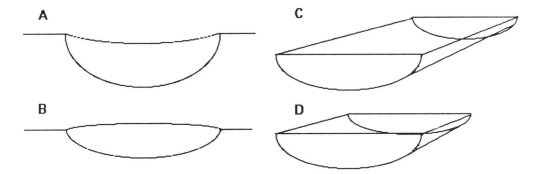

FIGURE 11-3 The classical view of the resorption lacuna is as a pit (A). Early termination of osteoclastic resorption might turn a negative balance (A) into a positive balance (B) if the osteoblast replaced the same amount of bone into a shallower pit. If the lacuna instead resembled a trench (C), it would still have the appearance of a pit on cross-section, but early termination of osteoclastic resorption would shorten the trench instead of making it shallower (D).

left behind? If resorption lacunae are frequently located at sites of microfracture or fatigue damage, then the net result of long-term inhibition of the osteoclast might be an accumulation of damaged or fatigued bone, which might not be recognizable morphologically in biopsies. If the agent were a bisphosphonate, then each region of inferior bone would be guarded against future resorption by the layer of bisphosphonate, which will remain buried under the new bone packet for many months. It is not predictable a priori how much net gain in bone mass would be needed to outweigh any adverse effect of this accumulation of microfracture damage.

Other unknowns have to do with osteoblast function. It is not certain that either the number of osteoblasts to arrive at a given resorption site or the amount of bone they will synthesize is preprogrammed. Osteoblast synthetic activity might somehow be influenced by or tailored to the size or volume of the resorption cavity, so that a smaller lacuna will elicit less bone formation. This would serve as a protective mechanism to prevent osteosclerosis from developing under normal conditions, but would prevent antiresorptive agents from being able to increase bone mass without an independent stimulation of osteoblast function.

Much more knowledge of the normal remodeling process is needed before the full effects of antiresorptive agents are understood. Nonetheless, clinical studies with antiresorptive agents have been underway. Those that have used bisphosphonates are reviewed.

Published Studies of Bisphosphonate Treatment of Osteoporosis

ADFR Regimens with Phosphate and Etidronate

Many of the studies of ADFR therapy have used phosphate and etidronate as the activator and depressor, respectively (Table 11-2).

In a prospective pilot study with 14 osteoporotic women already stabilized on estrogen replacement therapy (ERT), we used a regimen of oral neutral phosphate (1500 mg/d) for 7 days followed by a short (5-day) pulse of high-dose etidronate (900 mg/d), with the cycle repeated every 60 days. Patients were on a low-calcium diet during the phosphate and etidronate phases and were given a modest calcium supplement during the free phase (500 mg as the carbonate, b.i.d.). Spine bone mineral density (BMD) increased by 7.2% at 6 months and by 8.2% at 12 months (30). A concurrent control group of healthy postmenopausal women on ERT showed no change in lumbar BMD. No conclusion could be made about whether etidronate or phosphate was the important factor.

TABLE 11-2 Trials of Cyclic Phosphate and Etidronate

Reference	Number Patients on Etidronate	Concurrent Treatment	Increase in Spine BMD at One Year	Increase in BMD at Other Sites	Days of Phosphate/Etidronate /Cycle	Years of Treatment
Pacifici (33)	30	Calcium*	−8.0%[†]	Radius(−5%)	3/14/73	2
Mallette (30)	14	Estrogen, calcium	8.2%	Not done	7/5/60	1
Hodsman (32)	37	Calcium	8.4%	Not done	4/14/90	2
Woodson (35)	17	Estrogen, calcium	6.6%	"Forearm" (2.6%)	3/14/47	1
Watts (34)	107	Calcium	5.2%	Trochanter	3/14/90	2
Miller (36)	47	Calcium/vitamin D	13.0%	Not done	3/14/91	2
Pallot-Prades (37)	20	Calcium/vitamin D	Not done[‡]	Not done	3/14/90	1
Silberstein (38)	42	Calcium	6.6%	Neck and trochanter	3/14/101	3

*In this study instructions were not given to avoid taking etidronate and calcium at the same time, and the calcium supplement was given during all 90 days of each cycle.

[†]Change in the vertebral centrum measured by quantitative computed tomography. The measurements in the other studies were of the whole vertebra (usually L-2 to L-4) by dual energy absorptiometry.

[‡]No change in iliac crest trabecular bone volume by histomorphometry

BMD, bone mineral density

Bisphosphonates for the Treatment of Osteoporosis

Two patients showed a poor response of bone mass, and each also had only a minimal increase in serum PTH during phosphate administration, suggesting that the induced secondary hyperparathyroidism may have been an important factor. We concluded either that this set of patients happened to have had high turnover osteoporosis, with a large remodeling space at baseline to be filled in, or that the regimen at least transiently was able to place the remodeling sequence into positive balance.

The short pulse of etidronate was chosen in hopes of minimizing the volume of bone that might incorporate the drug long term. Other trials of this type of therapy have used a similar sequence, but with a shorter duration of phosphate administration and a 14-day duration of etidronate treatment (see Table 11-2). The rationale for the 14 days of etidronate administration is not clear. One published summary states that it was based on the length of time needed to see a biochemical response of resorption in Paget's disease (3), but data are not given or referenced.

While our work was in progress, Anderson and coworkers reported a trial of cyclic phosphate and etidronate therapy in five women treated for 9 to 24 months (31). Improvement in bone mass and remodeling parameters on biopsy encouraged an extension of these studies to 37 osteoporotic women with symptomatic spine fractures, reported by Hodsman (32). The regimen comprised phosphate (2 to 3 g/d) for 4 days, followed by etidronate (7.5 mg/kg/d) for 14 days, with cycles of 90 days. Spine bone mass increased by 8.4% after 12 months, but no increase was seen thereafter for up to 30 months. Vertebral fractures assessed by radiography were reduced by 67% after 15 months of therapy, compared with the fracture rate during the first 15 months of treatment.

Bone histomorphometry done 3 months after the seventh phosphate pulse showed highly variable changes from baseline. Mean wall thickness of new bone packets was unchanged, but erosion depth was not measured, so bone balance at the cellular level could not be estimated. The amount of eroded surface increased significantly, but osteoclast number was not changed. The number of osteoblasts per millimeter of bone perimeter decreased. This suggests that osteoclastic resorption under these conditions did not always call forth the expected osteoblast cohort (or had not yet done so at the time of the biopsy 3 months later). Mineral apposition rate was reduced, mineralization lag time prolonged, and the apparent duration of the remodeling cycle was prolonged from 290 to 492 days (Table 11-3). It is not clear whether the apparent uncoupling, the slowing of mineralization, and the prolongation of remodeling time are features of ADFR therapy or a response to etidronate (which is known in high doses to inhibit mineralization), but similar changes occur after intermittent administration of etidronate alone (see below). The slowed apposition rate and prolonged

TABLE 11-3 Effect of Cyclic or Intermittent Treatment on the Total Time for Completion of Bone Remodeling (Sigma, days)

Regimen	Reference	Sigma pre	Sigma post
Phosphate-etidronate	Hodsman (32)	290	492
Triiodothyronine-etidronate	Steiniche (28)	132	206
Etidronate alone	Steiniche (28)	119	407
PTH-(1–38) alone	Hodsman (27)	142	111
PTH-(1–38)-calcitonin	Hodsman (27)	154	111

remodeling time, however, would lessen the chances that bone mass would continue to increase long term.

▶319

A trial of a similar phosphate and etidronate regimen in a group of 30 women with postmenopausal osteoporosis found that spine and radius BMD decreased more rapidly in the etidronate group than in control women treated with calcium supplements alone or with hormone replacement therapy (33). This is the only negative study of etidronate effects on BMD reported to date. Two possible reasons for this negative result were poor drug absorption and insufficient stimulation of PTH secretion. These patients were given daily calcium supplements throughout the study, including the phosphate and etidronate phases. For adequate absorption etidronate must be taken on an empty stomach. Concomitant oral calcium will prevent its absorption. The course of phosphate was shorter (3 days versus 4 or 7 days), and the calcium supplement would have blunted any increase in PTH.

A large multicenter trial used oral neutral phosphate (1.0 g twice daily) for 3 days and etidronate (400 mg/d) for 14 days, in cycles of 90 days. It enrolled 429 postmenopausal women with compression fractures who were not on ERT (34). Patients were placed into four treatment groups: control, phosphate only, etidronate only, and phosphate plus etidronate. Spine BMD increased 5.2% in the phosphate-etidronate group; measurements at the hip did not change. The phosphate–etidronate group developed marginally fewer new spine deformities than the placebo group.

An uncontrolled open trial in 17 postmenopausal women with osteoporosis or osteopenia confirmed that spine bone mass would increase in estrogen-replaced subjects during administration of a cyclic phosphate-etidronate regimen (35). The patients were receiving conjugated estrogen, with medroxyprogesterone added when appropriate. Etidronate (400 mg/d) was given for 14 days and repeated cyclically every 45 days. Half the patients took neutral phosphate (2 g/d) for 3 days before each etidronate course. At one year, spine BMD had increased by 6.6% and proximal femoral BMD by 2.6%. Unlike our study, in which all women were stabilized on ERT for at least 6 months before the baseline bone mass measurement and first round of therapy, 10 of the 17 patients in this study were started on conjugated ERT simultaneously with the cyclic regimen. Thus, an antiresorptive effect of the estrogen may have been responsible for some of the increase in bone mass.

A group of 47 women with at least one idiopathic vertebral compression who were 12 ± 4 SD years postmenopausal received oral neutral phosphate (2000 mg/d) for 3 days, etidronate (400 mg orally at bedtime) for 14 days, and calcium supplements (to a total dietary calcium of 1500 mg) during the free period, with cycles repeated every 91 days (36). None received ERT, but all were instructed to receive 400 to 800 units vitamin D per day. They showed an increase of 13.0% in vertebral BMD after one year and a further 2.7% increase in the second year. No new vertebral compression deformities developed during the 2 years, and no patient lost height. A matched control group of 15 patients (15 ± 6 years postmenopausal) was "assigned" to treatment with only the above doses of calcium and vitamin D. Their vertebral BMD did not change significantly (as expected 15 years after the menopause), and six of the 15 developed a new vertebral compression deformity and lost 1.0 to 1.5 inches of height during the 2 years. Although the study was not randomized, the results in the phosphate-etidronate group were so striking that they could not have resulted simply from bias in group assignment.

Twenty patients with vertebral fracture at average age 65 years received phosphate (1500 mg/d) for 3 days, then etidronate (400 mg/d) for 14 days in 90 day cycles (37). Calcium carbonate with 400 units vitamin D was given daily, including the phosphate and etidronate days, again possibly minimizing any secondary hyperparathyroidism from the phosphate and possibly reducing etidronate absorption. BMD values were not measured. Bone biopsies performed before and after one year (four cycles) showed no change in bone mass or trabecular thickness or density. Remodeling was slowed, as demonstrated by a two-thirds reduction in eroded surface and osteoclast number, and a 50% fall in bone formation rate. Mean wall thickness of new bone packets was reduced from 38.7 μm to 36.4 μm, but resorption depth was not measured. The length of the remodeling cycle was not reported. The authors concluded that bone resorption and formation, which they thought to be uncoupled originally, were once more coupled, leading to a better quality of bone. Precisely what structural feature represented the better quality was not stated. Why eroded surface decreased here, but increased in Hodsman's study, is not known.

Silberstein and Schnur treated 42 postmenopausal osteoporotic women for 3 years with sequential oral phosphate (1 g/d) for 3 days, etidronate (10 mg/kg per day) for 14 days, with cycles repeated every 101 days (38). After the first four cycles the etidronate dosage was lowered to 5 mg/kg per day. A nonrandomized control group of 20 women received only calcium supplements. Of 27 women with evaluable spine density measurements, 25 showed a significant increase, averaging 6.6% at one year, with no further increase after the first year. BMD of the hip was evaluable in all 42 women, and increased in 28 patients at the femoral neck, 21 at Ward's triangle, and 24 at the trochanter, respectively. Approximately one fourth of the women showed a significant decrease at each site in the hip, however. The mean changes at each site for each group were not given, so the responses are difficult to compare with those in other studies. The etidronate group developed 83% fewer new lumbar vertebral deformities than the controls. This study confirms that spine BMD will increase only during the first 6 to 12 months of a regimen of phosphate and etidronate. The study also suggests that some women will show an increase in the hip as well. It does not, however, allow us to identify prospectively which women will respond positively, or to explain the variable result at the hip.

Thus, several studies have shown clearly that cyclic phosphate and etidronate will produce a significant increase in lumbar bone mass. Based on the large multicenter study, the first 3 days of phosphate seems to add little. A longer duration of phosphate administration was associated with greater increases in bone mass and should be tested directly in a cyclic regimen against intermittent bisphosphonate alone. The duration of etidronate administration for optimum results is also not established, one of the best responses being obtained with 5 days at a higher dosage. The increase in bone mass seems limited to the first 12 months, with values remaining stable thereafter. How much of the increase is due to filling in of the remodeling space is not clear, but there is not yet any evidence from biopsy studies to show that the remodeling sequence has been placed into positive balance. Etidronate seems to slow overall remodeling and perhaps doubles the length of time needed to complete remodeling (see Table 11-3). These observations suggest that future trials of cyclic therapy might better use a different bisphosphonate with less tendency to inhibit mineralization.

Other ADFR Regimens

Triiodothyronine (100 µg/d) for 7 days was used as the activating agent in a study of 15 women with postmenopausal osteoporosis (28). Etidronate (400 mg/d) for 14 days was used as the depressing agent, and cycles were repeated every 15 weeks. A control group given only intermittent etidronate will be described below. The ADFR regimen decreased serum alkaline phosphatase, but urinary calcium and hydroxyproline were unchanged. Bone histomorphometry before and after 60 weeks showed no change in resorption depth or mean wall thickness of new bone packets, and lumbar BMD did not increase. Eroded surfaces, activation frequency, bone formation rate, and mineral apposition rate were also unchanged. The remodeling period increased from 132 to 206 days,

▶ 321

but the change was not statistically significant due to high variability. Triiodothyronine administration seemed to lessen the prolongation of remodeling time seen with intermittent etidronate, but was not associated with any improvement in bone balance at the cellular level.

Etidronate and PTH were used cyclically in a study of bone histomorphometry and metabolism in eight patients, aged 29 to 61 years (average 47 years), with low turnover osteoporosis, diagnosed on the basis of baseline histomorphometry (26). Synthetic PTH-(1–38) (400 units, route not specified) was used for 14 days as the activating agent, with oral etidronate (300 mg/d) for 14 days as the depressing agent started on day 8 of PTH. Cycles were repeated every 15 weeks. Calcium intake was not restricted during the etidronate phase. Six of the patients had received prior therapy with various agents, including calcitonin, sodium fluoride, vitamin D, and anabolic steroids, and no interim time appears to have been allowed for a return to the basal remodeling state before study entry. PTH caused a slight increase in blood calcium concentration, within the normal range, and increased the urinary excretion of cyclic adenosine monophosphate as expected. Only four patients showed an increase in urinary hydroxyproline excretion after PTH administration, and the changes in intestinal calcium absorption and estimated calcium balance were variable. The bone accretion rate, measured with radiocalcium, and serum alkaline phosphatase activity each increased in five patients. BMD was not measured, but radiographs showed no new vertebral deformities during the year of therapy. Iliac histomorphometry was reported separately (24). As expected, given the baseline heterogeneity of the group, histologic parameters changed in variable fashion. There was, however, no overall change in trabecular volume, trabecular thickness, or mean wall thickness of new bone packets. Two patients were on fluoride before entry, and their osteoid volume decreased markedly, as expected. The length of the remodeling cycle was not reported.

Intermittent Regimens

Clodronate (1200 to 1600 mg/d) was given intermittently to a group of 24 postmenopausal women with osteoporosis. Patients were given drug for one month, kept off for 3 months, on for 3, off for 3, and on for one month. The rationale for this unusual sequence was not stated. Total body bone mass by neutron activation analysis increased by about 3% at one year in 18 patients and about 6% at 18 months in nine women, versus a 2% loss in placebo-treated patients (39). Formal publication of the final results of this study is awaited.

In the large multicenter study described above, one group of patients received only etidronate (400 mg/d) for 14 days every 91 days. After a year, spine BMD increased by 4.2%, a change that was not statistically different from the

5.2% increase in the phosphate-etidronate group. Density of the femoral trochanter also increased significantly in the etidronate alone group. Phosphate seems to add little to the effects of etidronate alone, but this may not have been a fair test, because the dose and duration of phosphate were less than in the two earlier studies that had showed greater increases in lumbar mass. The degree of hypocalcemia and increase in serum PTH induced by phosphate were not reported. Data from the etidronate only and phosphate-etidronate groups were pooled for a post hoc analysis of fracture incidence. The largest effect on fracture incidence was in the subgroup with baseline bone mass below the 50th percentile of those enrolled, suggesting the need for a prospective study to test whether antiresorptive therapy might be especially effective in patients with critically low bone mass.

▶ 323

Storm and coworkers (40) studied 66 early postmenopausal women with spine compression fractures, randomized to receive either etidronate (400 mg/d) or placebo for 2 weeks out of each 15 weeks, without any activating agent. Both groups were treated daily with oral calcium (500 mg/d) with a vitamin D supplement (400 U/d), but not estrogen. The etidronate group showed an increase in lumbar bone mass of approximately 5% that became significant only after 10 courses of etidronate (3 years), versus a 4% loss in controls. Forearm BMD was not decreased by etidronate. No evidence of osteomalacia appeared on bone biopsy. Beyond week 60, the etidronate group developed fewer new spinal deformities (6 versus 54) and lost less height. Histomorphometric data reported separately showed that bone balance per remodeling cycle improved by approximately the thickness of one lamella (41). The bone formation rate decreased by two thirds and mineralization lag time increased almost threefold. The duration of the remodeling period was not reported.

In the trial of triiodothyronine activation summarized above, the control group of 15 osteoporotic women received intermittent etidronate (400 mg/d) for 14 days out of each 15 weeks (28). Serum alkaline phosphatase and urinary calcium excretion decreased, but urinary hydroxyproline excretion was unchanged. Bone histomorphometry before and after 60 weeks showed that resorption depth decreased from 52 μm to 44 μm with no change in the mean wall thickness of new bone packets. The shift toward a more positive bone balance per cycle was not statistically significant, however, and lumbar BMD did not increase significantly during the 14 months of the study, confirming the results of Storm and coworkers. Activation frequency, bone formation rate, and mineral apposition rate were all reduced, but osteoid thickness was not increased. The remodeling period increased from 119 to 407 days, but the change was not statistically significant due to high variability. Eroded surface did not change.

Pamidronate (250 to 300 mg/d) was given orally during alternate 2-month periods to a group of women with postmenopausal osteoporosis and crush fractures (42). Lumbar BMD by dual photon absorptiometry increased by 2.4% the first year and by 2.5% the second year (43). Density of the mid–shaft radius was also increased, by 3.4% the first year and 1.8% the second year. No changes occurred in lumbar or forearm bone mass in the third, fourth, or fifth year (43). Formal publication of these results is awaited.

Pamidronate was given intravenously (20 mg/d for 10 days) to 15 patients with Paget's disease, and spine and proximal radius monitored for one year by dual or single photon absorptiometry (44). There was a transient rise in spine mineral of about 2% at 6 months, which failed to reach statistical significance, followed by a decline back to or below the starting value. Radial BMD showed a nonsignificant decline at one year of about 3%. At least in nonosteoporotic patients, a single short course of intravenous pamidronate had only transient and minor effects in either the axial or appendicular skeleton. Because the patients had a disease marked by a great increase in skeletal turnover, secondary hyperparathyroidism may have developed after treatment and would have contributed to a loss of cortical bone.

Alendronate was given intravenously (5 mg/d) on 2 consecutive days every 3 months for one year to women with postmenopausal osteoporosis. A randomized control group received oral calcium supplements (1000 mg/d) (45). Lumbar BMD increased 9%, and radial cortical density increased 5%, whereas both values declined in the controls. Alendronate lowered urinary hydroxyproline by 25%, and measures of bone formation (serum osteocalcin and alkaline phosphatase) were reduced by 15% to 20%. The pain score improved more in the bisphosphonate group. An acute phase reaction occurred in three of the 20 patients after the first dose of alendronate, as expected (46). Results beyond one year were not reported.

Continuous Regimens

In an early study, etidronate (20 mg/kg per day) was given orally daily for 6 to 12 months to 20 osteoporotic patients (47) and produced a slightly positive whole body calcium balance, but both bone resorption and formation, measured by isotope kinetic studies, were decreased, suggesting that any positive skeletal balance was minimized by the induced decline in bone formation. Bone mass and histology were not assessed, but the same course of etidronate was found in separate studies of Paget's disease to be associated with an increased incidence of fracture, presumably because of an induced mineralization defect (48,49).

Bone mineral content (BMC) of the spine and proximal radius was monitored by dual photon absorptiometry in 18 patients who received etidronate orally (5 mg/kg/d) for 6 months for treatment of Paget's disease (44). Spinal BMC increased by about 4% by 6 months and tended to decline slightly thereafter. BMC was lost from the wrist (4% decline at 6 months). The gain in the spine may have been at the expense of cortical bone elsewhere. It is not stated whether a calcium supplement was given or whether any subjects developed secondary hyperparathyroidism (50), which would have accelerated endocortical bone loss.

It was observed over a decade ago that oral administration of pamidronate for treatment of Paget's disease of bone led to a positive whole body calcium balance (51) and an increase in BMD of the midshaft radius (52). The major increase in calcium balance on a dosage of 600 mg/d was transient, as the remodeling space was filling in, but a small positive balance (approximately 20 mg/d) was still found after 9 months (51). These observations suggested that lower doses of pamidronate that did not totally arrest remodeling might allow a long-term positive balance. Trials of lower doses of continuous pamidronate for osteoporosis are now being reported.

▶ 325

Oral pamidronate (150 mg/d as an enteric-coated tablet) was given for an average of 3.7 years to 24 osteoporotic women, who showed a steady increase in lumbar BMD at an estimated 3.1% per year (53). A later reanalysis of the data with a more conservative statistical method confirmed that bone mass was increasing rather steadily over at least 4 years, at an estimated rate of 2.4% per year (5). The rate of increase was as great in the third year as in the first. The individual increases in bone mass were unrelated to the basal hydroxyproline excretion, suggesting that the increase did not simply represent filling of the remodeling space. There was no loss of cortical bone mass over the 2 years it was monitored. A retrospective control group receiving conventional therapy showed no change in lumbar bone mineral. New spine fractures occurred only in five subjects, each of whom had already sustained five or more compression deformities at entry and thus had severe osteoporosis (54). Formal metabolic balance studies confirmed the findings in Paget's disease: calcium balance at baseline was -14 mg/d, after one week was $+110$ mg/d, and after one year was $+26$ mg/d. The dose of pamidronate decreased urinary hydroxyproline excretion by only 23% suggesting that bone remodeling was reduced but not prevented. Bone histomorphometry was not reported. These encouraging results contrast with the effects of a larger dose of pamidronate given in alternate 2-month periods, outlined above, where the increase in bone mass continued only during the first 2 years. Further work will be needed to confirm these results and to determine whether the lower dosage or the continuous regimen was the important factor in sustaining the improvement in bone mass.

Pamidronate (200 mg/d as an enteric-coated tablet, taken one hour or more before breakfast) was given an average of 14 months to 36 postmenopausal women with osteoporosis and at least one vertebral compression (55). Lumbar BMD increased 5.5% per year, density of the femoral neck by 3.8% per year, and whole body bone mass by 3.2% per year. Spinal and femoral neck BMD in a calcium-treated control group decreased at one year by 0.7% and 1.1% respectively. Plasma osteocalcin values rose from 4.3 to 5.2 ng/mL, while alkaline phosphatase fell from 164 to 118 U/L, so changes in osteoblast function were unclear. Urinary calcium excretion decreased by 30% and hydroxyproline excretion by 40%. Bone histomorphometry was not assessed. Results beyond one year have not been reported.

One year of daily oral administration of pamidronate (4.8 to 6.0 mg/kg per day) to 35 postmenopausal women with one or more vertebral fracture produced a 5.3% increase in lumbar spine BMD (56). Density of the trochanter also increased by 5.3%, but no change in density occurred in the femoral neck, Ward's triangle, or radial shaft. Bone histomorphometry and changes in bone mass beyond one year were not reported.

The acute effects of a 4-week course of enteric-coated pamidronate (75 or 150 mg orally at bedtime) on biochemical parameters of bone remodeling were assessed in a placebo-controlled, randomized, double-blind, dose-ranging study (57). Sixty patients aged 53 to 76 years with a recent forearm fracture were entered. Both doses of pamidronate produced a significant decline in measures of bone resorption, including urinary hydroxyproline, pyridinoline, and deoxypyridinoline excretion. The decreases were already present by one week and reached a nadir at 2 to 4 weeks. The higher dosage of pamidronate also reduced serum osteocalcin significantly and produced mild secondary hyperparathyroidism. The dosage of 75 mg/d reduced resorptive parameters but not osteocalcin, so would seem to be more likely to produce a long-term positive remodeling balance. It is possible, however, that longer administration of the lower dosage would eventually slow turnover enough to reduce bone formation. These results should encourage longer studies of lower dosage ranges.

Special Applications

Prevention of Postmenopausal Bone Loss

Women entering natural menopause begin to remodel their skeleton at an accelerated rate and are placed into a negative remodeling balance so that bone is lost rapidly for the first 6 to 8 years. Loss is even more rapid after surgical menopause. In women with a low peak bone mass, the menopause may reduce bone mass sufficiently to place them at risk of fracture. Although ERT can prevent the loss of bone, many women are not able to take estrogen, so that an alternative is needed. Bisphosphonates, by slowing remodeling, might be expected to slow or prevent postmenopausal bone loss.

Etidronate (400 mg/d) or placebo was given daily for 3 months to 20 otherwise healthy women who had undergone oophorectomy for nonmalignant conditions (58). Etidronate suppressed the increase in bone resorption, as assessed by changes in serum and urine calcium and urinary hydroxyproline values. Etidronate also caused an insignificant fall in bone formation parameters: serum alkaline phosphatase and osteocalcin. Radial bone mass was not changed, but the duration of observation was too short to expect to see any change in cortical mass.

In a randomized, placebo-controlled, double-blind study, tiludronate (100 mg/d orally) was given daily for 6 months to 38 healthy women less than 96 months postmenopausal and on no other treatment (59). Lumbar BMD increased after 12 months by 1.3% ± 0.8% in the tiludronate group, versus a 2.1% fall in the controls (P<.01). Urinary hydroxyproline excretion fell in both groups, but the decline was significant only in the tiludronate group. Urinary calcium excretion did not change. A longer duration of tiludronate administration and assessment of changes in bone histomorphometry to determine resorption depth and mean wall thickness would be of interest to determine whether this apparently low dosage will continue to increase bone mass over the long term.

▶ 327

Steroid-Induced Osteoporosis

In a randomized study of 16 long-term glucocorticoid treated patients, one year of pamidronate (150 mg/d orally in an enteric-coated tablet) produced a 19.6% increase in BMD of the vertebral centrum, whereas the 19 controls showed a 9% decrease (60,61). Metacarpal cortical area also increased 1.2% in the treated group, but declined by 1.2% in the calcium-treated controls. Biochemical parameters and bone biopsy both suggested that bone remodeling was slowed by pamidronate. A further year of pamidronate treatment in 5 of the patients did not further increase bone mass, but 9 controls on placebo showed a further loss of density of the vertebral centrum, totaling 30% by the end of the second year (60,61). Pamidronate thus prevented the development of steroid osteoporosis, at the expense of a markedly slowed remodeling rate. The lack of a continued rise in bone mass during the last 18 months of this study is discouraging, but it is possible that inhibition of osteoblast synthetic activity by the glucocorticoid might have prevented a positive balance from developing.

Immobilization Osteoporosis

Etidronate (5 or 20 mg/kg per day) given to volunteers during 20 weeks of continuous bed rest did not alter the rate of calcaneal bone loss, but whole body calcium balance did become positive (62). Vertebral bone mass measurements were not available at the time of this study.

Clodronate (400 to 1600 mg/d orally) was given to 7 patients at each dosage level for 3.5 months starting within 30 days of spinal cord injury. It completely inhibited bone loss from the distal tibia at 3 and 6 months (63). Placebo-treated controls lost 7% of tibial mineral content by 6 months. Tibial bone mass and iliac crest trabecular bone volume were equally well maintained at each dose of clodronate, but the higher dosage gave a greater suppression of urinary hydroxyproline and calcium.

Fifteen healthy male volunteers, aged 33 ± 5 years, placed at bed rest for 120 days showed a marked increase in resorptive surface (115%) and osteoclast number (95%) in iliac crest biopsies (64). Daily treatment with etidronate (900 mg/d) throughout the 120-day bed rest period lessened the increase in resorptive surface by two thirds and caused a fall (by 75%) rather than a rise in the number of trabecular osteoclasts. It is discouraging that etidronate did not decrease the number of cortical (endosteal plus Haversian) osteoclasts (65). Endosteal and Haversian osteoclasts were not reported separately, perhaps because there were only small numbers in each separate compartment. If the goal is to thicken the cortex, however, inhibition of endosteal osteoclasts is the important step. One can speculate that Haversian osteoclasts, being sequestered at the tip of cutting cones, might not be exposed to effective levels of etidronate. Osteoid thickness and surface extent were both decreased by etidronate, suggesting an inhibition of osteoblast function. Remodeling time was not reported. No significant loss of bone volume was detected in the biopsies from either group, but radiographic bone mass measurements were not done. Further studies to include radiographic and densitometric cortical bone mass measurements are needed to determine the net effect of etidronate and of other bisphosphonates on the cortex over a longer time frame.

Pamidronate (intravenously in doses of 10 to 45 mg over 4 hours) effectively relieves immobilization hypercalcemia and hypercalciuria, with a duration of response of several weeks and continued responsiveness on second dosing on recurrence (66). Bone mass was not measured, but the relief of hypercalcemia must reflect the antiresorptive effect of pamidronate that would be expected to reduce bone loss.

Etidronate Versus Other Bisphosphonates

The initial increases in bone mass with phosphate–etidronate or intermittent etidronate protocols were encouraging, but the increase was limited to the first three or four cycles in most of the studies. This pattern is approximately the one that would be expected from a reduction in the remodeling space without a positive shift in the balance between bone removed and replaced at each remodeling site. Histomorphometric data have confirmed that etidronate greatly reduces the number of active remodeling sites. Data from at least two laboratories in three groups of patients suggest that etidronate also prolongs the time to complete remodeling, independently of whether phosphate is given, suggesting a long-term effect on osteoblast activity (see Table 11-3). The thickness of new bone packets was not reduced, suggesting that the osteoblasts simply take longer to complete the same amount of bone synthesis. This lengthening of the remodeling period could contribute to the limited ability of etidronate to increase bone mass after the first 6 to 12 months. No histomorphometric data on remodeling time in patients treated with an aminobisphosphonate or clodronate were found, so it is not clear whether this lengthening of remodeling is characteristic of bisphosphonates in general or is specific to etidronate. It is not a feature of ADFR or intermittent therapy because groups treated intermittently with PTH or cyclically with PTH followed by calcitonin as the depressing agent (27) did not show a prolongation (see Table 11-3).

▶ 329

The spatial distribution of etidronate in bone could differ from that of the aminobisphosphonates. Autoradiographic studies were done of the distribution of the aminobisphosphonate, alendronate, in animals with bone remodeling accelerated by injections of PTH-related peptide. After 24 hours the alendronate was concentrated on the bone surface in the immediate vicinity of and underneath osteoclasts (67). The osteoclasts were attached but showed an inactive ruffled border and appeared not to be resorbing bone. Apparently the drug bound only to areas where the bone surface was exposed around active osteoclasts. It did not penetrate the bone cell lining layer in significant amounts. When the osteoclast later moved over bone to which alendronate was bound, it became immobilized, probably by releasing a very high concentration of drug into the ruffled border space. Thus, the currently functioning crops of osteoclasts would be caused to cease resorption.

The less polar structure of etidronate might allow it to penetrate the bone cell lining layer better than do the aminobisphosphonates. It might eventually be deposited in significant amounts over the entire surface of bone, including areas where osteoblasts are laying down bone. To test this hypothesis, autoradiographic studies of the distribution of etidronate in bone are needed, as are histomorphometric estimates of remodeling time after intermittent treatment with an aminobisphosphonate. If the prolongation of remodeling time is unique to etidronate, use of an aminobisphosphonate together with an activating agent such as phosphate or PTH might still allow the promise of the ADFR concept to be fulfilled.

Bisphosphonates for the Treatment of Osteoporosis

Limitations of Available Data

The desired outcome of osteoporosis treatment is fracture prevention. We have no data on bisphosphonate effects on nonvertebral fracture rates. Data from one study (34) suggested a decrease in new vertebral deformities after intermittent etidronate, but this was a post hoc subgroup analysis that cannot prove the point. Studies of fracture incidence require large numbers of subjects, so that measurement of bone mass has often been used as a surrogate. A rise in bone mass may or may not be associated with a reduced risk of fracture, depending on the quality and location of the new bone. The available data on bone mass changes cover only one to 4 years and generally suggest only a limited regain of lost bone. What will eventually be required are truly long-term studies of bone mass, fracture rate, and histomorphometry, covering perhaps 10 years of therapy. Smaller pilot studies of bone mass might first be used to find agents and regimens that will produce a steady increase in bone mass continuing over at least 5 years. The increase should exceed that expected from a regain of the remodeling space and should be accompanied by a positive balance morphologically. Thus the overall task of finding the optimum regimen will require at least another 15 to 20 years of study.

The safety profile of the bisphosphonates thus far seems favorable. The effects of bisphosphonates on nonmineralized tissues, while less marked than their skeletal effects, have not been studied in the long term. Since bisphosphonates are released slowly from the skeleton with a half-life measured in months, each bisphosphonate must be regarded as potentially capable of producing its own set of rare or delayed adverse effects. It will be important to establish programs for long-term surveillance for each bisphosphonate.

Summary

Suggestive, but not conclusive, evidence indicates that bisphosphonates may reduce fracture incidence among those with severely reduced bone mass, perhaps by simply reducing the number of resorption lacunae. Continuous long-term usage or high doses are probably not needed for this effect, but the optimum regimen and agent are unknown and will take years to discover. There is not yet any evidence for a beneficial effect on fracture rate in subjects with mildly or moderately reduced bone mass, even with prior fractures. The long-term consequences of slowing bone remodeling are unknown, and fracture incidence conceivably could even increase as the skeleton ages as a result of not being renewed by normal remodeling.

Osteoporosis is a common disorder with enormous financial and emotional cost. This should provide motivation for new studies to cover a longer time frame and enroll larger numbers of subjects in various treatment protocols with each new bisphosphonate. The knowledge base is not yet available, however, on which to base an everyday use of bisphosphonates for osteoporosis in clinical practice. I agree with Dr. N. Hamdy (4) that "Until the beneficial effects of the newer bisphosphonates, or indeed any of the available ones, administered cyclically or continuously, are firmly established, their use in the treatment of osteoporosis should clearly remain the domain of the clinical investigator."

Unfortunately, first-generation bisphosphonates are already being prescribed to large numbers of osteoporotic women. This premature use of an unproved therapy may be viewed as inappropriate and potentially hazardous. It also leaves fewer women available for entry into proper trials of newer bisphosphonates. In my opinion, the prescription of bisphosphonates for osteoporosis can currently be justified clinically only for the patient with a diagnosis of osteoporosis firmly established by the occurrence of spontaneous spine fracture, with extremely reduced lumar bone mass, who is not able (for geographic or psychosocial reasons) to be enrolled in a prospective research trial, and who has failed to improve bone mass satisfactorily with available approved agents such as calcium, estrogen, vitamin D supplements, or calcitonin. Informed consent should be obtained for such a "compassionate usage" of bisphosphonate.

▶ 331

References

1. Parfitt AM. Use of bisphosphonates in the prevention of bone loss and fractures. Am J Med 1991;91(5B):42S-46S.

2. Attie MF. Bisphosphonate therapy for osteoporosis. Hosp Pract (Off Ed) 1991; 26:87–90.

3. Watts NB. Bisphosphonate therapy for postmenopausal osteoporosis. South Med J 1992;85:2S31–2S33.

4. Hamdy NA. Perspectives in the use of newer bisphosphonates in the management of established osteoporosis. South Med J 1992;85:2S52–2S54.

5. Papapoulos SE, Landman JO, Bijvoet OL, et al. The use of bisphosphonates in the treatment of osteoporosis. Bone 1992;1:S41–S49.

6. Eriksen EF. Normal and pathological remodeling of human trabecular bone: three dimensional reconstruction of the re-modeling sequence in normals and in metabolic bone disease. Endocr Rev 1986;7:379–408.

7. Parfitt AM. Surface specific bone remodeling in health and disease. In: Kleerekoper M KS, ed. Clinical disorders of bone and mineral metabolism. New York: Mary Ann Liebert Inc., 1989: 7–14.

8. Heaney RP, Recker RR, Saville PD. Menopausal changes in bone remodeling. J Lab Clin Med 1978;92:964–970.

9. Steiniche T, Hasling C, Charles P, Eriksen EF, Mosekilde L, Melsen F. A randomized study on the effects of estrogen/ gestagen or high dose oral calcium on trabecular bone remodeling in postmenopausal osteoporosis. Bone 1989;10:313–320.

10. Darby AJ, Meunier PJ. Mean wall thickness and formation periods of trabec-

ular bone packets in idiopathic osteoporosis. Calcif Tissue Int 1981;33:199–204.

11. Chow J, Tobias JH, Colston KW, Chambers TJ. Estrogen maintains trabecular bone volume in rats not only by suppression of bone resorption but also by stimulation of bone formation. J Clin Invest 1992;89:74–78.

12. Fang MA, Frost PJ, Iida KA, Hahn TJ. Effects of nicotine on cellular function in UMR 106-01 osteoblast-like cells. Bone 1991;12:233–286.

13. Ramp WK, Lenz LG, Galvin RJ. Nicotine inhibits collagen synthesis and alkaline phosphatase activity, but stimulates DNA synthesis in osteoblast-like cells. Proc Soc Exp Biol Med 1991;197:36–43.

14. Friday KE, Howard GA. Ethanol inhibits human bone cell proliferation and function in vitro. Metabolism 1991;40:562–565.

15. Horsman A, Jones M, Francis R, Nordin C. The effect of estrogen dose on postmenopausal bone loss. N Engl J Med 1983;309:1405–1407.

16. Riis B, Thomsen K, Christiansen C. Does calcium supplementation prevent postmenopausal bone loss? A double-blind controlled clinical study. N Engl J Med 1987;316:173–177.

17. Dawson-Hughes B, Dallai GE, Krall EA, Sadowski L, Sahyoun N, Tannenbaum S. A controlled trial of the effect of calcium supplementation on bone density in postmenopausal women. N Engl J Med 1990;323:878–883.

18. Mallette LE. An unusual morphologic evolution of Paget's disease of bone. Arthritis Rheum 1981;24:1544–1549.

19. Villareal DT, Murphy WA, Teitelbaum SL, Arens MQ, Whyte MP. Painful diffuse osteosclerosis after intravenous drug abuse. Am J Med 1992;93:371–381.

20. Parfitt AM. Morphologic basis of bone mineral measurements: transient and steady state effects of treatment in osteoporosis. Miner Elect Metab 1980;4:273–287.

21. Frost HM. The pathomechanics of osteoporosis. Clin Orthop 1985;200:198–225.

22. Frost HM. The ADFR concept and monitoring it. Metab Bone Dis Rel Res 1980;2S:317–321.

23. Frost HM. The ADFR concept revisited. Calcif Tissue Int 1984;36:349–353.

24. Delling G, Dreyer T, Hahn M, Vogel M, Rittinghaus EF, Hesch RD. Morphologic study of iliac crest spongiosa in patients with osteoporosis treated according to the ADFR (activation, depression of resorption, formation, repeat the cycle) with parathyroid hormone and diphosphonates (Hannover PTH I study). Z Orthop 1990;128:1–5.

25. Delling G, Dreyer T, Hesch RD, Schulz W, Ziegler R, Bressel M. Morphologic changes in iliac crest trabecular bone in primary hyperparathyroidism and their significance for diagnosis. Klin Wochenschr 1987;65:643–653.

26. Hesch RD, Heck J, Delling G, et al. Results of a stimulatory therapy of low bone metabolism in osteoporosis with (1–38)hPTH and diphosphonate EHDP. Protocol of study I, osteoporosis trial Hannover. Klin Wochenschr 1988;66:976–984.

27. Hodsman AB, Steer BM, Fraher LJ, Drost DJ. Bone densitometric and histomorphometric responses to sequential human parathyroid hormone (1–38) and salmon calcitonin in osteoporotic patients. Bone Miner 1991;14:67–83.

28. Steiniche T, Hasling C, Charles P, Eriksen EF, Melsen F, Mosekilde L. The effects of etidronate on trabecular bone remodeling in postmenopausal spinal osteoporosis: a randomized study comparing intermittent treatment and an ADFR regime. Bone 1991;12:155–163.

29. Passeri M, Palummeri E, Barbagallo M, et al. Sequential calcitriol-calcitonin in the therapy of osteoporosis. Minerva Endocrinol 1989;14:57–62.

30. Mallette LE, LeBlanc AD, Pool JL, Mechanick JI. Cyclic therapy of osteoporosis with neutral phosphate and brief, high-dose pulses of etidronate. J Bone Miner Res 1989;4:143–148.

31. Anderson C, Cape RDT, Crilly RG, Hodsman AB, Wolfe BM. Preliminary observations of a form of coherence therapy

/for osteoporosis. Calcif Tissue Int 1984; 1984:341–343.

32. Hodsman AB. Effects of cyclical therapy for osteoporosis using an oral regimen of inorganic phosphate and sodium etidronate: a clinical and bone histomorphometric study. Bone Miner 1989;5:201–212.

33. Pacifici R, McMurtry C, Vered I, Rupich R, Avioli LV. Coherence therapy does not prevent axial bone loss in osteoporotic women: a preliminary comparative study. J Clin Endocrinol Metab 1988;66:747–753.

34. Watts NB, Harris ST, Genant HK, et al. Intermittent cyclical etidronate treatment of postmenopausal osteoporosis. N Engl J Med 1990;323:73–79.

35. Woodson GC. Concurrrent therapy with etidronate and estrogen increases bone mass in osteoporosis and osteopenia. In: Christiansen C, Overgaard K, eds. Osteoporosis 1990 Proceedings of the Third International Symposium on Osteoporosis. October 14–18, 1990. Vol 3. Copenhagen: Osteopress ApS, 1990:1476–1478.

36. Miller PD, Neal BJ, McIntyre DO, Yanover MJ, Anger MS, Kowalski L. Effect of cyclical therapy with phosphorus and etidronate on axial bone mineral density in postmenopausal osteoporotic women. Osteoporosis Int 1991;1:171–176.

37. Pallot-Prades B, Chappard D, Tavan P, Prallet B, Riffat G, Alexandre C. Bone histomorphometric study in involuted fractured osteoporosis treated with 1-ethane-1-hydroxybiphosphonate (etidronate) during one year. Rev Rhum Mal Osteoartic 1991;58:771–776.

38. Silberstein EB, Schnur W. Cyclic oral phosphate and etidronate increase femoral and lumbar bone mineral density and reduce lumbar spine fracture rate over three years. J Nucl Med 1992;33:1–5.

39. Chesnut CH III. Synthetic salmon calcitonin, diphosphonates and anabolic steroids in the treatment of postmenopausal osteoporosis. In: Christiansen C, Arnaud CD, Nordin BEC, et al., eds. Osteoporosis. Vol 2. Copenhagen: Aalborg Stiftsbogtrykkeri, 1984: 549–555.

40. Storm T, Thamsborg G, Steiniche T, Genant HK, Sorensen OH. Effect of intermittent cyclical etidronate therapy on bone mass and fracture rate in women with postmenopausal osteoporosis. N Engl J Med 1990;322:1265–1271.

41. Steiniche T, Hasling C, Thamsborg G, et al. A histomorphometric analysis of iliac crest bone biopsies from patients treated with intermittent, cyclical etidronate therapy for postmenopausal osteoporosis. In: Christiansen C, Johansen C, Riis BJ, ed. Osteoporosis 1987. Vol 2. Copenhagen: Osteopress ApS, 1987:1182–1187.

42. Devogelaer JP, Huaux JP, Nagant de Deuxchaisnes C. Bisphosphonates therapy with APD in involutional osteoporosis with vertebral crush fractures. In: Christiansen C, Johansen C, Riis BJ, eds. Osteoporosis 1987. Vol 2. Copenhagen: Osteopress ApS, 1987:950–952.

43. Devogelaer JP, Nagant de Deuxchaisnes C. Treatment of involutional osteoporosis with the bisphosphonate APD (disodium pamidronate): non-linear increase of lumbar bone mineral density. In: Christiansen C, Overgaard K, eds. Osteoporosis 1990 Proceedings of the Third International Symposium on Osteoporosis. October 14–18, 1990. Vol 3. Copenhagen: Osteopress ApS, 1990:1507–1609.

44. Geusens P, Wouters C, Jijs J, Dequeker J. Effect of the bisphosphonates EHDP and APD on bone mineral density in patients with Paget's disease. In: Christiansen C, Overgaard K, eds. Osteoporosis 1990 Proceedings of the Third International Symposium on Osteoporosis. October 14–18, 1990. Vol 3. Copenhagen: Osteopress ApS, 1990:1451–1452.

45. Passeri M, Baroni MC, Pedrazzoni M, et al. Intermittent treatment with intravenous 4-amino-1-hydroxybutylidene-1,1-bisphosphonate (AHBuBP) in the therapy of postmenopausal osteoporosis. Bone Miner 1991;15:237–247.

46. Adami S, Bhalla AK, Dorizzi R, et al. The acute-phase response after bisphosphonate administration. Calcif Tissue Int 1987;41:326–331.

47. Heaney RP, Saville PD. Etidronate disodium in postmenopausal osteoporosis. Clin Pharmacol Ther 1976;20:593–604.

48. Khairi MRA, Altman RD, DeRosa GP, Zimmermann J, Schenk RK, Johnston CC. Sodium etidronate in the treatment of Paget's disease of bone. A study of long-term results. Ann Intern Med 1977;87:656–663.

49. Krane SM. Etidronate disodium in the treatment of Paget's disease of bone. Ann Intern Med 1982;96:619–625.

50. Harris ST, Neer RM, Segre GV, et al. Secondary hyperparathyroidism associated with dicholoromethane diphosphonate treatment of Paget's disease. J Clin Endocrinol Metab 1982;55:1100–1107.

51. Frijlink WB, te Velde J, Bijvoet LLM, Heynen G. Treatment of Paget's disease with (3-amino-1-hydroxypropylidene)-1,1-bisphosphonate (APD). Lancet 1979;i:799–803.

52. Nagant de Deuxchaisnes C, Devogelaer JP, Esselinckx W, Depresseux G, Rombouts-Lindemans C, Huaux JP. Non-hormonal-treatment of osteoporosis. Br Med J 1983;286;1648.

53. Valkema R, Vismans FJ, Papapoulos SE, Pauwels EK, Bijvoet OL. Maintained improvement in calcium balance and bone mineral content in patients with osteoporosis treated with the bisphosphonate APD. Bone Miner 1989;5:183–192.

54. Papapoulos SE, Bijvoet OLM, Valkema R, et al. New bisphosphonates in the treatment of osteoporosis. In: Christiansen C, Overgaard K, eds. Osteoporosis 1990 Proceedings of the Third International Symposium on Osteoporosis. October 14–18, 1990. Vol 3. Copenhagen: Osteopress ApS, 1990:1294–1300.

55. Zanchetta JR, del Valle E, Bogado CE, Spivacow FR, Perez Lloret A. Improvement in bone mineral content in patients with osteoporosis treated with the bisphosphonate APD. In: Christiansen C, Overgaard K, eds. Osteoporosis 1990 Proceedings of the Third International Symposium on Osteoporosis. October 14–18, 1990. Vol 3. Copenhagen: Osteopress ApS, 1990:1461–1463.

56. Fromm GA, Vega E, Plantalech L, Galich AM, Mautalen CA. Differential action of pamidronate on trabecular and cortical bone in women with involutional osteoporosis. Osteoporosis Int 1991;1:129–133.

57. Mallmin H, Ljunghall S, Larsson K, Lindh E. Short-term effects of pamidronate on biochemical markers of bone metabolism in osteoporosis—a placebo-controlled dose-finding study. Ups J Med Sci 1991;96:205–212.

58. Smith ML, Fogelman I, Hart DM, Scott E, Bevan J, Leggate I. Effect of etidronate disodium on bone turnover following surgical menopause. Calcif Tissue Int 1989;44:74–79.

59. Reginster JY, Lecart MP, Deroisy R, et al. Prevention of postmenopausal bone loss by tiludronate. Lancet 1989;2:1469–1471.

60. Reid IR, King AR, Alexander CJ, Ibbertson HK. Prevention of steroid-induced osteoporosis with (3-amino-1-hydroxypropylidene)-1,1-bisphosphonate (APD). Lancet 1988;1:143–146.

61. Reid IR, Heap SW, King AR, Ibbertson HK. Two-year follow-up of bisphosphonate (APD) treatment in steroid osteoporosis. Lancet 1988;2:1144. Letter.

62. Lockwood TR, Vogel JM, Schneider VS, Hulley SB. Effect of the diphosphonate EHDP on bone mineral metabolism during prolonged bed rest. J Clin Endocrinol Metab 1975;41:533–541.

63. Minaire P, Depassio J, Berard E, et al. Effects of clodronate on immobilization bone loss. Bone 1987;8:S63–S68.

64. Chappard D, Alexandre C, Palle S, et al. Effects of a bisphosphonate (1-hydroxyethylidene-1,1 bisphosphonic acid) on osteoclast number during prolonged bed rest in healthy humans. Metabolism 1989;38:822–325.

65. Chappard D, Petitjean M, Alexandre C, Vico L, Minaire P, Riffat G. Cortical osteoclasts are less sensitive to etidronate than trabecular osteoclasts. J Bone Miner Res 1991;6:673–680.

66. Gallacher SJ, Ralston SH, Dryburgh FJ, et al. Immobilization-related hypercal-

caemia—a possible novel mechanism and response to pamidronate. Postgrad Med J 1990;66:918–922.

67. Sato M, Grasser W, Endo N, et al. Bisphosphonate action. Alendronate localization in rat bone and effects on osteoclast ultrastructure. J Clin Invest 1991;88:2095–2105.

▶ 335

12 ▸ Nonpharmacologic Management of Osteoporosis

▸ ▸ ▸ Michael R. McClung

Osteoporosis is a disorder of skeletal fragility characterized by low bone mass and an increased risk of nontraumatic fractures. It is a chronic disorder which, at present, is irreversible. This is not to say, however, that osteoporosis is not treatable. The mainstays of current therapy are orthopedic management of nonvertebral fractures and pharmacologic therapy aimed at suppressing osteoclastic bone resorption and preventing further bone loss and fractures. Following a fracture, pain and impaired physical function often become the major concerns for patients and their families. Standard pharmacologic therapy is effective in slowing bone loss and decreasing fracture frequency but has little effect on the patient's symptoms or level of function. However, the intensity of the symptoms can be diminished, the functional status of patients can be improved, and their ability to cope with their chronic illness can be enhanced by other management strategies.

This chapter focuses on the nonorthopedic and nonpharmacologic issues of clinical management that arise in patients who are suspected of having or who are referred for the treatment of osteoporosis. Because the approach to rehabilitation of patients following surgical management of hip fracture has been so well reviewed, this chapter deals primarily with the management of osteoporotic vertebral fractures. Most of the management issues apply similarly to patients with primary and secondary forms of osteoporosis.

Objectives of Management

When initially presented with a patient suspected of having osteoporosis, a physician considers the following four principal clinical objectives:

1. Establish the correct diagnosis.
2. Lessen the patient's symptoms.

3. Improve functional capacity.
4. Reduce frequency of subsequent fractures.

No single approach to therapy will accomplish all of these objectives. Osteoporosis, like other chronic and debilitating illnesses, requires a comprehensive, multifaceted approach to management for maximum benefit.

Diagnostic Evaluation

At the time of the first evaluation, an attempt is made to establish the appropriate diagnosis. This evaluation has two components. In some patients, it is important to confirm that the diagnosis of osteoporosis is correct and that the patient's signs and symptoms are not caused by other clinical disorders. In patients found to have osteoporosis, correctable factors that may contribute to bone loss and skeletal fragility must be identified.

Confirming the Diagnosis of Osteoporosis

In routine practice, the diagnosis of osteoporosis is generally made on clinical grounds. The condition is often suspected when a postmenopausal woman or an older man presents with a history of back pain, height loss, and vertebral compression fractures. However, other degenerative diseases of the spine are also common in older individuals and may be the cause of the patient's symptoms.

Degenerative disease involving several intervertebral disks may also present with height loss and back pain. Disk space narrowing and its associated symptoms occur most commonly in the lumbar spine, but the thoracic region may be affected as well. Idiopathic scoliosis and kyphosis are conditions that usually begin in adolescence and often become more marked with advancing age. Scoliosis is associated with both back pain and height loss. Even mild to moderate scoliosis can be recognized by carefully examining the back while the patient is standing. In scoliotic patients, x-rays will reveal the curvature, the associated facet joint arthropathy, and the sclerosis and osteophyte formation along the inner or weight-bearing margin of the scoliotic curve (1). Radiographic and densitometric features of vertebral demineralization may be evident. Attempting to determine whether vertebral fracture has occurred is more difficult in the presence of significant scoliosis. Idiopathic kyphosis, which begins in adolescence, may cause progressive rounding of the thoracic spine, height loss, and back pain (2). The deformity of idiopathic kyphosis is generally a very smooth curve without the angulation of the spine that often accompanies a thoracic vertebral fracture. Radiographs demonstrate uniform anterior height loss of several mid-thoracic vertebral bodies, not associated with skeletal demineralization or true vertebral fractures.

These other degenerative conditions may be the sole clinical problem or may be confusing additions to osteoporosis as a cause of the patient's symptoms. Bone density testing may be helpful in determining whether osteoporosis coexists with these deformities. Regardless of whether osteoporosis is present, the presence of other degenerative diseases of the spine must be recognized so that appropriate analgesic, anti-inflammatory, or rehabilitative therapy can be instituted.

When it is determined that a patient's back pain and height loss are related to a vertebral fracture, it is imperative that causes of fractures other than osteoporosis be excluded. Fractures can occur following a fall or injury in patients without osteoporosis. Bone density testing is helpful in determining whether osteoporosis is a predisposing factor in a traumatic fracture. Metastatic disease of the spine is usually easily distinguished from generalized osteoporosis on routine radiographs by noting destructive changes in the vertebral body or pedicles. At the time of the initial fracture, however, these radiographic signs may not be obvious. Computed tomography of the spine may demonstrate the metastatic involvement more readily than do routine radiographs. Magnetic resonance imaging (MRI) most clearly distinguishes metastatic involvement from uncomplicated osteoporosis. Replacement of marrow by tumor results in loss of marrow signal on T1-weighted images and a more intense signal in T2-weighted scans. Other focal skeletal diseases such as Paget's disease of bone, bone cysts, infections, and benign bone tumors may present with acute vertebral fracture and must be distinguished from osteoporosis (3)

Identification of Correctable Factors Contributing to Bone Loss

After the diagnosis of osteoporosis is confirmed, treatable medical problems or other factors that contribute to bone loss must be identified. Smoking and excessive alcohol ingestion have been identified as important risk factors for osteoporosis. Careful inquiry may be required to elicit a history of excessive alcohol ingestion. Assistance with strategies to discontinue ethanol consumption or smoking may substantially augment an individual's skeletal response to pharmacologic treatment for osteoporosis. Endocrine abnormalities including endogenous or exogenous hyperthyroidism and cortisol excess, hyperparathyroidism, and androgen deficiency in men should be evaluated if clinical clues to these problems are noted. Glucocorticoid and anticonvulsant therapy need to be recognized. Chronic liver or renal insufficiency may contribute to bone loss, and the presence of these problems will alter the pharmacologic management of the patient. Multiple myeloma or other hematopoietic malignancies may present with generalized bone loss, vertebral fractures, and pain. Almost always, other clinical features such as weight loss or anorexia, anemia, hypercalcemia, or renal insufficiency are noted on routine evaluation of patients with myeloma. Serum or urine protein electrophoresis is indicated if the diagnosis is suspected.

A thorough laboratory evaluation including serum chemistry and hematology studies is indicated in every patient with osteoporosis. The need to perform laboratory screening for specific medical problems that may cause bone loss depends on the comfort of the clinician with the clinical recognition of these abnormalities.

Alterations in vitamin D metabolism and calcium balance are common in ▶ 339
the elderly and probably predispose to bone loss and, perhaps due to independent effects on muscle function, to increased frequency of falls and fractures. Lack of solar exposure and the effects of aging on skin reduce cutaneous vitamin D production. Gastrointestinal absorption of vitamin D becomes less efficient with aging, and the renal conversion of vitamin D to its active metabolite calcitriol is impaired in the elderly, including those with osteoporosis (4). Together these factors reduce the efficiency of calcium absorption. When coupled with restricted calcium intake, which is quite common in elderly women, negative calcium balance develops and is the probable explanation of the secondary hyperparathyroidism known to occur in older individuals. When defects of vitamin D metabolism are more pronounced, osteomalacia may occur. In its classical, severe form, osteomalacia is recognized by the presence of diffuse skeletal tenderness, muscle weakness, hypocalcemia, hypophosphatemia, and elevated serum alkaline phosphatase activity. Vitamin D deficiency may exist, however, without obvious clinical signs or routine laboratory abnormalities. In older individuals with risk factors for vitamin D deficiency, measurement of serum 25-hydroxyvitamin D (25-(OH)D) provides useful information about the adequacy of vitamin D stores. Even mild vitamin D deficiency unmasks inefficient renal activation of vitamin D. Patients with serum concentrations of 25-(OH)D below 30 mg/mL should receive vitamin D replacement therapy. Vitamin D deficiency may also indirectly contribute to bone loss. Muscle weakness or musculoskeletal pain caused by vitamin D deficiency often causes decreased physical activity, which results in increased bone resorption. Correction of calcium and vitamin D deficiency is effective in decreasing the fracture frequency in elderly patients with osteoporosis (5).

Renal calcium wasting may also be an important contributing factor in patients with osteoporosis. Both secondary hyperparathyroidism and osteopenia have been described in individuals with a renal calcium leak (6). In our osteoporosis clinic, between 5% and 10% of women with idiopathic postmenopausal osteoporosis are demonstrated to have hypercalciuria (more than 250 mg daily or 4 mg/kg per day). The recognition of hypercalciuria due to decreased renal calcium resorption may warrant therapy with thiazide diuretics.

Management of Patients with Acute Vertebral Fracture

Vertebral fractures are the most common complications in patients with osteoporosis. The true incidence of vertebral fracture is difficult to ascertain because many fractures occur without significant symptoms or with only transient back discomfort attributed to muscle strain. These patients do not routinely undergo evaluation to document the occurrence of a fracture. The incidence of vertebral fractures that were diagnosed clinically in Rochester, Minnesota was 145/ 100,000 person-years in women and 73/100,000 person-years in men (7). In a radiographic survey of 103 Swedish patients, aged 70 to 75, without a history of hip fracture, 22% were found to have vertebral deformities defined as a loss of anterior or central vertebral height of more than 33% (8). In a Dutch study, Symmons and coworkers evaluated women between the ages of 54 and 73 by spinal x-rays (9). Evidence of vertebral fracture was noted in 17%. Of those with fractures, 47% to 57% did not have a history of back pain.

Vertebral fractures most commonly occur near the thoracolumbar junction or in the mid-back. Between 10% and 15% of vertebral fractures happen as a consequence of a fall from a standing position or an automobile accident (7). Others may follow episodes of unusually strenuous activity for that individual. Most fractures, however, occur following routine activities of daily living. Nine of 30 acute vertebral episodes described by Patel and colleagues occurred while the patient was in bed (10). Fractures that occur with a fall usually cause intense pain of acute onset which is localized to the site of fracture and is associated with tenderness over the spinous process of the fractured vertebra. A similar pattern of symptoms may accompany acute fractures not associated with a fall, but many vertebral fractures present with a subacute course in which pain gradually develops over several days to a few weeks. The pain tends not to be as intense as that associated with traumatic fracture, but it is otherwise similar in nature. The pain is initially localized to the site of fracture but may be diffusely felt above and below the fracture site. The back is tender to percussion and palpation of the spinous processes, and the tenderness is most intense at the site of fracture.

Sitting, standing, or other body motion often aggravates the pain. Many patients find weight bearing impossible for the first few days after an acute fracture. The pain is improved and often relieved by lying down. Sitting in a well-supported reclining chair is more comfortable than lying flat in bed for some patients. Cramping or spasm of the paravertebral muscles adjacent to the fracture is a common complication and may dominate the clinical picture. With spasm, severe pain is experienced over a broader area of the back than is the pain of the fracture itself. Attempts to turn, sit, or stand may acutely initiate a muscle spasm and severe pain. Palpable tightness and tenderness of the paravertebral muscles are evident on examination of the back. Nausea and anorexia often accompany the acute fracture. Ileus, abdominal bloating, and constipation may be the result of bed rest and inactivity or, more commonly, of analgesic therapy.

Radiation of pain around the chest wall is commonly associated with severe muscle spasm. This may reflect sympathetic muscle contraction or, more rarely, a true radiculopathy due to nerve root compression. The back pain may radiate into the leg, usually to the iliopsoas band of the lateral thigh. Signs of ▶ 341 nerve root pressure occur infrequently because actual entrapment or compression of nerve roots occurs only rarely, even after fractures with significant deformity. This probably is related to the fact that nerve roots exit the vertebral column posteriorly, and the posterior elements of the spine are rarely affected with uncomplicated vertebral body compression fractures. A small proportion of patients with acute vertebral fractures, generally those with traumatic fractures, experience a compound fracture with displacement of fragments of the vertebral body (11). Posterior displacement of fragments, especially with fractures of the thoracic spine, may impinge on the spinal canal and cause unilateral or bilateral signs of cord compression. Prompt evaluation with MRI is indicated. This is a serious circumstance that may require surgical intervention, including posterior stabilization and anterior decompression of the fracture. Although such therapy may be considered aggressive for frail, elderly patients, the risk of permanent neurologic deficit is high with either operative or nonoperative management when signs of cord compression exist.

Except for patients whose fractures are complicated by nerve root or spinal cord compression, the symptoms associated with acute fracture begin to improve after a few days as the fracture begins to heal (12). Most often, symptoms resolve completely within 3 months following the fracture. The aims of management of an acute fracture are to relieve symptoms and to maximize long-term functional status.

Strict bed rest may be required for 2 to 7 days in patients with marked symptoms, although many patients are comfortable sitting or ambulating. More prolonged bed rest is to be strongly discouraged because of the rapid muscular deconditioning that occurs as well as the potential for compounding the osteoporosis by the added element of immobilization bone loss. Ambulation at the earliest possible time is advocated. Lying flat on the bed with the knees flexed is often the position of most comfort for patients with lumbar spine fractures. Those with mid-thoracic fractures frequently experience the most comfort while lying on their side with a pillow supporting their back. Assisting patients from the bed to sit in an adjacent chair can usually be accomplished without difficulty. Patients should draw their knees toward their chest and roll over onto their side. They can then be gently lifted into a sitting position on the bed and helped into a chair. A thoracolumbar corset may be helpful in stabilizing the patient's back and providing a sense of support and strength.

Sitting may be particularly uncomfortable for some patients with lumbar fractures, since intervertebral pressure is higher while sitting than it is with standing or recumbent positions. Sneezing, coughing, and the Valsalva maneuver may accentuate the pain. Assisting patients from recumbency to a standing position with support may need to be the first step in reambulation. Here, too, a lumbar support corset is often useful. Walking can then follow, initially with assistance and later with a walker or four-point cane. When muscle spasm magnifies pain, physical therapy modalities may be required. For severe spasms, ultrasound therapy, massage, or cooling of the muscles with ice packs may provide temporary relief. Transcutaneous electrical stimulation units are frequently used but rarely afford benefit at this stage.

Orthotic back supports are useful in some patients. Extension braces can be used to unload the thoracic spine in patients with recent fractures. These braces may be poorly tolerated by patients with scoliosis, severe kyphosis, or fractures of the lower lumbar spine. Molded body jackets can provide support for the lower thoracic and lumbar spine region, but these devices are bulky, heavy, and expensive. The brace or body jacket needs to be carefully fitted and adjusted by the therapist or orthotist to ensure proper stabilization and maximal comfort. If the support device is not effective in improving symptoms, its use should be discontinued. The best "back brace" is, of course, strong extensor musculature of the spine. An external brace is a temporizing measure to help patients with acute symptoms following a fracture. Use over an extended time may be counterproductive, limiting a patient's work on extensor muscle reconditioning. Except in situations of marked spinal instability, the use of a solid back support device for more than a few weeks is to be discouraged. Its use should be replaced with an appropriate back strengthening exercise program.

Lumbar support corsets or belts may be helpful during rehabilitation after a vertebral fracture. These devices are easy to use, and quite comfortable and provide a sense of support without causing significant disuse of lower back musculature. Lumbar supports with rigid stays are supplied by a therapist or orthotist. Our patients frequently use a simple, inexpensive lumbar belt obtained at a sporting goods store. The belt reminds them to attend to their posture and to work on muscle strengthening.

Muscle relaxants are generally ineffective at this stage. Therapy with analgesics is frequently prescribed but is usually only minimally helpful. Acetaminophen, salicylates, and nonsteroidal anti-inflammatory drugs may be given.

Codeine and other narcotics may be useful in individual patients and should be administered if pain is severe. Adequate fluid intake should be maintained and stool softeners given to all patients who require bed rest or are given narcotics, especially in the very elderly. If altered mental status occurs or if no symptomatic benefit is noted after treatment is begun, narcotic therapy should be decreased or discontinued.

Calcitonin has been recommended as an analgesic agent for patients with acute vertebral fractures. In the few controlled trials evaluating its use, patients receiving 50 to 100 units salmon calcitonin subcutaneously daily had somewhat more rapid improvement in symptoms than did those who received placebo (13,14). In clinical practice, some patients seem to respond dramatically to therapy whereas others experience no response. An empiric trial of 7 to 10 days of therapy may be warranted in patients whose back pain significantly limits their activity and is not responsive to standard measures.

▶ 343

Management of Chronic Symptoms

Following an acute vertebral fracture, many patients experience complete resolution of back symptoms despite persistence of the vertebral deformity. Other patients, however, continue to have chronic symptoms, primarily pain associated with activity, especially forward bending (15,16). It is difficult to know what proportion of patients with osteoporotic fractures are symptomatic. The symptoms these patients experience are nonspecific and similar to back discomfort seen in many older individuals who do not have evidence of osteoporotic fracture. It is estimated that as many as 50% of women over the age of 85 have chronic back discomfort (17). On the other hand, many women with vertebral fractures and obvious kyphosis do not experience significant back pain (18,19). In patients with vertebral fractures, Leidig and colleagues found that physical limitations and the intensity of pain were correlated with an index of spine deformity (20). Ross and his colleagues, reassessing the data of Ettinger with risk analysis, concluded that subjects with obvious, multiple vertebral fractures had an increased risk of back pain, disability, and other adverse outcomes (21).

The etiology of the chronic back pain is also not well understood and is probably multifactorial. Bone tenderness or pain is uncommon. Fortunately, nerve compressive syndromes are uncommon in patients with vertebral fractures. Facet joint arthropathy may be the chronic result of vertebral deformity. Concomitant degenerative disk disease may be a major contributor to symptoms in some patients. In our clinic, the most common cause of back discomfort is muscle dysfunction related to vertebral deformity. Most patients experience little or no pain when at rest, either lying in bed or sitting in a comfortable chair.

On attempting to rise from bed or a chair, acute pain in the lower back is experienced. The pain occurs over a wide area across the back and is not localized to a discrete area like the pain of an acute fracture. After a short time, the intensity of the pain diminishes. Walking is usually accomplished without difficulty. However, standing in one position for any length of time, particularly if coupled with forward bending such as over the stove, sink, or bed to perform regular household chores, precipitates recurrence of an ache and feeling of tightness across the lower back and often a burning, painful sensation between the shoulder blades. Unless the activity is curtailed, the intensity of the symptoms continues to increase. Ultimately, muscle spasm and severe pain occur. On sitting or lying down, the symptoms gradually subside over a few minutes. The individual can then resume the activities for another, shorter interval of time before symptoms recur.

Examination of these individuals usually demonstrates diminished musculature in the upper mid-back. Tightness and tenderness is frequently observed in the paravertebral muscles of the lower back and in the interscapular region. Muscle weakness in older women is a common phenomenon. Studies by Sinaki and others have demonstrated that women with osteoporosis have decreased extensor muscle strength in their back compared to age-matched controls (22). It is not clear whether this weakness is a characteristic of the patients with osteoporosis or the result of deconditioning of back muscles in patients who have decreased their activity following a vertebral fracture. This muscle weakness is a major factor in the back pain experienced by older osteoporotic patients. Decreased strength causes muscle fatigue and aching with only modest activity. Patients then curtail their activity to alleviate the backache, and the decreased activity accentuates the muscle weakness. Individuals who have had vertebral deformity may be particularly susceptible to the muscle dysfunction associated with regular daily activities. Pronounced kyphosis increases the work of extensor muscles of the mid-back and decreases ability to perform functions requiring forward bending. Thoracic fractures and kyphosis also cause a reciprocal accentuation of lumbar lordosis, resulting in increased work and decreased stamina of lower back extensor muscles.

Whether the pain is due primarily to muscle dysfunction, to facet joint arthropathy, or to degenerative disk disease, a program of extensor muscle strengthening and stretching can be of value. Most of the studies evaluating exercise therapy in patients with osteoporosis have focused on the trophic effects of exercise on bone (23-25). It is well recognized that mechanical unloading of the skeleton results in an acceleration of bone loss. Attempts to retard age-related bone loss or to augment bone mass with exercise have been evaluated in several settings. Even with intense exercise programs, the changes in vertebral bone density are at best modest and transient, being quickly lost when the exercise

Osteoporosis

program is curtailed (26). Therapy with calcium and antiresorptive drugs is much more effective for the preservation of bone mass than is exercise in older individuals.

The principal benefit from a program of exercise in any patient should be to increase muscle strength and endurance. Osteoporotic patients are usually eager to be physically active but are reluctant to engage in a program of exercise for fear of aggravating symptoms or experiencing a new fracture. Health care providers contribute to that anxiety by prescribing restricted activity. In individuals with muscle dysfunction, many exercises and activities evoke pain, which is interpreted as being harmful or destructive. For these reasons, the frequency and intensity of physical activity gradually diminishes in patients with back discomfort. This decreased activity results in progressive muscle weakness and increases susceptibility to muscle fatigue and pain with even less exertion. It is this vicious cycle of weakness contributing to pain that contributes to weakness that must be addressed in the symptomatic management of this group of patients. Explanation about the nature of the symptoms and the rationale for an exercise program are important for the patient's acceptance of the program.

▶ 345

In our program, patients with back discomfort are referred to an experienced physical therapist for the initiation of a comprehensive rehabilitative program. The therapist is an important and integral part of the team caring for patients with osteoporosis. In that capacity, the physical therapist has several roles.

1. Provide additional assessment of the patient's symptoms and their cause.
2. Use modalities such as ultrasound, heat, and massage for the transient relief of symptoms related to muscle tightness and spasm
3. Design a program of exercise based on the nature and location of the patient's symptoms, the location of the vertebral fractures, and the patient's history of exercise and daily activity. The intensity of the exercise program may be varied according to the severity of osteoporosis as determined by bone densitometry.
4. Instruct the patient to perform the exercises correctly and safely with the goal of discharging the patient to a home exercise program, which is used daily.
5. Monitor the symptomatic response of such therapy.
6. Participate in educating the patient about osteoporosis and approaches to its symptomatic management.

Local measures such as massage or the application of heat or ultrasound may provide transient relief of muscle tightness and pain. A heating pad or other devices with chemical heat may be helpful. These can be used even before the patient gets out of bed in the morning or when episodes of symptoms occur during the day. Following such treatment, extensor muscle stretching exercises to retrain those muscle groups and to minimize the recurrence of muscle tightness and spasm are used. Strengthening exercises are not begun until the intensity of the muscle tightness has diminished. Beginning strengthening exercises while muscle tightness exists only exacerbates the tendency for muscle spasm.

We use exercises aimed at the extensor muscles of the upper, middle, and lower back, similar to a program described by Dr. Sinaki and her colleagues (27). Flexion exercises, particularly those involving flexion of the mid-thoracic spine, should be avoided. Such exercises increase the mechanical strain on the anterior portion of the vertebral body and increase the occurrence of fractures in patients with severe skeletal fragility. We use simple resistance devices such as the Theraband as an aid to strengthening the upper back and shoulders. Isometric strengthening of the abdominal muscles, pectoral stretching, and strengthening of the muscles of respiration are also objectives of the exercise program, especially in patients with pronounced kyphosis. Examples and illustrations of these exercises are available in the paper by Dr. Sinaki or in publications from the National Osteoporosis Foundation (28).

The effects of muscle strengthening programs and rehabilitative programs in patients with osteoporosis have only just begun to be evaluated. Experience with rehabilitation of other elderly individuals provides encouragement for such an approach. The effectiveness of exercise in improving muscle strength is as good in older women as it is in younger women (29). Furthermore, the intensity of the exercise program does not need to be marked. It is encouraging to note that the gains in muscle strength and endurance achieved with an exercise program can be maintained by short sessions of exercise two to three times each week (30).

Another advantage of a rehabilitation program is that it engages the patient directly in the therapeutic process. Patients with osteoporosis are, as a group, a highly motivated set of individuals who are eager to be active participants in a program of improvement. The combination of education regarding the role and importance of exercise coupled with individualized instruction so that their fears of performing exercises incorrectly are allayed are important aspects of this rehabilitation program. It is also important to involve other family members in this process. Very often, other members of the family are overly protective of patients with chronic debilitating illnesses and resist efforts of these patients to care for themselves. Explanation of the rationale and importance of maintaining physical activity should be directed at both the patients and their families.

Our exercise program is provided in one of several settings. Most patients see a physical therapist for four to six visits in the outpatient rehabilitation department. At the end of that experience, patients are able to perform their exercises at home on a regular and consistent basis. Assessment of their progress is made at regular intervals. Patients who are too infirm or handicapped to come to the outpatient department are seen initially by the physical therapist from the home health department. Instruction in exercise, the application of ultrasound, heat, and massage and instructions in activities, such as transferring from the bed to the chair, can be given at home. In addition, a group exercise program for women with osteoporosis has been established. These groups meet twice each week for one hour of supervised instruction. Having a designated appointment time for the exercise program improves compliance and consistency of the exercise regimen. Performing the exercise under the guidance and in the presence of the physical therapist provides added confidence and assurance for those individuals afraid of further injury. Finally, the socialization of the group setting is of substantial value to these individuals.

▶ 347

In addition to the exercise program focused on the back, a program of general exercise and rehabilitation is appropriate. Many individuals are initially unable to walk or to be involved in significant aerobic activities because of their back discomfort. Once their back pain has diminished, a program of walking can be more easily instituted. The benefits of this program include improved cardiovascular function and decreased back pain, increased stamina, an improved sense of well-being and decreased risk of falling or injury (31).

Injury Prevention

Osteoporotic fractures usually occur as a result of an injury in a patient with skeletal frailty. Fractures of the spine may occur spontaneously but most often are associated with injuries involving lifting, especially if associated with a bent or twisted position, but may also occur while turning over in bed or after a cough or a fall. Falls are the most frequent cause of fractures of the femoral neck and wrist. The incidence of hip fracture increases exponentially with aging, whereas the rate of bone loss decreases linearly with aging. One interpretation of these data is that progressive bone loss is associated with a geometrically increasing degree of fragility. Alternatively, these data suggest that the factors associated with aging contribute to the risk of hip fracture over and above the bone loss that occurs. It is well accepted that falls are an important risk factor for osteoporotic fracture. Some studies have suggested that fall frequency and the inability to protect oneself from falls is of greater importance in determining the likelihood of hip fractures than is bone loss. More recent prospective studies, however, document that osteoporosis is a risk factor for fractures independent of injury (32). The most appropriate model of the pathogenesis of fractures is that an increasing gradient of risk of fracture is associated with decreasing bone mass. In patients at risk for fracture (ie, with osteoporosis), injuries and falls are more likely to result in fracture. Reversing the osteoporotic process is not possible currently. In individuals who have already experienced bone loss, a major focus of management should be the prevention of injuries leading to fractures.

Several studies have evaluated the many factors associated with increased risk of falling (33-35). Factors pertaining to the health and vigor of the individual and to his or her environment or activities are recognized to correlate with fracture frequency. Falls most commonly occur in individuals with several risk factors. Age, cognitive impairment, and diminished sensory input including decreased vision, hearing, and proprioception are associated with an increased likelihood of falls. Medications, especially sedative and antidepressant drugs, predispose to falling (36). Excessive alcohol intake is related to fall frequency in younger individuals, but this has not been documented in older subjects. Impaired balance, vertigo, postural hypotension, nocturia, and muscle weakness are associated with increased fall frequency (37). Other debilitating illnesses such as arthritis, foot disease, neuropathy, Parkinson's disease, and heart disease increase the likelihood of falls, perhaps related to the deconditioning associated with chronic illness as well as other factors. Although sophisticated tests of gait and balance are available in many medical centers, simple tests such as the ability to stand from a chair and tandem walking can identify persons frail or unsteady enough to be at high risk for falling. Of importance, however, is the observation that even healthy, active older adults fall frequently. In a study of elderly persons living in the community, 17% of vigorous subjects fell at least once during the year of evaluation (38). Thus, attention to injury prevention should be a part of the management of all persons with osteoporosis, not just the very frail.

The environment may also influence the likelihood of fracture. Most injuries and falls occur in the home in the course of regular daily activities. Only a very small proportion of injuries are associated with particularly hazardous activity such as falling from a stool or ladder. Ten percent to 15% of falls occur while ascending or especially descending stairs. Tripping over loose carpet, wires, or furniture, and slipping on icy sidewalks or in the bathtub are described by patients as frequent contributors to falls. Wearing unsteady shoes with high heels increases the possibility of loosing balance. Environmental causes of falls may be more important for those patients with modest functional impairment than severely handicapped persons. The extremely frail patients, who ambulate infrequently and who are unable to climb stairs, do not often expose themselves to environmental hazards.

Feeble older adults are able to protect themselves less well when they fall. Despite this, the frequency with which falls are associated with significant injury is higher in younger, healthier, more mobile adults. Serious injury occurred in 33% of falls in vigorous older adults but in only 6% of falls in frail, even older subjects (38). Perhaps the force of the fall is diminished in older in-

348 ◀

dividuals who walk very slowly and, as a consequence, fall more gently. The lack of cushion in both the patient and in the surface on which the fall occurs has been implicated as factors related to the risk of injury from a fall.

From our understanding of the importance of injuries in causing fractures and our ability to identify the factors that predispose to falls and injuries, recommendations to prevent injuries and fractures have been proposed (39). Unfortunately, little data exist evaluating the usefulness of these approaches, some of which vary substantially. Many physicians advocate reducing physical activity, thereby minimizing the likelihood of serious falls or injuries. Although this may be advantageous in the short run, such an approach will ultimately be detrimental by contributing to further weakness, deconditioning, frailty, and isolation. Many experts recommend programs of generalized exercise such as walking, doing so with the knowledge that such activities might actually increase the frequency of falls and injuries. Increased strength and aerobic capacity and improved measures of balance have also been demonstrated in individuals who are engaged in regular exercise, resulting in improved stability and decreased falling.

▶ 349

Gait training, exercises specifically designed to promote balance, and the use of walking aids can be taught or arranged by the physical therapist. Reducing hazards in the home requires education of the patient and help from the family or health care professionals (40). Provision of adequate lighting, removing hazards for tripping and installing handrails on stairs and in the bathtub may lessen the opportunity for injury. Instruction in practical body mechanics including proper techniques for lifting, transferring out of bed, and accomplishing household chores is appropriate.

No program of fall prevention will be completely successful. Protecting frail patients from the effects of a fall is a strategy of management just now being evaluated (41). Wearing hip pads markedly reduced the incidence of hip fractures in nursing home residents.

There is great interest in this area of geriatric management and research. The determination of whether such a rehabilitation approach is of benefit in reducing the risk of fractures awaits the results of carefully planned prospective studies (42). The design of a program to prevent injuries must carefully balance the value of increasing activity to promote strength and endurance with the potential risk for injury that increased activity might cause. Severe restriction of activity results in muscular deconditioning. A carefully designed rehabilitation program should strive to promote muscle conditioning, increase the capacity for independent living, and enhance self-esteem. At the same time, the program may decrease the depression and frustration arising from their symptoms and functional impairment and reduce the anxiety associated with the fear of future disability. The coordinated efforts of the physical therapist with the other members of the management team are necessary to attain these objectives.

The effect of a comprehensive rehabilitative program on the psychological aspect of a patient's illness is another outcome that cannot be overemphasized. The exercise program for some becomes a focus which, in the least, serves as a distraction from their chronic illness and symptoms.

Psychosocial Function

Osteoporosis is one of several diseases limiting mobility and function that are associated with chronic pain. Responses of patients to these complications vary widely. Some patients cope with their illness and disabilities surprisingly well. They seem little affected and continue their activities, albeit in a relatively limited fashion, with acceptance and without complaint. Other patients, especially those with multiple vertebral fractures and many patients following hip fracture, experience a significant change in their physical activity and mental outlook. Either because of the physical limitations or because of a fear of falling and injury, activities outside the home are frequently curtailed. This results in an increasing isolation from family, friends, and social groups. Women with vertebral fractures exhibit more depression and anxiety than do healthy individuals of the same age. Osteoporosis, as a degenerative disease, is viewed as clear evidence of deterioration and aging. The image of physically shrinking and becoming stooped and deformed is a disturbing factor to many patients. Other frequent concerns include worry about loss of mobility, embarrassment because of dependence on others for assistance, transportation and household chores, and fear of recurrent injury, pain and progressive deformity. These concerns are magnified when patients are told that osteoporosis is simply a consequence of growing old and that nothing can be done for it.

These psychosocial effects of the illness can be addressed by several members of the health care team including the nursing staff, social workers, counselors, and physical therapists. The physician, however, must acknowledge and respond to these concerns of the patients. The simple act of recognizing and validating the patient's worries is often helpful. This process is particularly valuable when there is repetitive, consistent attention to the patient's concerns by each of several members of the health care team. Simple encouragement and empathy evoke positive and calmed responses. The experience of one multidisciplinary approach to management documents the improved psychosocial function of older patients with osteoporosis (44).

Education about osteoporosis, the nature of the symptoms and complications and the approaches to management will improve a patient's understanding of this clinical problem. This often results in decreased anxiety about the illness, in less depression and in better coping with chronic problems (45,46).

Patients and their families must be engaged in the process of rehabilitation (47). Goals of function and activity, realistic but challenging, should be set for the patient to work toward. Meeting other patients who have experienced and overcome similar problems is especially encouraging. In our program, this process is enhanced by the availability of a group exercise class and a support group. In these groups, patients become encouraged to help themselves.

Summary

Osteoporosis is a heterogeneous, multifactorial disorder characterized by dete- ▶351 rioration of skeletal integrity and function, especially in older individuals. In some patients the effects of osteoporosis are the most significant factors contributing to physical and psychological decline. Recent insights into the natural history of postmenopausal and age-related bone loss, coupled with the use of estrogen and other antiresorptive drugs, offer the promise of preventing osteoporosis and its complications. However, for many patients already afflicted with osteoporosis, management strategies to minimize discomfort, to enhance their level of activity and function, and to decrease the risk of further skeletal injury need to be used. With the combination of pharmacologic therapy, rehabilitation and exercise therapy, and appropriate attention to the psychologic aspects of this illness, improvements in the quality of life of these patients can be accomplished. This goal is likely best accomplished when the combined efforts of a health care team, including nurses, physical therapists, and counselors as well as the physicians, are brought to bear on the patients' problems and when both the patients and their families and support systems are actively involved in the process.

As our population continues to age, the management of symptomatic osteoporosis and other chronic debilitating diseases is becoming an increasing challenge. One of the most important and exciting tasks of clinicians caring for patients with osteoporosis will be to refine our strategies for nonpharmacologic management and to document the functional effects and outcomes of these approaches.

References

1. Robin GC, Span Y, Steinberg R, Menczel J. Scoliosis in the elderly, a follow-up study. Spine 1982;355–359.

2. Milne JS, Williamson J. A longitudinal study of kyphosis in older people. Age Ageing 1983;12:225–233.

3. Griffiths HE, Jones DM. Pyogenic infection of the spine: a review of twenty-

eight cases. J Bone Joint Surg [Br] 1971;53: 383–391.

4. Eastell R, Yergey AL, Vieira NE, Cedel SL, Kumar R, Riggs BL. Interrelationship among vitamin D metabolism, true calcium absorption, parathyroid function, and age in women: evidence of an age-related intestinal resistance to 1.25-dihydroxyvitamin D action. J Bone Miner Res 1991;6:125–132.

5. Chapuy MC, Arlot ME, Duboeuf F, et al. Vitamin D_3 and calcium to prevent hip fractures in elderly women. N Engl J Med 1992;327:1637–1642.

6. Fuss M, Pepersak T, VanGeel J, et al. Involvement of low-calcium diet in the reduced bone mineral content of idiopathic renal stone formers. Calcif Tissue Int 1990;46:9–13.

7. Cooper C, Atkinson EJ, O'Fallon WM, Melton LJ III. Incidence of clinically diagnosed vertebral fractures: a population-based study in Rochester, Minnesota, 1985–1989. J Bone Miner Res 1992;7:221–227.

8. Finsen V. Osteoporosis and back pain among the elderly. Acta Med Scand 1988;223:443–449.

9. Symmons DPM, Van Hemert AM, Vandenbroucke JP, Valkenberg HA. A longitudinal study of back pain and radiological changes in the lumbar spines of middle aged women. II. Radiographic findings. Ann Rheum Dis 1991;50:162–166.

10. Patel U, Skingle S, Campbell GA, Crisp AJ, Boyle IT. Clinical profile of acute vertebral compression fractures in osteoporosis. Br J Rheum 1991;30:418–421.

11. Kaplan PA, Orton DF, Asleson RJ. Osteoporosis with vertebral compression fractures, retropulsed fragments, and neurologic compromise. Radiology 1987;165:533–535.

12. Hazel WA, Jones RA, Morrey BF, Stauffer RN. Vertebral fractures without neurological deficit. A long-term follow-up study. J Bone Joint Surg [Am] 1988;70-A:1319–1321.

13. Levernieux J, Julien D, Caulin F. The effect of calcitonin on bone pain and acute resorption related to recent osteoporotic crush fractures: result of a double blind and an open study. In: Cecchetin M, Segre G, eds. Calciotropic hormones and calcium metabolism. Amsterdam: Elsevier BV, 1986:171–178.

14. Paul KK, Chan LWL. Analgesic effect of intranasal salmon calcitonin in the treatment of osteoporosis vertebral fractures. Clin Ther 1989;11:205–209.

15. Lyritas GP, Mayasis B, Tsakalakos N, et al. The natural history of the osteoporotic vertebral fracture. Clin Rheumatol 1989;8(suppl 2):66–69.

16. Young MH. Long-term consequences of stable fractures of the thoracic and lumbar vertebral bodies. J Bone Joint Surg [Br] 1973;55B-2:295–300.

17. Kanis JA, Pitt FA. Epidemiology of osteoporosis. Bone 1992;13:S7–S15.

18. Zetterberg C, Mannius S, Mellstrom D, Rundgren A, Astrand K. Osteoporosis and back pain in the elderly. A controlled epidemiologic and radiographic study. Spine 1990;15:783–786.

19. Ettinger B, Block JE, Smith R, Cummings RS, Harris ST, Genant HK. An examination of the association between vertebral deformities, physical disabilities and psychosocial problems. Maturitas 1988;10:283–296.

20. Leidig G, Minne HW, Sauer P, et al. A study of complaints and their relation to vertebral destruction in patients with osteoporosis. Bone Miner 1990;8:217–219.

21. Ross PD, Ettinger B, Davis JW, Melton LJ, Wasnich RD. Evaluation of adverse health outcomes associated with vertebral fractures. Osteoporosis Int 1991;1:134–140.

22. Sinaki M, McPhee MC, Hodgson SF, Merritt JM, Offord KP. Relationship between both mineral density of spine and strength of back extensors in healthy postmenopausal women. Mayo Clin Proc 1986;61:116–122.

23. Krølner B, Toft B, Nielsen SP, et al. Physical exercise as prophylaxis against involutional vertebral bone loss: a controlled trial. Clin Sci 1983;64:541–546.

24. Snow-Harter C, Marcus R. Exercise, bone mineral density, and osteoporosis. Exerc Sport Sci Rev 1991;19:351–388.

25. Forwood MR, Burr DB. Physical activity and bone mass: exercises in futility? Bone Miner 1993;21:89–112.

26. Dalsky GP, Stocke KS, Ehsani AA, Slatopolsky E, Lee WC, Birge SJ Jr. Weight bearing exercise training and lumbar bone mineral content in postmenopausal women. Ann Intern Med 1988;108:824–828.

27. Sinaki M, Mikkelsen BA. Postmenopausal spinal osteoporosis: flexion versus extension exercises. Arch Phys Med Rehabil 1984;65:593–596.

28. Boning up on osteoporosis: a guide to prevention and treatment. New York: National Osteoporosis Foundation, 1991.

29. Fiaterone M, Marks E, et al. High-intensity strength training in nonagenarians: effects on skeletal muscle. JAMA 1990;263:3029–3034.

30. Tucci JT, Carpenter DM, Pollock ML, Graves JE, Leggett SH. Effect of reduced frequency of training and detraining on lumbar extension strength. Spine 1992;17:1497–1501.

31. Harrison JE, Chow R, Dornan J, Goodwin S, Strauss A, and the Bone and Mineral Group of the University of Toronto. Evaluation of a program for rehabilitation of osteoporotic patients (PRO): 4-year follow-up. Osteoporosis Int 1993;3: 13–17.

32. Cummings SR, Black DM, Nevitt MC, et al. Bone density at various sites for prediction of hip fractures. Lancet 1993;341: 72–75.

33. Melton LJ, Riggs BL. Risk factors for injury after a fall. Clin Geriatr Med 1985;1:525–539.

34. Tinetti ME, Speechley M, Ginter SF. Risk factors for falls among elderly persons living in the community. N. Engl J Med 1988;319:1701–1707.

35. Grisso JA, Kelsey JL, Strom BL, et al. Risk factors for falls as a cause of hip fractures in women. N Engl J Med 1991; 324:1326–1331.

36. Ray WA, Griffin MR, Schaffner W, Baugh DK, Melton LJ. Psychotropic drug use and the risk of hip fracture. N Engl J Med 1987;316:363–369.

37. Stewart RB, Moore MT, May FE, Marks RG, Hale WE. Nocturia: a risk factor for falls in the elderly. J Am Geriat Soc 1992;40:1217–1220.

38. Speechley M, Tinetti M. Falls and injuries in frail and vigorous community elderly persons. J Am Geriat Soc 1991;39: 46–52.

39. Tinetti ME, Speechley M. Prevention of falls among the elderly. N Engl J Med 1989;320:1055–1059.

40. Tideiksaar R. Preventing falls: home hazard checklists to help older patients protect themselves. Geriatrics 1986;41:26–28.

41. Lauritzen JB, Petersen MM, Lund B. Effect of external hip protectors on hip fracture. Lancet 1993;341:11–13.

42. Hornbrook MC, Stevens VJ, Wingfield DJ. Seniors' program for injury control and education. J Am Geriat Soc 1993;41:309–314.

43. Silverman SL. The clinical consequences of vertebral compression fracture. Bone 1992;13:S27–S31.

44. Gold DT, Stegmaier BS, Bales CW, Lyles KW, Westlund RE, Drezner MK. Psychosocial functioning and osteoporosis in late life: results of a multidisciplinary intervention. J Women's Health 1993;2: 149–155.

45. Gold DT, Bales CW, Lyles KW, Drezner MK. Treatment of osteoporosis: the psychologic impact of a medical education program on older patients. J Am Geriatr Soc 1989;37:417–422.

46. Gold DT, Lyles KW, Bales CW, Drezner MK. Teaching patients coping behaviors: an essential part of successful management of osteoporosis. J Bone Miner Res 1989;4:799–801.

47. Giloth BE. Promoting patient involvement: educational, organizational, and environmental strategies. Patient Education and Counseling 1990;15:29–38.

13 ▸ In Vivo Animal Models
in Osteoporosis Research

▶ ▶ ▶ Donald B. Kimmel

This chapter establishes criteria for evaluating animal models of osteoporosis and then applies them within today's knowledge framework. The criteria are based on (1) knowledge about human osteoporosis, (2) basic facts about human and animal skeletons, and (3) experiments that use the same agent in different species. Both the criteria and the evaluation should be able to evolve with time as data about osteoporosis and each animal model accumulates.

Food and Drug Administration Recommendations for Animal Models of Osteoporosis

The Food and Drug Administration (FDA) has established guidelines for using animals in preclinical testing of agents intended to treat osteoporosis (1). These guidelines recommend the use of animals that are either losing bone or that have become osteopenic following ovariectomy, because of the firm linkage of osteoporosis to estrogen depletion. They require data from both the rat and a larger species after oophorectomy. Studies of all species must be of at least 16 months' duration, ostensibly equivalent to 4 years of human treatment, and include histologic evaluation. The guidelines also suggest measuring bone density, biochemical markers of bone turnover, and bone strength by biomechanical testing, the last as a surrogate for the propensity to develop fragility fractures.

A Perspective on In Vivo Animal Experimentation

In vivo animal models are often overused in osteoporosis research. This may signal nothing more than an imbalance in the numbers of clinical and bench investigators. However, it may also mark the existence of misconceptions about efficient experimentation. In vivo adult human experimentation is desirable because its results require minimal extrapolation to predict the outcome in adult individuals. Huge epidemiologic data bases with information about human osteoporosis should be frequently and thoroughly tapped (2,3), and opportunities to add information to those data bases should always be sought. When agents already approved for human use have a sound basis for efficacy in *new* clinical situations, a thorough and unbiased examination of existing human data and a phase I human trial, *not* an animal experiment, are likely to be the next logical steps. Investigators should heed the short adage, "When possible, do it in humans," more often.

▶ 355

However, when experimental designs or new agents that pose overt toxicity risks or threaten subtle longer term adverse effects are to be evaluated, in vivo animal experimentation is the only choice. When animal experimentation must be used and convenient in vivo animal models accurately reproduce human data and offer significant time savings, they are the best solution. The lack of such a strategy, including proper use of animal models in the late 1970s, might have played a role in the unfavorable impression left by a recent multicenter osteoporosis treatment trial (4,5). That outcome played a pivotal role in the FDA's requirement that investigators of future osteoporosis treatment agents demonstrate both bone mass increases and antifracture efficacy in clinical trials.

Criteria for Animal Models in Osteoporosis: A Time for Compromise

Expecting full parallelism of human symptoms with in vivo animal models is unrealistic. The criteria below are intended to be flexible, occasionally creatively applied, and able to evolve as new evidence or new needs appear. They place a higher value on animal models that match the clinically apparent behavior of osteoporosis, than on providing a complete match of detailed mechanisms.

It is in the best interests of all bone researchers to participate in the refinement of these criteria. Clinical investigators can facilitate the development of in vivo animal models by ranking the importance of various clinical characteristics of osteoporosis. In vivo animal investigators should be quick to do experiments that show how their models may better fit human symptoms. The recent history of the ovariectomized rat model is a textbook example of bench scientists doing experiments to validate a highly relevant preclinical in vivo animal model (6–9). The effort to develop tests of bone fragility in small animals is another example that is currently evolving (10,11).

In vivo animal scientists can also develop better animal models by confining themselves to using relevant, easily applicable physiologic conditions to create consistent symptoms. For example, when the goal is to characterize better an *adult* disease process, choosing a growing animal with more active metabolic processes, simply to see a condition develop quickly, makes little sense. Doing nerve resection to study disuse (12,13) may really model only the motionless, *denervated* limb, not the motionless limb. Combining extreme calcium deprivation with estrogen depletion to accelerate (or even just to permit) bone loss, may create a confused physiologic environment that bears little resemblance to the clinical picture (14). For osteoporosis research, a consistent, incomplete set of symptoms produced by relevant methods in an adult animal model is more acceptable than using nonphysiologic circumstances to develop a full set of symptoms. A model that gives sporadic results in the hands of numerous competent investigators or requires convoluted manipulations that are not widely practiced is not likely to become widely accepted.

Unlike a decade ago, with today's current knowledge of animal models and osteoporosis, using an irrelevant animal model in osteoporosis research is inexcusable and wasteful. Using a costly, relevant model is necessary when unique features are under study. Decisions should continually be reviewed to improve the mix of cost and relevance. Imposing nonphysiologic conditions to create desired symptoms is frequently not necessary and always decreases the model's relevance.

The Criteria

Application of in vivo animal models for the skeleton has been reviewed elsewhere in several excellent articles (15–17). This chapter not only emphasizes many of their important points, but also widens the perspective by encompassing other animal models. Its approach is to match outward symptoms and tissue behaviors, rather than to ensure identical cellular mechanisms.

EXISTENCE OF GROWTH AND ADULT PHASES

An in vivo animal model of osteoporosis should exhibit both growing and adult skeletal phases of significant duration. This requirement stems from the importance of peak bone mass in the development of osteoporosis (18). Peak bone mass is a concept that has received too little attention, because of the long-term nature of studying it (19,20) (see Chapter 4). Bone mass measurement at menopause is the best predictor of future fracture in healthy persons (21–23). That value approximates peak bone mass because bone mass changes before menopause are minor (24–28).

Osteoporosis

Growth processes, principally bone modeling, and its modifiers like nutrition and physical activity (20,29), determine peak bone mass. Adult phase skeletal processes (predominantly bone remodeling, but some bone modeling to effect shape changes in response to changing physical activity patterns) determine bone mass trends after attainment of peak bone mass (30). The best animal models of osteoporosis would have both growth and adult phases in lengths that allow both accuracy and time frame compression.

MENSTRUAL/ESTRUS CYCLICITY

Human beings not only have a menarche and regular, frequent ovulatory cycles, but also experience bone loss at cessation of menses. The linkage of these two facts on the surface seems weak, but a strong hint of its importance is the low bone mass that exists in amenorrheic individuals (32–38) and the bone accumulation that occurs on resumption of normal menses (38,39). Mammals that have regular, frequent ovulatory cycles with high peaks of estradiol may be the only ones that suffer estrogen-depletion bone loss. Some hold that regularly cycling female mammals accumulate an estrogen-related component of bone that is integrated into the skeleton (40,41) and lost summarily at menopause, as if estrogen regulates bone mass (31). It would then follow that animals with infrequent cycles and low estradiol peaks might develop only a small estrogen-related bone compartment and show little estrogen-depletion bone loss.

NATURAL MENOPAUSE

Most women experience a natural menopause that occurs over a 2- to 7-year period (42); about 25% to 30% of women experience surgical menopause (43). Most animal skeletal models of estrogen depletion invoke surgical or medical oophorectomy (6,44,45). No meaningful differences in bone behavior between surgical and natural menopause are known (46,47). Animals with a natural menopause with hormone changes like human beings might be the best models for human osteoporosis. For instance, the gradual cessation of estrogen peaks and increasing intermittency over a long period may elicit a different bone adaptive response than the precipitous removal of ovaries without estrogen replacement.

BONE LOSS AND RISE IN TURNOVER RATE
AFTER ESTROGEN DEPLETION

Following estrogen depletion, bone loss accelerates (48–51) for a time in multiple sites (52), then decelerates and enters a semiplateau phase (53,54). These changes are most pronounced in cancellous regions and at endocortical surfaces

(55,56). Estrogen status plays a much more important role in determining bone quantity in the aged skeleton than does age itself (57–59). Estrogen-depletion changes in intracortical (Haversian) remodeling are poorly documented. This cancellous and endocortical bone loss is accompanied by an increase in bone turnover (60,61) and a marked, though transiently negative calcium balance (62). Histomorphometric changes of increased turnover across menopause are readily demonstrable within individuals (63). These behaviors should be easily demonstrable in an accurate animal model of postmenopausal osteoporosis. It is even reasonable to think that the same measuring techniques applied in human beings to define these end points might work for animals.

358 ◄

SKELETAL RESPONSE TO ESTROGEN REPLACEMENT

Oophorectomized or menopausal women given prompt estrogen replacement experience a smaller rise in turnover (60,64), less bone loss (65–67), and fewer fractures (65,68–70) than those who do not receive estrogen replacement (71). This response is demonstrated well by histomorphometric techniques (64) and is so stereotyped in adult women that one should expect an accurate ovariecto-mized animal model to experience an identical response to estrogen replacement.

DEVELOPMENT OF OSTEOPOROTIC FRACTURES AND STEADY-STATE OSTEOPENIA

Osteoporosis is marked by the development of low-trauma fractures of the spine and hip (72–74). An accurate animal model should develop fragility fractures.

Women with osteoporotic fractures tend to be osteopenic (75–77). Current goals for conservative or aggressive treatment, respectively, are to stabilize patients at their current bone mass or substantially increase that bone mass. An accurate animal model should develop convincing estrogen depletion osteopenia in a time that gives considerable time frame compression when compared to the human being.

BONE LOSS AND DECREASED FORMATION AFTER DECREASED MECHANICAL USAGE

Older individuals lose cancellous and cortical bone and experience declines in bone formation unrelated to estrogen depletion (78,79). These changes come during a life phase when general declines in physical activity also occur. Extreme physical inactivity, as during bed rest or paraplegia, causes marked bone loss (80–82). This bone behavior should also be easily demonstrable in an accurate animal model of osteoporosis.

Cancellous: Adult men and women have cancellous bone remodeling, the in situ removal and replacement of aged cancellous bone tissue (30). This process is expressed at endocortical surfaces as tunneling initiated from marrow cavities (56). An accurate animal model would display such activity in its skeleton.

Cortical: Adult individuals have Haversian or intracortical bone remodeling, the process of in situ removal and replacement of aged cortical bone tissue (30). Although this process does not seem to be strongly affected by estrogen depletion and postmenopausal osteoporosis is usually characterized by only minimal cortical porosity, an accurate animal model should display Haversian remodeling.

    ▶ 359

Cortical bone plays a dominant role in determining skeletal strength. The main reason for an animal model to have Haversian remodeling is to be able to prove that agents with favorable effects at cancellous and endocortical surfaces cause no deleterious effects on Haversian remodeling. Accelerating Haversian remodeling might lower cortical strength by creating additional porosity as it enlarges the remodeling space. Slowing Haversian remodeling might lower cortical strength by allowing fatigue damage to accumulate.

TIME FRAME COMPRESSION

In adult, estrogen-depleted women, the phase of accelerated estrogen-depletion bone loss lasts 5 to 8 years. The time from attainment of peak bone mass until the development of fragility fractures is 30 or more years. An effective animal model known to experience peak bone mass followed by postovariectomy bone loss should compress those times by an order of magnitude or more.

CONVENIENCE

Convenience for animal models is denominated as animal cost, availability, housing requirements, and handling difficulties, and the necessity for designing, implementing, or validating new analytical procedures. Using an animal model with the highest degree of accuracy can be so inconvenient that it is not worthwhile. It may occasionally be worse than doing a human study. For example, if an intervention requires active subject cooperation, animals may not be capable of that cooperation. On the other hand, in animal experiments, recruitment and compliance, both nagging problems in clinical research, are not issues.

Animals that seem convenient to some investigators because they possess specialized facilities and expertise, are not the best choice for others lacking those tools. In today's scientific environment, investigators tempted to maintain familiar techniques that have become outdated often impede their own progress in the name of convenience. New enterprises, with the opportunity to freshly allocate resources, enjoy the advantages and burdens of the chance to define their own level of convenience. However one views it, the worst scenario is to have wasted scarce resources on an irrelevant model in the name of convenience.

Animal Models for Human Osteoporosis

Animals that should receive initial consideration in osteoporosis research are bird, mouse, rat, dog, pig, sheep, and nonhuman primate species. Because the above criteria are directed at clinical symptoms and outcomes in human beings, the animal models will generally be evaluated on their ability to duplicate those outcomes. Dissimilarities from the human condition in detailed mechanisms of development of one or more of the conditions may well exist. The fit of each animal model to the criteria above is summarized in Table 13-1.

Bird

Birds have growing and adult skeletal phases. Certain adult female birds have daily egg-laying cycles that correspond to the alternating deposition and resorption of medullary bone during cyclic oviposition and egg calcification (83). The bone accumulation phase occurs with a rising serum estradiol level. Estradiol treatment of male birds also causes medullary bone accumulation (84).

The bird skeleton experiences localized bone loss during immobilization and increased bone mass during applied mechanical loads (85–87). Although avian models of decreased and increased loading have broken new ground in understanding bone responses to the mechanical environment, they are not models for studying the estrogen/fracture-centered disease of osteoporosis. Furthermore, current data, mostly observational in nature, suggest that birds normally have little cancellous or Haversian remodeling.

The interesting bone response to estrogen in birds provides many opportunities for experiments that bear on bone biology (88), but the estrogen-related bone buildup suggests a fundamental dissimilarity to adult mammalian physiology. It can be loosely inferred that hypoestrogenemia in birds is associated with medullary bone *loss,* just as estrogen depletion in mammals is associated with bone loss, but the course of bone mass following oophorectomy, an event more relevant to osteoporosis and osteopenia, is not known in birds. The estrogen-related bone accumulation may actually be important in pubertal hu-

TABLE 13-1   Summary of In Vivo Animal Models for Osteoporosis

Attribute	Human	Bird	Mouse	Rat	Dog	Pig	Sheep	Primate
Growth and Adult Phases?	Yes	±Yes	±Yes	±Yes	Yes	Yes	Yes	Yes (Late)
Menstrual/Estrus Cyclicity	28 d	Daily	Inducible	4–5 d	205 d	21 d	21 d seasonal	21–28d
Natural Menopause	Yes	No	No	±Yes	No	?	?	Yes
Bone Loss after Estrogen Depletion	Yes	?	Probably	Yes	Not consistent	Weak	Weak	Yes
Response to Estrogen	Turnover↓	Formation↑	Formation↑	Turnover↓	Not consistent	?	?	Turnover↓
Development of Osteoporotic Fractures	Yes	No	No	No	No	?	?	No
Cancellous Remodeling	Yes	No	No	Some	Yes	Yes	Yes	Yes
Haversian Remodeling	Present (study site difficult)	No	No	Low levels; inducible	Yes	Yes	Yes	Present (study site difficult)
Time Frame Compression	No	?	Yes	Yes	No	Some	Some	Some
Convenience	±Yes	Yes	Yes	Yes	Weak	Poor	Poor	±No
Drug Dose Range like Humans?	Yes	?	No	No (1/100)	Close	?	?	Yes
Cost Effectiveness	Yes	No	Yes	Yes	Weak	?	?	?

▶ 361

In Vivo Animal Models in Osteoporosis Research

mans (40–41,89–90), but seems likely to hinder the proper interpretation of experiments about osteoporosis, an adult disease.

Birds are an example of a model that is convenient with low cost, but largely irrelevant for osteoporosis research because their skeletal behavior does not mimic features commonly associated with adult human osteoporosis.

Mouse

Past success with mice in skeletal research has been encouraging. The mouse has been very useful for studies of osteoporosis and osteoclast ontogeny (91–95). Lately, the mouse has become even more popular for the ease with which its genome can be manipulated (96). It is logical that the mouse be considered as an animal model of osteoporosis.

However, data that would validate the mouse as an in vivo model for osteoporosis research are in short supply. The few existing studies suggest that cancellous (97–98), but not cortical (99) bone loss occurs soon after ovariectomy. Estrogen-depletion bone loss appears to be prevented by estrogen replacement (97). Ectopic bone ossicles are preserved in male mice by estradiol treatment, due to combined increased formation and decreased resorption (100). Mice experience cancellous and cortical bone loss in the vertebrae (101–102) and femur (103) during the second year of life. However, increased bone formation with deposition of new woven bone after estrogen administration, as in birds, is a routine finding (97,99,104–107) and may depend upon the presence of the uterus (108). The mouse's inducible estrus cycle, rather than a pituitary regulated cycle as found in larger rodents, is another important dissimilarity to human beings.

Validation of the mouse as a model for osteoporosis will take some targeted experimental work. The few available reports suggest that the mouse suffers estrogen-depletion bone loss, which is stopped by estrogen replacement. Its time course and the site specificity for the development of estrogen-depletion osteopenia must be established, as it has been for the rat (6). The aberrant formation response to injected estradiol at endocortical surfaces must be considered. It resembles the avian skeletal estradiol response more closely than that of mammals. This unique estrogen responsiveness of bone may be age related; an aged mouse given estradiol may show no such response. Until it is either shown that an older mouse has no such anabolic response to estradiol or that estradiol can elicit a bone formation response in adult human beings, the chances for a universally accepted murine model for osteoporosis seem remote. Furthermore, the similar life span of mice and rats, the smaller though adequate bone specimens provided by the mouse, and the overall similar cost for experimentation suggest that osteoporosis investigators should have in mind a specific goal, like genetic manipulation, when they choose the mouse.

The Senescence-Accelerated Mouse

The senescence-accelerated mouse (SAM) has lifelong osteopenia and develops fractures in old age (109–111). It is the *only* experimental animal with documented fragility fractures of aging. The SAM needs a full genetic, hormonal, and biomechanical characterization. If it does not suffer from collagen defects like those in osteogenesis imperfecta (112), it may provide an opportunity to study the role of low peak bone mass in causing late-life osteopenia and fractures ▶ 363 with a drastically reduced time frame. It may also provide opportunities to study treatments to enhance peak bone mass. Such studies must include testing of the material properties of the bone tissue itself, as has been done for MOV-13 osteogenesis imperfecta mice (113).

Rat

The rat has a long history of providing accurate fundamental data about the adult human skeleton. It gave the first evidence that osteoclasts ingest bone substance (114) and early evidence about osteoclast origin (115). The rat skeleton was once held unsuitable as an adult human skeletal model because many epiphyseal growth cartilages in *male* rats remain open past age 30 months (116). The past unintentional focus on male rats masked important sex differences in epiphyseal closure times. For osteoporosis research, attention should be paid to female rats. Anatomically identical growth cartilages close earlier in females than in males (117–120). Studies of the effects of gonadal hormones on growing male and female rats also suggest that intact females cease growing earlier than males (121).

Bone elongation ceases and effective epiphyseal closure ensures at important sampling sites in female rats by age 6 to 9 months, an age after which much useful experimental life span remains (122). Peak bone mass for the adult female rat skeleton occurs around age 10 months, as periosteal expansion continues (123,124). The mean healthy life span for these rats is 21 to 24 months. Thus, the rat has an appreciable life span both before and after attainment of adult skeletal status. The relatively lengthy bone accumulation period in the rat presents ample untapped opportunities for the study of both internal and external determinants of peak bone mass attainment. Past opinions about the inappropriateness of the rat as a model of adult human skeletal disease because of its "continuous growth and lack of remodeling," have now been modified. They now include only a caution to use female rats of 6 to 9 months age and to avoid studying Haversian remodeling (125).

Adult female rats have a regular estrus cycle in which estradiol levels spike to 50 to 90 pg/mL for 18 hours every 4 days (126). During the second year of life, the fraction of female rats found in constant diestrus rises gradually (127), and cancellous bone loss is also frequently observed (123). Although this is not a true menopause, spikes in estradiol cease as cancellous bone loss occurs, making a linkage of rat "menopause" to cancellous bone loss possible.

Following ovariectomy, loss of cancellous bone and strength occurs (7,128–136) for several months, then decelerates and enters a plateau phase (6). This cancellous bone loss is accompanied by an increase in the rate of bone turnover (7,130,137). These features mimic very well the bone changes that follow oophorectomy or natural menopause in human beings. Although not all cancellous bone sites in the rat experience such bone loss (138), the heterogeneity tightens the parallel of the rat and the human skeletons, since it is well known that osteoporotic fragility fractures and osteopenia are limited to a few sites in human beings (2,52). Dual energy x-ray absorptiometry, the current state of the art for measuring bone mass in patients, can be readily applied for rats (132,139).

Ovariectomized rats given prompt estrogen replacement experience no rise in turnover (9,140–142) and no bone loss (9,142–144). This response fully parallels that seen in postmenopausal women receiving estrogen replacement. Agents like bisphosphonates (135,145,146) and calcitonin (147,148) also block the rise in turnover and bone loss in rats, just as they do in human beings (149–155). Data from one laboratory suggest that high doses of estradiol stimulate bone formation in the rat, as it does in birds and mice (156,157). These data and their interpretation have not been confirmed in other laboratories. It is likely that the use of growing rats and an unusually long fluorochrome labeling interval played a role in the interpretation of the data.

The rat, like other experimental animal models of osteoporosis, has no fragility fractures associated with the development of osteopenia. This apparent shortcoming can be overcome by carefully designed mechanical tests. Such tests now exist for vertebral bodies (10,11,136) and the proximal femur (11). Additional experiments using treatments known to decrease fracture frequency in adult human beings, that show improved bone strength in rats, will provide further validation.

Rats lose bone following immobilization. Several methods of permanent and temporary immobilization are available (12,13,158–161). Acute phase (160), chronic phase (162), and recovery phase (161,163,164) bone changes related to disuse are easily studied. Rats are a weak model of glucocorticoid osteopenia. Although they exhibit decreased bone formation after glucocorticoid treatment, they do not consistently develop osteopenia (165–167).

Adult rats have adequate amounts of cancellous bone remodeling to permit useful experiments (125,168–169). Controversy exists as to the frequency of modeling and remodeling activity in the rat. Classic reversal lines at the base of cancellous osteons are not present in 4-month-old rats (156), perhaps suggesting that modeling predominates in rats of this age. Although modeling would be expected to predominate in such young rats, as in all younger animals, studies of older rats are needed to confirm that rats, like other aged animals undergo a transition to remodeling activity (30).

However, indirect reasoning strongly supports the existence of remodeling in rat cancellous bone. Many regions of cancellous bone in adult rats, like that in long bone metaphyses and vertebral bodies, maintain a stable bone mass for long periods of time while showing abundant bone formation and resorption. This signifies a neutral balance for resorption and formation (6,131), suggestive of remodeling. Whether the activity is locally linked or nonlocally linked resorption and formation, the mass preservation in the whole region is more suggestive of remodeling than modeling, which is usually associated with bone mass changes (30).

▶ 365

In most of its cortical bone, the rat displays low levels of Haversian remodeling often not detectably different from zero. However, processes resembling intracortical remodeling are induced by strong anabolic agents (170) or stressful metabolic conditions (171,172). Unfortunately, it is not known whether these same agents and conditions also accelerate Haversian remodeling in human beings. Current data suggest that the rat has such low levels of Haversian remodeling that it is impractical to use it for analysis of Haversian remodeling behavior, especially when evaluating agents that may suppress Haversian remodeling. However, regions of cortical bone that surround cancellous bone, as in long bone metaphyses, are a reasonable, and currently uninvestigated, place to look in rats to find higher levels of Haversian remodeling.

In 3-month-old ovariectomized rats, the phase of accelerated estrogen-depletion bone loss lasts 3 to 4 months (6), at least an order of magnitude time frame compression when compared with newly estrogen-depleted women. The rat reaches peak bone mass in less than one year, a thirtyfold time frame compression when compared with the adult woman. The rat is also among the most convenient of experiment animals to handle and house.

SUMMARY

The FDA has made a wise choice in requiring rat work during osteoporosis research. The ovariectomized rat is an excellent model that correctly models the most important clinical features of the estrogen-depleted adult human skeleton that malfunction in osteoporosis. Its site-specific development of cancellous osteopenia is one of the most certain physiologic responses in skeletal research.

Ample time exists to either prevent estrogen–depletion bone loss or restore bone lost after estrogen depletion. Its response to estrogen replacement parallels the human response closely. The rat's low levels of Haversian remodeling present little immediate problem when testing agents for the ability to prevent the loss of cancellous bone or rebuild lost cancellous bone. It appears that investigators can compensate for the lack of fragility fractures by biomechanical testing. Rats are convenient for most investigators. Existing laboratory measurement tools of biochemistry, histomorphometry, and densitometry are readily applicable.

Guinea Pig, Rabbit, and Cat

Although occasional reports using guinea pigs, rabbits, and cats in osteoporosis research have appeared (173–175), few studies of estrogen-depletion bone loss exist. Too few experiments exist to assess properly their validity. Seven-month-old ovariectomized guinea pigs do not lose bone by 4 months postsurgery (174). Adult rabbits have active Haversian remodeling and might serve as a model for testing Haversian remodeling after treatment with agents that have strong anabolic effects on cancellous bone. Their reproductive (estrus) cycle is *not* similar to that of human beings. Rabbits are an excellent model of glucocorticoid-induced osteopenia (173). The success of the rabbit and dog (176), animals with significant Haversian remodeling, as models for glucocorticoid-induced osteopenia, coupled with the failure of a rat, an animal with minimal Haversian remodeling, suggests that glucocorticoid osteopenia is a disease of deranged Haversian remodeling.

Dog

The adult dog has always been a reliable model for the adult human skeleton. It is generally similar to the human skeleton in both metabolic and structural characteristics. Autoradiographic studies of ^{239}Pu-injected beagles first proved the existence of adult cancellous bone remodeling (114). Beagle studies also contributed one of the earliest indications of the hematogenous origin of osteoclasts (177). The ratio of cortical to cancellous bone is similar to that in human beings (178–180). Haversian and cancellous osteons remodel with similar morphology, though more rapidly in dogs (181,182). Skeletal responsiveness of the adult beagle parallels the adult human for corticosteroids (176,183), uremia (184,185), bisphosphonates (186,187), and disuse (80–82,188–191).

In contrast to all other applications for adult beagles as a model of the adult human skeleton, the oophorectomized beagle is controversial as a choice for studying estrogen-depletion bone loss. Data from nine laboratories compare skeletal end points in over 100 oophorectomized to nearly 100 sham-operated adult female beagles from 1 to 31 months postsurgery (192). Few studies report significant skeletal changes after oophorectomy. Many of these make type II errors by using histomorphometry, a measurement tool offering 20% to 25% precision, to attempt to detect bone loss of about 15%. Power calculations show that sample sizes of 25 in both experimental and sham-operated groups are required to demonstrate this degree of bone loss with histomorphometry. Unfortunately, group sizes of 6 to 8 were used.

Other experiments using human beings and dogs also indicate that sample size is a serious problem for many oophorectomized dog studies. The early histomorphometric studies that found significant age-related changes in bone mass in patients had hundreds of subjects (193–196). Calcium kinetic studies in over 200 women show a more negative calcium balance and elevated remodeling transmenopausally (60,62). In fact, in one study of 109 beagles, a significant secular trend in spinal bone loss was detectable (197). Furthermore, when studies in oophorectomized beagles used precise tools of bone mass measurement like dual photon absorptiometry, an 8% to 10% loss of cancellous bone (198–200) and strength (201,202) after estrogen depletion, coupled with an early phase of elevated turnover were noted (203). Despite the lack of significant findings in many individual studies, an overall look at the data in a meta-analysis fashion is instructive (204).

BONE MASS IN THE ESTROGEN-DEPLETED BEAGLE

The preponderance of evidence suggests that estrogen-depletion bone loss occurs in oophorectomized beagles. This conclusion is based on the three most prominent types of studies: (1) those that find a significant decline (198, 200,205–208) (2) those that find a nonsignificant decline (45,201,202,209), and (3) those that find no bone mass or strength change (14,203,210–216). Increases rarely occur (218,219), and then in experiments of very small sample size (n = 3). One paper with strongly positive results showing bone loss (198) used spinal densitometry, a tool of high precision (220). A report with mildly positive results found some decline in vertebral trabecular strength by mechanical testing, a tool with good specificity, although weak precision for trabecular bone evaluation (201,202).

BONE FORMATION IN THE
ESTROGEN-DEPLETED BEAGLE

The pattern of bone formation over time after oophorectomy suggests an early rise followed by a return to baseline or sub-baseline levels. Work from one group (205–207) suggests that formation falls rapidly to 50% of baseline, with no detectable phase of increased turnover. This finding suggests the possibility of a marked dissimilarity to histomorphometric findings in transmenopausal women, where the early rise in both formation and individual cell activity (134) that accompanies rapid bone loss, has been documented (60).

THE CANINE ESTRUS CYCLE COMPARED TO HUMAN BEINGS AND OTHER ANIMAL MODELS

Estradiol levels are usually very low (less than 20 pg/mL) in the dog, rising *twice yearly* for several weeks to 45 to 75 pg/mL (221–223). In rats, estradiol shows phasic increases to 50 to 90 pg/mL for 18 hours every 4 days (126). Women experience estradiol levels of 300 to 400 pg/mL for one or 2 days each month (224,225). The estrus cycle in monkeys has a similar frequency to that in human beings, but reaches estradiol peaks only about half as high (226). Integrated estrogen exposure in dogs, though only marginally less than in rats, is only one fourth that in human beings. It is similar to that in primates, except during the peak periods. Estradiol peaks in canines are one sixth as frequent and one sixth as high as in women. This difference could contribute to the dog's developing a smaller estrogen-dependent compartment of cancellous bone.

Because of the inconsistency of the ovariectomized dog model, understanding its response to estrogen is also difficult. The data suggest that estrogen suppresses turnover but that its bone mass-sparing effects are uncertain (214–216).

SUMMARY

There is wide agreement that the adult beagle is an excellent model of the adult human skeleton except for estrogen depletion. Its principal advantage over smaller animals is its Haversian remodeling. Although the oophorectomized beagle has estrogen-depletion osteopenia, poor interlaboratory reproducibility in finding significant bone loss accompanied by transient rises in bone formation has caused many investigators to be skeptical about its relevance to human beings. Most of the individual studies using histomorphometry contain insufficient power to detect the amount of bone loss expected (199–219). Beagles are less estrogen replete than women and may have a smaller estrogen-dependent compartment of bone in their skeleton. Despite the inconsistency for development of estrogen-depletion bone loss, the dog remains an excellent candidate model for testing the effects on Haversian remodeling of agents that have strong anabolic effects on cancellous bone.

Osteoporosis

Pig

The oophorectomized pig has been tested in one study (227). Although minor structural deterioration was noted, no change in bone mass, either by densitometry or histomorphometry, was seen. The pig has a regular estrus cycle that is somewhat shorter than the human menstrual cycle. Porcine species have been used successfully to study fluoride and exercise effects on the skeleton (228,229). More work will be necessary before swine can gain acceptance as a model of estrogen–depletion bone loss.

Sheep

The ewe has both growing and adult skeletal phases, but the age of peak bone mass is not known. Ewes have a regular estrus cycle during the short days of winter, but experience seasonal anestrus when days are longer (230,231). The ewe has also been used to study fluoride effects in the adult skeleton. The findings seem to parallel histologic changes in human beings, that is, frequent signs of increased formation in association with sluggish mineralization and toxicity to bone forming cells (232–234). Skeletal behavior after oophorectomy has not been documented but is likely to be subject of interest during the next few years. Sheep cannot be housed readily at most university-based animal quarters. However, in the correct setting, they pose little problem for handling. More data are needed to validate the usefulness of the adult ewe as an in vivo model of osteoporosis.

Nonhuman Primate

The nonhuman primate has both growing and adult skeletal phases. It appears that peak bone mass occurs around age 10 years in cynomolgous and rhesus monkeys and baboons. Nonhuman primates have a regular menstrual cycle with an approximate duration of 28 days, and are an excellent analog of human beings. Primates experience a natural menopause near the end of the second decade of life.

Primates experience decreased bone mass (236–239) with increased turnover (239) after ovariectomy. They also experience reversible bone loss after gonadotropin-releasing hormone agonist treatment (44). The response to estrogen replacement has not been well characterized. Nonhuman primates experience bone loss after immobilization of long duration (240). Histomorphometric studies of primates and human beings yield remarkably similar values (238,239, 241,242).

Baboons experience osteopenia (242), but no vertebral compression fractures during late life that would suggest similarity to the human osteoporotic syndrome (244). Late life spinal pathology in baboons (244) and rhesus monkeys (245) is mostly osteoarthritis. This may signal some trouble for nonhuman primates as a model of fragility fractures, because in patients osteoarthritis and osteoporosis tend to be mutually exclusive conditions (246–248). In addition, spinal bone mass measurements in older primates may be affected because the osteophytes that occur in osteoarthritis have enough calcium artifactually to change spinal bone mass values and obscure proper interpretation (249–252). Like the dog, nonhuman primates offer cancellous and Haversian remodeling that is directly comparable to that found in the adult human skeleton. The time course of bone loss after ovariectomy has not been well characterized but appears to offer significant time frame compression when compared to the human being.

Extreme requirements for housing and care of nonhuman primates limits their use to relatively small numbers of facilities. However, when handled by experienced staff in an appropriate environment, they present few care problems.

Summary of All In Vivo Animal Models

When an in vivo osteoporosis research project cannot be done in human beings, the 10-month-old ovariectomized female rat is the first animal model of choice. It has reached peak bone mass and accurately simulates most clinical findings of osteoporosis in the adult female skeleton. Methods like serum biochemistry, histomorphometry, and densitometry that are routinely used in patients, are likewise applicable in rats. Like all animal models of osteoporosis, the rat develops no fragility fractures. However, mechanical testing of rat bones seems to substitute well as a detector of bone fragility. When studied before age 10 months, the female rat also has skeletal growth and maturation phases that are useful for various experiments about peak bone mass.

However, the rat's low levels of Haversian remodeling do not permit accurate evaluation of intracortical bone behavior. A larger animal known to have Haversian remodeling must be selected. The dog is generally an accurate model of the adult human skeleton, but the ovariectomized dog has yielded inconsistent results for skeletal behavior in the acutely estrogen-depleted state that are possibly different from those found in patients. Data on oophorectomized swine and sheep are currently scarce. Estrogen-depleted primates are the in vivo large animal of choice when Haversian remodeling outcomes are to be studied.

Birds have a metabolically active skeleton whose behavior does not seem directly relevant to osteoporosis research. Data about estrogen-deplete mice now seem promising, but the current high state of development of the ovariectomized rat model suggests that work to develop an ovariectomized mouse model is not urgently needed. Mice may become more useful as osteoporosis studies involving gene manipulation grow more important.

References

1. Guidelines for preclinical and clinical evaluation of agents used in the prevention or treatment of postmenopausal osteoporosis. Division of Metabolism and Endocrine Drug Products, Food and Drug Administration, 1993.

2. Cummings SR. Epidemiologic studies of osteoporotic fractures: methodologic issues. Calcif Tissue Int 1991:49(suppl): S15–S20.

3. Kiel DP, Felson DT, Anderson JJ, Wilson PWF, Moskowitz MA. Hip fracture and the use of estrogens in postmenopausal women. The Framingham study. N Engl J Med 1987;317:1169–1174.

4. Kleerekoper M, Peterson EL, Nelson DA, et al. A randomized trial of sodium fluoride as a treatment for postmenopausal osteoporosis. Calcif Tissue Int 1991;49: 155–161.

5. Riggs BL, Hodgson SF, O'Fallon WM, et al. Effect of fluoride treatment on the fracture rate in postmenopausal women with osteoporosis. N Engl J Med 1990;322: 802–809.

6. Wronski TJ, Dann LM, Scott KS, Cintron M. Long-term effects of ovariectomy and aging on the rat skeleton. Calcif Tissue Int 1989;45:360–366.

7. Wronski TJ, Cintron M, Dann LM. Temporal relationship between bone loss and increased bone turnover in ovariectomized rats. Calcif Tissue Int 1988;42: 179–183.

8. Wronski TJ, Dann LM, Scott KS, Crooke LR. Endocrine and pharmacological suppressors of bone turnover protect against osteopenia in ovariectomized rats. Endocrinology 1989;125:810–816.

9. Wronski TJ, Cintron M, Doherty AL, Dann LM. Estrogen treatment prevents osteopenia and depresses bone turnover in ovariectomized rats. Endocrinology 1988; 123:681–686.

10. Mosekilde LI, Sogaard CH, Danielsen CC, Torring O, Nilsson MHL. The anabolic effects of human parathyroid hormone (hPTH) on rat vertebral body mass are also reflected in the quality of bone, assessed by biomechanical testing: a comparison study between hPTH-(1-34) and hPTH-(1-84) Endocrinology 1991;129: 421–428.

11. Toolan BC, Shea M, Myers ER, et al. Effects of 4-amino-1-hydroxybutylidene bisphosphonate on bone biomechanics in rats. J Bone Miner Res 1992;7:1399–1406.

12. Svesatikoglou JA, Mattson S. Changes in composition and metabolic activity of the skeletal parts of the extremity of the adult rat following resection of the sciatic nerve. Acta Chir Scand 1976; (suppl 476):16–29.

13. Wakley GK, Baum BL, Hannon KC, Turner RT. The effects of tamoxifen on the osteopenia induced by sciatic neurotomy in the rat: a histomorphometric study. Calcif Tissue Int 1988;43:383–388.

14. Geusens P, Schot LPC, Nijs J, Dequeker J. Calcium-deficient diet in ovariectomized dogs limits the effects of 17-β-estradiol and nandrolone decanoate on bone. J Bone Miner Res 1991;6:791–798.

15. Rodgers JB, Monier-Faugere MC, Malluche HH. Animal models for the study of bone loss after cessation of ovarian function. Bone 1993;14:369–377.

16. Vanderschueren D, Van Herck E, Schot P, et al. The aged male rat as a model for human osteoporosis: evaluation by nondestructive measurements and biomechanical testing. Calcif Tissue Int 1993;53: 342–347.

17. Cesnjaj M, Stavljenic A, Vukicevic S. In vivo models in the study of osteopenias. Eur J Clin Chem Clin Biochem 1991;29: 211–219.

18. Chesnut CH. Theoretical overview: bone development, peak bone mass, bone loss, and fracture risk. Am J Med 1991;91(suppl 5B):2S–4S.

19. Matkovic V, Fontana D, Tominac C, Goel P, Chesnut CH III. Factors that influence peak bone mass formation: a study of calcium balance and the inheritance of bone mass in adolescent females. Am J Clin Nutr 1990;52:878–888.

20. Matkovic V. Calcium intake and peak bone mass. N Engl J Med 1992;327: 119–120.

21. Hui SL, Slemenda CW, Johnston CC Jr. Baseline measurement of bone mass predicts fracture in white women. Ann Intern Med 1989;111:355–361.

22. Gärdsell P, Johnell O, Nilsson BE. Predicting fractures in women by using forearm bone densitometry. Calcif Tissue Int 1989;45:235–242.

23. Ross PD, Wasnich RD, Vogel JM. Detection of prefracture spinal osteoporosis using bone mineral absorptiometry. J Bone Miner Res 1988;3:1–11.

24. Recker RR, Lappe JM, Davies KM, Kimmel DB. Change in bone mass immediately before menopause. J Bone Miner Res 1992;7:857–862.

25. Rodin A, Murby B, Smith MA, et al. Premenopausal bone loss in the lumbar spine and femoral neck: a study of 225 caucasian women. Bone 1990;11:1–5.

26. Schlechte J, Walkner L, Kathol M. A longitudinal analysis of premenopausal bone loss in healthy women and women with hyperprolactinemia. J Clin Endocrinol Metab 1992;75:698–703.

27. Marcus R, Kosek J, Pfefferbaum A, Horning S. Age-related loss of trabecular bone in premenopausal women: a biopsy study. Calcif Tissue Int 1983;35:406–409.

28. Meema HE, Meema S. Longitudinal microradioscopic comparisons on endosteal and juxtaendosteal bone loss in premenopausal and postmenopausal women, and in those with end stage renal disease. Bone 1988;8:343–350.

29. Jones HH, Priest JD, Hayes WC, Tichenor CC, Nagel DA. Humeral hypertrophy in response to exercise. J Bone Joint Surg 1977;59A:204–208.

30. Frost HM. The skeletal intermediary organization. Metab Bone Dis Rel Res 1983;4:281–290.

31. Frost HM. The mechanostat: a proposed pathogenic mechanism of osteoporoses and the bone mass effects of mechanical and nonmechanical agents. Bone Miner 1987;2:73–85.

32. Drinkwater BL, Nilson K, Chesnut CH, Brenner WJ, Shainholtz S, Southworth MB. Bone mineral content of amenorrheic and eumenorrheic athletes. N Engl J Med 1984;311:277–281.

33. Marcus R, Cann C, Madvig P, et al. Menstrual function and bone mass in elite women distance runners. Ann Intern Med 1985;102:158–163.

34. Cann CE, Martin MC, Genant HK, Jaffe RB. Decreased spinal mineral content in amenorrheic women. JAMA 1984;251: 626–629.

35. Klibanski A, Greenspan SL. Increase in bone mass after treatment of hyperprolactinemic amenorrhea. N Engl J Med 1986;315:542–546.

36. Biller BMK, Baum HBA, Rosenthal DI, Saxe VC, Charpie PM, Klibanski A. Progressive trabecular osteopenia in women with hyperprolactinemic amenorrhea. J Clin Endocrinol Metab 1992;75: 692–697.

37. Rico H, Arnanz F, Revilla M, et al. Total and regional bone mineral content in women trated with GnRH agonists. Calcif Tissue Int 1993;52:354–357.

38. Dawood YM, Lewis V, Ramos J. Cortical and trabecular bone mineral content in women with endometriosis: effect of gonadotropin-releasing hormone agonist and danazol. Fertil Steril 1989;52:21–27.

39. Drinkwater BL, Nilson K, Ott S. Bone mineral density after resumption of menses in amenorrheic athletes. JAMA 1986;256:380–382.

40. Garn SM. The early gain and later loss of cortical bone. Springfield, Ill: CC Thomas, 1970:26–30.

41. Gilsanz V, Gibbens DT, Roe TF, et al. Vertebral bone density in children: effect of puberty. Radiology 1988;166:847–850.

42. Treloar AE. Menstrual cyclicity and the pre-menopause. Maturitas 1981;3:249–264.

43. McMahon B, Worcester B. Age at menopause. National Center for Health Statistics, 1966; Series 11:19.

44. Mann DR, Gould KG, Collins DC. A potential primate model for bone loss resulting from medical oophorectomy or menopause. J Clin Endocrinol Metab 1990; 71:105–110.

45. Martin RB, Butcher RL, Sherwood LL, et al. Effects of ovariectomy in beagle dogs. Bone 1987;8:23–31.

46. Cann CE, Genant HK, Ettinger B, Gordan GS. Spinal mineral loss in oophorectomized women. JAMA 1980;244: 2056–2059.

47. Hartwell D, Riis BJ, Christiansen C. Changes in vitamin D metabolism during natural and medical menopause. J Clin Endocrinol Metab 1990;71:127–132.

48. Nordin BEC, Horsman A, Brook R. Williams DA. The relationshp between oestrogen status and bone loss in postmenopausal women. Clin Endocrinol 1976;5:353S–361S.

49. Lindquist O, Bengtsson C, Hansson T, Jonsson R. Changes in bone mineral content of the axial skeleton in relation to aging and the menopause. Scand J Clin Lab Invest 1983;43:333–338.

50. Gallagher JC, Goldgar D, Moy A. Total bone calcium in normal women: effect of age and menopause status. J Bone Miner Res 1987;2:491–496.

51. Hedlund LR, Gallagher JC. The effect of age and menopause on bone mineral density of the proximal femur. J Bone Miner Res 1989; 4:639–642.

52. Wasnich R, Yano K, Vogel J. Postmenopausal bone loss at multiple skeletal sites: relationship to estrogen use. J Chron Dis 1983;36:781–790.

53. Lindsay R, Hart DM, MacLean A. Bone response to termination of estrogen treatment. Lancet 1978;1:1325–1327.

54. Horsman A, Simpson M, Kirby PA, Nordin BEC. Non-linear bone loss in

oophorectomized women. Br J Radio 1977; 50:504–507.

55. Nilas L, Borg J, Christiansen C. Different rates of loss of trabecular and cortical bone after the menopause. In: Christiansen C, Arnaud CD, Nordin BEC, Parfitt AM, Peck WA, Riggs BL, eds. Osteoporosis I. Copenhagen: Glostrup Hospital, 1984:161–163.

56. Keshawarz NW, Recker RR. Expansion of the medullary cavity at the expense of cortex in postmenopausal osteoporosis. Metab Bone Dis Rel Res 1984;5:223–228.

57. Richelson LS, Wahner HW, Melton LJ, Riggs BL. Relative contributions of aging and estrogen deficiency to postmenopausal bone loss. N Engl J Med 1984;311: 1273–1275.

58. Dequeker J, Geusens P. Contributions of aging and estrogen deficiency to postmenopausal bone loss. N Engl J Med 1985;313:453.

59. Nilas L, Christiansen C. Bone mass and its relationship to age and the menopause. J Clin Endocrinol Metab 1987;65: 697–702.

60. Recker RR, Heaney RP, Saville PD. Menopausal changes in remodeling. J Lab Clin Med 1978;92:964–971.

61. Stepan JJ, Pospichal J, Presl J, Pacovsky V. Bone loss and biochemical indices of bone remodeling in surgically-induced postmenopausal women. Bone 1987;8: 279–284.

62. Heaney RP, Recker RR, Saville PD. Menopausal changes in calcium balance performance. J Lab Clin Med 1978;92: 953–963.

63. Recker RR, Lappe JM, Kimmel DB. Longitudinal transmenopausal skeletal changes measured by histomorphometry. Proceedings of IVth International Osteoporosis Workshop. Hong Kong, March, 1993, #155.

64. Steiniche T, Hasling C, Charles P, Eriksen EF, Mosekilde L, Melsen F. A randomized study on the effects of estrogen/gestagen or high dose oral calcium on trabecular bone remodeling in postmenopausal osteoporosis. Bone 1989;10:313–320.

65. Jensen GF, Christiansen C, Transbøl I. Fracture frequency and bone preservation

in postmenopausal women treated with estrogen. Obstet Gynecol 1982;69:493–496.

66. Christiansen C, Christensen MS, McNair P, Hagen C, Stocklund KE, Transbøl I. Prevention of early postmenopausal bone loss: controlled 2-year study in 315 normal females. Eur J Clin Invest 1980;10:273–279.

67. Meema S, Meema HE. Menopausal bone loss and estrogen replacement. Isr J Med Sci 1976;12:601–606.

68. Ettinger B, Genant HK, Cann CE. Long-term estrogen replacement therapy prevents bone loss and fractures. Ann Intern Med 1985;102:319–324.

69. Lindsay R, Hart DM, Aitken JM. Long-term prevention of osteoporosis by estrogen. Lancet 1976;1:1038–1041.

70. Weiss NS, Ure CL, Ballard JH. Decreaased risk of fractures of the hip and lower forearm with post-menopausal use of estrogen. N Engl J Med 1980;303:1195–1202.

71. Christiansen C, Lindsay R. Estrogens, bone loss and preservation. Osteoporosis Int 1990;1:7–13.

72. Kanis JA, McCloskey EV. Epidemiology of vertebral osteoporosis. Bone 1992;13:S1–S10.

73. Cummings SR, Kelsey JL, Nevitt MC, O'Dowd KJ. Epidemiology of osteoporosis and osteoporotic fractures. Epidemiol Rev 1985;7:178–208.

74. Jensen GF, Christiansen C, Boesen J, Hegedus V, Transbøl I. Epidemiology of postmenopausal spinal and long bone fractures. Clin Orthop Rel Res 1982;166:75–81.

75. Nilsson BE, Westlin NE. Bone mineral content and fragility fractures. Clin Orthop Rel Res 1977;125:196–199.

76. Aloia JF, Vaswani A, McGowan D, Ross P. Preferential osteopenia in women with osteoporotic fractures. Bone Miner 1992;18:51–63.

77. Eventon I, Frisch B, Cohen Z, Hamel I. Osteopenia, hematopoiesis, and bone remodeling in iliac crest and femoral biopsies: a prospective study of 102 cases of femoral neck fractures. Bone 1991;11:1–6.

78. Schaadt O, Bohr H. Different trends of age-related diminution of bone mineral content in the lumbar spine, femoral neck, and femoral shaft in women. Calcif Tissue Int 1988;42:71–76.

79. Riggs BL, Melton LJ III. Heterogeneity of involutional osteoporosis: evidence for two osteoporosis syndromes. Am J Med 1983;75:899–901.

80. Donaldson CL, Hulley SB, Vogel JM, Hattner RS, Bayers JH, McMillan DE. Effect of prolonged bedrest on bone mineral. Metabolism 1970;19:1071–1084.

81. Minaire P, Meunier PJ, Edouard C, Bernard J, Courpron P, Bourret J. Quantitative histologic data on disuse osteoporosis. Calcif Tissue Res 1974;17:57–73.

82. Krolner B, Toft B. Vertebral bone loss: an unheeded side effect of therapeutic bed rest. Clin Sci 1983;64:537–540.

83. Bloom W, Bloom MA, McLean FC. Calcification and ossification. Medullary bone changes in the reproductive cycle of female pigeons. Anat Rec 1941;79:443–466.

84. Miller SC, Bowman BM. Medullary bone osteogenesis following estrogen administration to mature male Japanese quail. Dev Biol 1981;87:52–63.

85. Rubin CT, Lanyon LE. Regulation of bone formation by applied dynamic loads. J Bone Joint Surg 1984;66A:397–402.

86. Rubin CT, Lanyon LE. Regulation of bone mass by mechanical strain magnitude. Calcif Tissue Int 1985;37:411–417.

87. Lanyon LE, Rubin CT, Baust G. Modulation of bone loss during calcium insufficiency by controlled dynamic loading. Calcif Tissue Int 1986;38:209–216.

88. Miller SC. Osteoclast cell-surface changes during the egg-laying cycle in Japanese quail. J Cell Biol 1977;75:104–118.

89. Attie KM, Ramirez, NR, Conte FA, Kaplan SL, Grumbach MM. The pubertal growth spurt in eight patients with true precocious puberty and growth hormone deficiency: evidence for a direct role of sex steroids. J Clin Endocrinol Metab 1990;71:975–983.

90. Bonjour JP, Theintz G, Buchs B, Slosman D, Rizzoli R. Critical years and stages of puberty for spinal and femoral bone mass accumulation during adolescence. J Clin Endocrinol Metab 1991;73:555–563.

91. Walker DG. Congenital osteoporosis in mice cured by parabiotic union with normal siblings. Endocrinology 1972;91: 916–920.

92. Walker DG. Osteopetrosis cured by temporary parabiosis. Science 1973;180: 75.

93. Marks SC, Schneider GB. Evidence for a relationship between lymphoid cells and osteoclasts: bone resorption restored in ia (osteopetrotic) rats by lymphocytes, monocytes and macrophages from a normal littermate. Am J Anat 1978;152:331–342.

94. Walker DG. Bone resorption restored in osteopetrotic mice by transplants of normal bone marow and spleen cells. Science 1975;190:784–785.

95. Walker DG. Spleen cells transmit osteoporosis in mice. Science 1975;190:785–786.

96. Koretsky AP. Investigation of cell physiology in the animal using transgenic technology. Am J Phys 1992;262:261–275.

97. Suzuki HK. Effects of estradiol-17-β-n-valerate on endosteal ossification and linear growth in the mouse femur. Endocrinology 1958;60:743–747.

98. Balena R, Costantini F, Yamamoto M, et al. Mice with IL-6 gene knock-out do not lose cancellous bone after ovariectomy. J Bone Miner Res 1993;8(suppl 1);S130 (#56).

99. Edwards MW, Bain SD, Bailey MC, Lantry MM, Howard GA. 17-β-estradiol stimulation of endosteal bone formation in the ovariectomized mouse: an animal model for the evaluation of bone-targeted estrogens. Bone 1992;13:29–34.

100. Hashimoto J, Takaoka K, Yoshikawa H, Miyamoto S, Suzuki S, Ono K. Preservation of ectopically-induced bone in the mouse by estradiol. Bone 1991;12:249–255.

101. Bar-Shira-Maymon B, Coleman R, Cohen A, Steinhagen-Thiessen E, Silbermann M. Age-related bone loss in lumbar vertebrae of CW-1 female mice: a histomorphometric study. Calcif Tissue Int 1989;44:36–45.

102. Bar-Shira-Maymon B, Coleman R, Steinhagen-Thiessen E, Silbermann M. Correlation between alkaline and acid phosphatase activities and age-related osteopenia in murine vertebrae. Calcif Tisue Int 1989;44:99–207.

103. Weiss A, Arbell I, Steinhagen-Thiessen E, Silbermann M. Structural changes in aging bone: osteopenia in the proximal femurs of female mice. Bone 1991;12:165–172.

104. Urist MR, Budy AM, McLean FC. Endosteal bone formation in estrogen-treated mice. J Bone Joint Surg 1950;32A: 143–162.

105. Bain SD, Bailey MC, Celino DL, Lantry MM, Edwards MW. High dose estrogen inhibits bone resorption and stimulates bone formation in the ovariectomized mouse. J Bone Miner Res 1993;8: 435–442.

106. Bain SD, Bailey MC, Edwards MW. The anabolic effect of estrogen on endosteal bone formation in the mouse is attenuated by ovariohysterectomy: a role for the uterus in the skeletal response to estrogen? Calcif Tissue Int 1992;51:223–228.

107. Bain SD, Jensen E, Celino DL, Bailey MC, Lantry MM, Edwards MW. High-dose gestagens modulate bone resorption and formation and enhance estrogen-induced endosteal bone formation in the ovariectomized mouse. J Bone Miner Res 1993;8:219–230.

108. Bain SD, Bailey MC, Edwards MW. The anabolic effect of estrogen on endosteal bone formation in the mouse is attenuated by ovariohysterectomy: a role for the uterus in the skeletal response to estrogen? Calcif Tissue Int 1992;51:223–228.

109. Tsuboyama T, Takahashi K, Matsushita M, et al. Decreased endosteal formation during cortical bone modeling in SAM-P/6 mice with a low peak bone mass. Bone Miner 1989;7:1–12.

110. Tsuboyama T, Matsushita M, Okumura H, Yamamuro T, Hanada K, Takeda T. Modification of strain-specific femoral bone density by bone marrow chimerism in mice: a study on the spontaneously osteoporotic mouse (SAM-P/6). Bone 1989;10:269–277.

111. Matsushita M, Tsyboyama T, Kasai R, et al. Age-related changes in bone mass

in the senescence-accelerated mouse (sam) Am J Pathol 1986;125:276–283.

112. Spotila LD, Constantinou CD, Sereda L, Ganguly A, Riggs BL, Prockop DJ. Mutation in a gene for type I procollagen (COL1A2) in a woman with postmenopausal osteoporosis: evidence for phenotypic and genotypic overlap with mild osteogenesis imperfecta. Proc Natl Acad Sci 1991;88:5423–5427.

113. Altschuler RA, Dolan DF, Ptok M, Gholizadeh G, Bonadio J, Hawkins JE. An evaluation of otopathology in the MOV-13 transgenic mutant mouse. Ann N Y Acad Sci 1991;630:249–252.

114. Arnold JS, Jee WSS. Bone growth and osteoclastic activity as indicated by radioautographic distribution of [239]Pu. Am J Anat 1957;101:367–417.

115. Gothlin G, Ericsson JLE. On the histogenesis of the cells in fracture callus. Virchows Arch B 1973;12:318–329.

116. Dawson AB. The age order of epiphyseal union in the long bones of the albino rat. Anat Rec 1925;31:1–17.

117. Acheson RM, MacIntyre MN, Oldham E. Techniques in longitudinal studies of the skeletal development of the rat. Br J Nutr 1959; 13:283–296.

118. Joss EE, Sobel EH, Zuppinger KA. Skeletal maturation in rats with special reference to order and time of epiphyseal closure. Endocrinology 1963;72:117–122.

119. Spark C, Dawson AB. The order and appearance of centers of ossification in the fore and hind limbs of the albino rat, with reference to the possible influence of the sex factor. Am J Anat 1928;41:411–445.

120. Swanson HE, van der Werff Ten Bosch JJ. Sex differences in growth of rats, and their modification by a single injection of testosterone propionate shortly after birth. J Endocrinol 1963;26:197–207.

121. Turner RT, Hannon KS, Demers LM, Buchanan J, Bell NH. Differential effects of gonadal function on bone histomorphometry in male and female rats. J Bone Miner Res 1989;4:557–563.

122. Kimmel DB. Quantitative histologic changes in the proximal tibial epiphyseal growth cartilage of aged female rats. Cells Materials 1992;1(suppl):11–18.

123. Schapira D, Lotan-Miller R, Barzilai D, Silbermann M. The rat as a model for studies of the aging skeleton. Cells Materials 1992;1(suppl):181–188.

124. Li XJ, Jee WSS, Ke HZ, Mori S, Akamine T. Age related changes of cancellous and cortical bone histomorphometry in female Sprague-Dawley rats. Cells Materials 1992;1(suppl):25–37.

125. Frost HM, Jee WSS. On the rat model of human osteopenias and osteoporosis. Bone Miner 1992;18:227–236.

126. Butcher RL, Collins WE, Fugo NW. Plasma concentration of LH, FSH, prolactin, progesterone, and estradiol-17-β throughout the four day cycle of the rat. J Endocrinol 1974;94:1704–1708.

127. Lu KH, Hopper BR, Vargo TM, Yen SSC. Chronological changes in sex steroid, gonadotropin, and prolactin secretion in aging female rats displaying different reproductive states. Biol Reprod 1979;21:193–203.

128. Kalu DN. The ovariectomized rat as a model of postmenopausal osteopenia. Bone Miner 1991;15:175–191.

129. Wronski TJ. The ovariectomized rat as an animal model for postmenopausal bone loss. Cells Materials 1992;1(suppl 1):69–74.

130. Wronski TJ, Walsh CC, Ignaszewski LA. Histologic evidence for osteopenia and increased bone turnover in ovariectomized rats. Bone 1986;7:119–124.

131. Wronski TJ, Dann LM, Horner SL. Time course of vertebral osteopenia in ovariectomized rats. Bone 1989;10:295–301.

132. Kimmel DB, Wronski TJ. Nondestructive measurement of bone mineral in femurs from ovariectomized rats. Calcif Tissue Int 1990;46:101–110.

133. Geusens P, Dequeker J, Nijs J, Bramm E. Effect of ovariectomy and prednisolone on bone mineral content in rats: evaluation by single photon absorptiometry and radiogrammetry. Calcif Tissue Int 1990;47:243–250.

134. Eskandar E, Kimmel DB, Wronski TJ. Rapid determination for cancellous

bone mineral loss in ovariectomized rats by a subtraction technique. Anat Rec 1991; 230:169–174.

135. Seedor JG, Quartuccio HA, Thompson DD. The bisphosphonate alendronate (MK-217) inhibits bone loss due to ovariectomy in rats. J Bone Miner Res 1991;6:339–346.

136. Mosekilde Li, Danielsen CC, Knudsen UB. The effect of aging and ovariectomy on the vertebral bone mass and biomechanical properties of mature rats. Bone 1993;14:1–6.

137. Black D, Farquharson C, Robins SP. Excretion of pyridinium cross-links of collagen in ovariectomized rats as urinary markers for increased bone resorption. Calcif Tissue Int 1989;44:343–347.

138. Ito H, Ke HZ, Jee WSS, Sakou T. Anabolic responses of an adult cancellous bone site to prostaglandin E_2 in the rat. Bone Miner 1993;31:219–236.

139. Amman P, Rizzoli R. Slosman D, Bonjour JP. Sequential and precise in vivo measurement of bone mineral density in rats using dual energy x-ray absorptiometry. J Bone Miner Res 1992;7:311–317.

140. Turner RT, Vandersteenhoven JJ, Bell NH. The effects of ovariectomy and 17-β-estradiol on cortical bone histomorphometry in growing rats. J Bone Miner Res 1992;2:115–122.

141. Kalu DN, Liu CC, Salerno E, Hollis BW, Echon R, Ray M. Skeletal response of ovariectomized rats to low and high doses of 17-β-estradiol. Bone Miner 1991; 14:175–187.

142. Wronski TJ, Yen CF, Scott KS. Estrogen and diphosphonate treatment provide long-term protection against osteopenia in ovariectomized rats. J Bone Miner Res 1991;6:387–394.

143. Beall PT, Misra LK, Young RL, Spjut HJ, Evans HJ, BeBlanc A. Clomiphene protects against osteoporosis in the mature ovariectomized rat. Calcif Tissue Int 1991;36:123–125.

144. Garner SC, Anderson JJB, Mar MH, Parikh I. Estrogens reduce bone loss in the ovariectomized, lactating rat model. Bone Miner 1992;15:19–31.

145. Schenk R, Merz WA, Fleisch HA, Muhlbauer RC, Russell RGG. Effects of ethane-1-hydroxy-1,1-diphosphonate (EHDP) and dichloromethylene disphosphonate (C12MDP) on the calcification and resorption of cartilage and bone in the tibial episphsis and metaphysis of rats. Calcif Tissue Res 1973;11:196–214.

146. Schenk R, Eggli P, Fleisch H, Rosini S. Quantitative morphometric evaluation of the inhibitory activity of new aminobisphosphonates on bone resorption in the rat. Calcif Tissue Int 1986;38:342–349.

147. Nakatsuka K, Nishizawa Y, Hagiwara S, et al. Effect of calcitonin on total body bone mineral contents of experimental osteoporotic rats determined by dual photon absorptiometry. Calcif Tissue Int 1990;47:378–382.

148. Mazzuoli GF, Tabolli S, Bigi F, et al. Effects of salmon calcitonin on the bone loss induced by ovariectomy. Calcif Tisue Int 1990;47:209–214.

149. Harris ST, Gertz BJ, Genant HK, et al. The effect of short term treatment with alendronate on vertebral density and biochemical markers of bone remodeling in early postmenopausal women. J Clin Endocrinol Metab 1993;76:1399–1406.

150. Watts NB, Harris ST, Genant HK, et al. Intermittent cyclical etidronate treatment of postmenopausal osteoporosis. N Engl J Med 1990;323:73–79.

151. Fromm GA, Vega E, Plantalech L, Galich AM, Mautalen CA. Differential action of pamidronate on trabecular and cortical bone in women with involutional osteoporosis. Calcif Tissue Int 1991;49: 129–133.

152. Smith ML, Fogelman I, Hart DM, Scott E, Bevan J, Leggate I. Effect of etidronate disodium on bone turnover following surgical menopause. Calcif Tissue Int 1989;44:74–79.

153. Reginster JY, Deroisy R, Denis D, et al. Prevention of postmenopausal bone loss by tiludronate. Lancet 1989;2:1469–1470.

154. MacIntyre I, Whitehead MI, Banks LM, Stevenson JC, Wimalawansa SJ, Healy MJR. Calcitonin for prevention of post-

menopausal bone loss. Lancet 1988;1:900–901.

155. Szucs J, Horvath C, Kollin E, Szathmari M, Hollo I. Three-year calcitonin combination therapy for postmenopausal osteoporosis with crush fractures of the spine. Calcif Tissue Int 1992;50:7–10.

156. Lean JM, Chow JWM, Chambers TJ. Estrogen induces bone formation on non-resorptive surfaces in the rat. Bone 1993;14:297–302.

157. Chow JWM, Lean JM, Chambers TJ. 17-β-estradiol stimulates cancellous bone formation in female rats. Endocrinology 1992;130:3025–3032.

158. Svesatikoglou JA, Larsson SE. Changes in composition and metabolic activity of the skeletal parts of the extremity of the adult rat following below-knee amputation. Acta Chir Scand 1976;(suppl 476):9–15.

159. Thomaidis VT, Lindholm TS. The effect of remobilization on the extremity of the adult rat after short-term immobilization in a plaster cast. Acta Chir Scand 1976;(suppl 476):36–39.

160. Thompson DD, Rodan GA. Indomethacin inhibition of tenotomy-induced bone resorption in rats. J Bone Miner Res 1988;3:409–414.

161. Lindgren JU, Mattson S. The reversibility of disuse osteoporosis. Calcif Tissue Res 1977;23:179–184.

162. Li XJ, Jee WSS, Chow SY, Woodbury DM. Adaptation of cancellous bone to aging and immobilization in the adult rat: a single photon absorptiometry and histomorphometry study. Anat Rec 1990;227:12–24.

163. Maeda H, Kimmel DB, Lane N, Raab D. The musculoskeletal response to immobilization and recovery. Bone 1993;14:153–159.

164. Mattson S. The reversibility of disuse osteoporosis. Acta Orthop Scand 1972;(suppl 144):59–88.

165. Young RH, Crane WAJ. Effect of hydrocortisone on the utilization of tritiated thymidine for skeletal growth in the rat. Ann Rheum Dis 1964;23:163–167.

166. Simons DJ, Kunin AS. Autoradiographic and biochemical investigations of the effect of cortisone on the bones of the rat. Clin Orthop Rel Res 1967;55:201–215.

167. Ferretti JL, Vazquez SO, Delgado CJ, Capozza R, Cointry G. Biphasic dose-response curves of cortisol effects on rat diaphyseal bone biomechanics. Calcif Tissue Int 1992;50:49–54.

168. Vignery A, Baron R. Dynamic histomorphometry of alveolar bone remodeling in the adult rat. Anat Rec 1980;196:191–200.

169. Baron R, Tross R, Vignery A. Evidence of sequential modeling in rat trabecular bone: morphology, dynamic histomorphometry, and changes during skeletal maturation. Anat Rec 1984;208:137–145.

170. Jee WSS, Mori S, Li XJ, Chan S. Prostaglandin E_2 enhnaces cortical bone mass and activates intracortical bone remodeling in intact and ovariectomized female rats. Bone 1990;11:253–266.

171. deWinter FR, Steendijk R. The effect of a low-calcium diet in lactating rats; observations on the rapid development and repair of osteoporosis. Calcif Tissue Res 1975;17:303–316.

172. Ruth E. An experimental study of the Haversian-type vascular channels. Anat Rec 1953;112:429–455.

173. Duncan H, Hanson CA, Curtiss A. The different effects of soluble and crystalline hydrocortisone on bone. Calcif Tissue Res 1973;12:159–168.

174. Vanderschueren D, Van Herck E, Suiker AKM, et al. Bone and mineral metabolism in the adult guinea pig: long-term effects of estrogen and androgen deficiency. J Bone Miner Res 1992;7:1407–1415.

175. Jowsey J, Gershon-Cohen J. Effect of dietary calcium levels on production and reversal of experimental osteoporosis in cats. Proc Soc Exp Biol Med 1964;116:437–441.

176. Jett S, Wu K, Duncan H, Frost HM. Adrenalcorticosteroid and salicylate actions on human and canine Haversian bone formation and resorption. Clin Orthop Rel Res 1970; 68:310–315.

177. Jee WSS, Nolan PD. Origin of osteoclasts from the fusion of phagocytes. Nature 1963;200:225–226.

178. Gong JK, Arnold JS, Cohn SH.

Composition of trabecular and cortical bone. Anat Rec 1964; 149:325–331.

179. Johnson LC. Composition of trabecular and cortical bone in humans. In: Frost HM, ed. Bone Biodynamics. Boston: Little-Brown, 1964;543–654.

180. Parks NJ, Jee WSS, Dell RB, Miller GE. Assessment of cortical and trabecular bone distribution in the beagle skeleton by neutron activation analysis. Anat Rec 1986; 215:230–250.

181. Frost HM. Tetracycline-based histological analysis of bone remodeling. Calcif Tissue Res 1969;3:211–239.

182. Kimmel BD, Jee WSS. A quantitative histologic study of bone turnover in young adult beagles. Anat Rec 1982;203: 35–51.

183. Bressot C, Meunier PJ, Chapuy MC, Lejeune E, Edouard C, Darby AJ. Histomorphometric profile, pathophysiology and reversibility of corticosteroid-induced osteoporosis. Metab Bone Dis Rel Res 1979;1:303–311.

184. Ritz E, Krempien B, Mehls O, Malluche HH. Skeletal abnormalities in chronic renal insufficiency before and during maintenance hemodialysis. Kidney Int 1973;4: 116–127.

185. Malluche HH, Faugere MC, Friedler RM, Matthews C, Fanti P. Calcitriol, parathyroid hormone and accumulation of aluminum in dogs with renal failure. J Clin Invest 1987;79:754–761.

186. Delmas PD, Charhon S, Chapuy MC, et al. Long-term effect of dichlormethylene disphosphonate on skeletal lesions in multiple myeloma. Metab Bone Dis Rel Res 1982;4:163–168.

187. Flora L, Hassing GS, Parfitt AM, Villanueva AR. Comparative skeletal effects of two diphosphonates in dogs. In: Jee WSS, Parfitt AM, eds. Bone Histomorphometry III. Paris: Armour Montagu, 1981:389-407.

188. Uhthoff HK, Sekaly G, Jaworski ZFG. Effect of long-term nontraumatic immobilization on metaphyseal spongiosa in young adult and old beagle dogs. Clin Orthop Rel Res 1985;192:278–283.

189. Uhthoff HK, Jaworski ZFG. Bone loss in response to long-term immobilisa-

tion. J Bone Joint Surg 1978;60B:420–429.

190. Jaworski ZFG, Liskova-Kiar M, Uhthoff HK. Effect of long-term immobilisation on the pattern of bone loss in older dogs. J Bone Joint Surg 1980;62B:104–110.

191. Jaworski ZFG, Uhthoff HK. Reversibility of nontraumatic disuse osteoporosis during its active phase. Bone 1986;7:431–439.

192. Kimmel DB. The oophorectomized beagle as an experimental model for estrogen-depletion bone loss in the adult human. Cells Materials 1992;(suppl)1: 75–84.

193. Merz WA, Schenk RK. Quantitative structural analysis of human cancellous bone. Acta Anat 1970;75:54–66.

194. Meunier P, Courpron P, Edouard C, Bernard J, Bringuier J, Vignon G. Physiological senile involution and pathological rarefaction of bone. Quantitative and comparative histological data. J Clin Endocrinol Metab 1973;2:239–256.

195. Delling G. Age-related bone changes. Curr Top Pathol 1974;58:118–147.

196. Melsen F, Melsen B, Mosekilde L, Bergman S. Histomorphometric analysis of normal bone from the iliac crest. APMIS 1978;86A:70–81.

197. Jee WSS, Kimmel DB, Hashimoto EG, Dell RB, Woodbury LA. Quantitative studies of beagle lumbar vertebral bodies. In: Jaworski ZFG, ed. Bone Morphometry. Ottawa: University of Ottawa Press; 1976:110–117.

198. Drezner MK, Nesbitt T. Role of calcitriol in prevention of osteoporosis: Part I. Metabolism 1990;39(suppl 1):18–23.

199. Barbier A, Bonjour JP, Geusens P, deVernejoul MC, Lacheretz F. Tiludronate: a bisphosphonate with a positive effect on bone quality in experimental models. J Bone Miner Res 1991;6(suppl 1):S217 (#531).

200. Shaw JA, Wilson, Paul EM, Bruno A. Vertebral trabecular bone volume in dogs: comparison of oophorectomized females, sham females, and males. Trans Orthop Res Soc 1992;17:(#135).

201. Lynch WR, Goldstein SA, Shulick AM, Mase CA. The effects of calcitonin on torsional properties of the long bones of

ovariohysterectomized beagles. Transactions of the 37th Annual Meeting of the Orthopaedic Research Society 1991;16:430. Abstract.

202. McCubbrey DA, Goulet RW, Goldstein SA, Shulick AM. Vertebral body architecture and mechanical properties alternations due to ovariectomy in the beagle. Transactions of the 37th Annual Meeting of the Orthopaedic Research Society 1991;16:284. Abstract.

203. Boyce RW, Franks AF, Jankowsky ML, et al. Sequential histomorphometric changes in cancellous bone from ovariohysterectomized dogs. J Bone Miner Res 1990;5:947–953.

204. Cumming RG. Calcium intake and bone mass: a quantitative review of the evidence. Calcif Tissue Int 1990;47:194–201.

205. Malluche HH, Faugere MC, Rush M, Friedler RM. Osteoblastic insufficiency is responsible for maintenance of osteopenia after loss of ovarian function in experimental beagle dogs. Endocrinology 1986;119:2649–2655.

206. Faugere MC, Fanti P, Friedler RM, Malluche HH. Bone changes occurring early after cessation of ovarian function in beagle dogs: a histomorphometric study employing sequential biopsies. J Bone Miner Res 1990;5:263–272.

207. Malluche HH, Faugere MC, Friedler RM, Fanti P. 1,25 dihydroxyvitamin D₃ corrects bone loss but suppresses bone remodeling in ovariohysterectomized beagle dogs. Endocrinology 1988;122:1998–2006.

208. Nakamura T, Nagai Y, Yamato H, Suzuki K, Orimo H. Regulation of bone turnover and prevention of bone atrophy in ovariectomized beagle dogs by the administration of $24R,25(OH)_2D_3$ Calcif Tissue Int 1992;50:221–227.

209. Dannucci GA, Martin RB, Patterson-Buckendahl P. Ovariectomy and trabecular bone remodeling in the dog. Calcif Tissue Int 1987;40:194–199.

210. Karambolova KK, Snow GR, Anderson C. Differences in periosteal and corticoendosteal bone envelope activities in spayed and intact beagles: a histomorphometric study. Calcif Tissue Int 1985;41: 665–668.

211. Shen V, Dempster DW, Birchman R, et al. Lack of changes in histomorphometric, bone mass, and biochemical parameters in ovariohysterectomized dogs. Bone 1992;13:311–316.

212. Karambolova KK, Snow GR, Anderson C. Surface activity on the periosteal and corticoendosteal envelopes following continuous progestogen supplementation in spayed beagles. Calcif Tissue Int 1986;38:239–243.

213. Karambolova KK, Snow GR, Anderson C. Effects of continuous 17-β-estradiol administration on the periosteal and corticoendosteal envelope activity in spayed beagles. Calcif Tissue Int 1987;40: 12–15.

214. Snow GR, Anderson C. The effects of 17-β-estradiol and progestagen on trabecular bone remodeling in oophorectomized dogs. Calcif Tissue Int 1986;39:198–205.

215. Snow GR, Anderson C. The effects of continuous estradiol therapy on cortical bone remodeling activity in the spayed beagle. Calcif Tissue Int 1985;37:437–440.

216. Snow GR, Anderson C. The effects of continuous progestogen treatment on cortical bone remodeling activity in beagles. Calcif Tissue Int 1985;37:282–286.

217. Snow GR, Cook MA, Anderson C. Oophorectomy and cortical bone remodeling in the beagle. Calcif Tissue Int 1984;36:586–590.

218. Koyama T, Uno H, Nagaami A, Makita T, Konno T, Takahashi H. Effects of active vitamin D₃ derivatives on bone remodeling in ovariectomized beagle dogs—two year study—II Histomorphometric analysis of trabecular bone. Jap Bone Miner 1984;2:268–275.

219. Koyama T, Nagaami A, Makita T, Konno T, Akazawa H, Takahashi H. Effect of 1-α,24(R)-dihydroxyvitamin D₃ on trabecular bone remodeling in adult beagle dogs. Jap J Bone Miner 1984;2:249–257.

220. Shipp CC, Berger PS, Deehr MS, Dawson-Hughes B. Precision of dual photon absorptiometry. Calcif Tissue Int 1988;42:287–292.

221. Concannon PW, Hansel W, Visek WJ. The ovarian cycle of the bitch: plasma

estrogen, LH and progesterone. Biol Reprod 1975;13:112–121.

222. Jones GE, Boyns AR, Cameron EHD, Bell ET, Christie DW, Parkes MF. Plasma oestradiol, luteinizing hormone and progesterone during the oestrous cycle in the beagle bitch. J Endocrinol 1973;57:331–332.

223. Bell ET, Christie DW, Younglai EV. Plasma oestrogen levels during the canine oestrous cycle. J Endocrinol 1971;51:225–226.

224. Baird DT, Guevara A. Concentration of unconjugated estrone and estradiol in peripheral plasma in nonpregnant women throughout the menstrual cycle, castrate and postmenopausal women and in men. J Clin Endocrinol 1969;29:149–156.

225. Reed MJ, Beranek PA, James VHT. Oestrogen production and metabolism in peri-menopausal women. Maturitas 1986; 8:29–34.

226. Longcope C, Hoberg L, Steuterman S, Baran D. The effect of ovariectomy on spine bone mineral density in rhesus monkeys. Bone 1989;10:341–344.

227. Mosekilde Li, Weisbrode SE, Safron JA, et al. Calcium-restricted ovariectomized Sinclair S-1 minipigs: an animal model of osteopenia and trabecular plate perforation. Bone 1993;14:379–382.

228. Kragstrup J, Richards A, Fejerskov O. Effects of fluoride on cortical bone remodeling in the growing domestic pig. Bone 1989;10:421–424.

229. Raab DM, Crenshaw T, Kimmel DB, Smith EL. Cortical bone response in adult swine after exercise. J Bone Miner Res 1991;6:741–749.

230. Webb R, Baxer G, McBride D, Ritchie M. Springbett AJ. Mechanism controlling ovulation rate in ewes in relation to seasonal anoestrus. J Reprod Fertil 1992; 94:143–151.

231. Malpaux B, Karsch FJ. A role for short days in sustaining seasonal reproductive activity in the ewe. J Reprod Fertil 1990;90:555–562.

232. Eriksen EF, Mosekilde L, Melsen F. Effect of sodium fluroide, calcium, phosphate, and vitamin D_2 on trabecular bone balance and remodeling in osteoporotics. Bone 1985;6:381–389.

233. Chavassieux P, Pastoureau P, Boivin G, Chapuy MC, Delmas PD, Meunier PJ. Dose effects on ewe bone remodeling of short-term sodium fluoride administration—a histomorphometric and biochemical study. Bone 1991;12:421–427.

234. Chavassieux P, Pastoureau P, Boivin G, et al. Fluoride-induced bone changes in lambs during and after exposure to sodium fluoride. Osteoporosis Int 1991;2:26–33.

235. Chavassieux P, Pastoureau P, Chapuy MC, Delmas PD, Meunier PJ. Glucocorticoid-induced inhibition of osteoblastic bone formation in ewes: a biochemical and histomorphometric study. Osteoporosis Int 1993;3:97–102.

236. Miller C, Weaver D. Bone loss in ovariectomized monkeys. Calcif Tissue Int 1986;38:62–65.

237. Miller LC, Weaver DS, McAlister JA, Koritnik DR. Effects of ovariectomy on vertebral trabecular bone in the cynomolgus monkey. Calcif Tissue Int 1986;38: 62–65.

238. Pope NS, Gould KG, Anderson DC, Mann DR. Effects of age and sex on bone density in the rhesus monkey. Bone 1989;10:109–112.

239. Jerome C, Kimmel DB, McAlister JA, Weaver DS. Effects of ovariectomy on iliac trabecular bone in baboons (*Papio anubis*). Calcif Tissue Int 1986;39:206–208.

240. Young DR, Niklowitz WJ, Steele CR. Tibial changes in experimental disuse osteoporosis in the monkey. Calcif Tissue Int 1983;35:304–308.

241. Schnitzler CM, Ripamonti U, Mesquita JM. Histomorphometry of iliac crest trabecular bone in adult male baboons in captivity. Calcif Tissue Int 1993;52: 447–454.

242. Recker RR, Kimmel DB, Parfitt AM, Davies KM, Keshawarz N, Hinders S. Static and tetracycline-based bone histomorphometric data from 34 normal postmenopausal females. J Bone Miner Res 1988;3:133–144.

243. Aufdemorte TB, Fox WC, Miller D, Buffum K, Holt GR, Carey KD. A

non-human primate model for the study of osteoporosis and oral bone loss. Bone 1993;14:581–586.

244. Kimmel DB, Lane NE, Kammerer CM, Stegman MR, Rice KS, Recker RR. Spinal pathology in adult baboons. J Bone Miner Res 1993;8(suppl 1):S279 (#652).

245. Grynpas MD, Huckell CB, Reichs KJ, Derousseau CJ, Greenwood C, Kessler MJ. Effect of age and osteoarthritis on bone mineral in rhesus monkey vertebrae. J Bone Miner Res 1993;8:909–917.

246. Dequeker J. The relationship between osteoporosis and osteoarthritis. Clin Rheum Dis 1985;11:271–296.

247. Pogrund H, Rutenberg M, Makin M, Robin GC, Steinberg R, Bloom R. Osteoarthritis of the hand and osteoporosis. Clin Orthop Rel Res 1986;203:239–243.

248. Ng KC, Revell PA, Beer M, Boucherf BJ, Cohen RD, Currey HLF. Incidence of metabolic bone disease in the rheumatoid arthritis and osteoarthritis. Ann Rheum Dis 1984;43:370–377.

249. Hopkins A, Zylstra S, Hreshchyshyn MM, Anbar M. Normal and abnormal features of the lumbar spine observed in dual energy absorptiometry scans. Clin Nucl Med 1989;14:410–414.

250. Orwoll ES, Oviat SK, Mann T. The impact of osteophytic and vascular calcifications on vertebral mineral density measurements in men. J Clin Endocrinol Metab 1990;70:1202–1207.

251. Reid IR, Evans MC, Ames R, Wattie DJ. The influence of osteophytes and aortic calcification on spinal mineral density in postmenopausal women. J Clin Endocrinol Metab 1991;72:1372–1374.

252. Drinka PJ, DeSmet AA, Bauwens SF, Rogot A. The effect of overlying calcification on lumbar bone deensitometry. Calcif Tissue Int 1992;50:507–510.

382 ◀

Index

Endometrial cancer, 119
Endometriosis, 293
Endplate sclerosis, DXA and, 57
Environmental influences, bone mass,
 80–84, 111
Epidemiologic studies, calcium intake and
 fractures, 239–241, 240f
Epidermal growth factor (EGF), 31, 32
ERT. *See* Estrogen replacement therapy
 (ERT)
17β-estradiol, 36, 300
Estrogen. *See also* Menopause
 animal models, criteria for, 357–358
 bone loss and, 10–11, 297
 bone remodeling and, 295–297, 312–313
 calcium balance and, 230, 295–297
 calcium intake and, 10–11
 deficiency, 89–90, 293–294, 312–313
 1,25-(OH)₂D and, 270–271
 fracture, effect on, 299–300
 inhibits IL-6 production, 36–37
 menopause, calcium balance/bone remodeling, 295–297
 skeletal effects, 298–299
 Turner syndrome and, 89–90
Estrogen replacement therapy (ERT)
 acquisitional osteopenia and, 89
 animal models, criteria for, 358
 bone loss, adult, 119
 cessation of, 302
 combination therapy, use of, 302–303
 drug choice/dose requirement, 300–301
 glucocorticoid-induced osteoporosis,
 216–217
 nonskeletal aspects, 303–304
 osteoporosis prevention, 11
 route of administration, 301
 skeletal effects, 297–298, 298f
 timing of, 301–302
Estrone, 296–297
Estrus cycle
 animal model criteria, 357
 canine, compared to menstruation, 368
Ethanol-induced bone disease. *See also*
 Alcohol use
 mechanisms, 170–173, 171f, 173f
 therapy, 173–174
Ethnicity. *See* Skeletal health and ethnicity
Etidronate
 ADFR regimens with phosphate, 316–
 321, 317t, 319t
 clinical trials, 327

osteoporosis therapy with bisphosphonate, 328–329
Exercise. *See also* Physical activity
 bone accretion and, 83–84
 chronic back pain, programs for,
 344–347
 mechanical force and bone mass,
 160, 232
 optimal types, osteogenic response, 8–9
 osteopenia of anorexia nervosa, 87
 resistance training, 8–9, 84
Exercise-induced amenorrhea
 acquisitional osteopenia and, 87–89
 bone loss and, 11
 bone mineral deficits, 294
Extensor muscle stretching exercises,
 back, 344, 345–346

F
Falls and falling
 alcohol use and, 114
 causes, 155
 ethnic differences and, 130
 as fracture determinants, 155
 prevention, 113, 347–350
 vertebral fractures and, 340
Fat content, marrow/surrounding tissues,
 49, 58
Fatigue properties of bone, 5, 50
FDA. *See* Food and Drug Administration
 (FDA)
Femur, skeletal composition, 2
Fiber, dietary, calcium balance and,
 83, 238
Fibroblast growth factor
 acidic (aFGF), 32
 basic (bFGF), 22
Fibronectin, 22
Fluoride therapy
 bone loss, adult, 120
 glucocorticoid-induced osteoporosis,
 217
Food and Drug Administration (FDA),
 animal model guidelines, 354, 365
Food sources of calcium, 135, 236–241,
 257–258, 259f
Forearm DXA, 59
Fractures. *See also* Hip fractures; Stress
 fractures; Vertebral fractures
 alcohol use as risk factor, 170
 animal models, criteria for, 358

▶ 389

bone density and, 5–6, 50, 154
bone loss as risk factor, 116–117
bone mass measurement as predictor of, 51
calcium intake and, studies of, 239–241, 240f, 242t
causes, bone architecture, 155, 156f
estrogen, effect on, 299–300
falls as risk factor, 155
incidence, 149–154, 151f, 153f, 241
compared men to women, 155–157, 157f
osteoporosis, men, 149–157, 151f
risk, estimating, 71

G

Gait training, 349
Gastrectomy, 175
Gastric acidity, calcium absorption and, 238–239, 257–258
Gastrointestinal disorders, osteoporosis and, 174–176
Gender. *See also* Osteoporosis in men; Postmenopausal osteoporosis
bone accretion and, 78–80, 79f
bone loss, adult, 107–108
fracture incidence and, 155–157, 157f
Genetic factors
bone accretion, 76–78
bone loss, adult, 110–111
peak bone mass acquisition, 147
Geometric/material properties and mass (of bone), 6, 50, 51, 71–72
Girls. *See* Bone acquisition, childhood/adolescence; Exercise-induced amenorrhea
Glucocorticoid-induced osteoporosis
bisphosphonate therapy, 327
causes, 88
childhood/adolescence, 94–95
clinical presentation, 209–210
Cushing's disease, monitoring, 219
epidemiology, 203–204
evaluation of the patient, 210–211
men, 162–163, 163f
overview, 202–203
pathophysiology, 204–209
prevention, 218t
therapy, 211–219, 218t
Glucocorticoids
administration, cytokines and, 217

alternate-day therapy, 212
bone loss, adult, 115
bone remodeling, effect on, 204–206
calcium absorption and, 207–208
gonadal dysfunction and, 209
inhaled, adverse effects, 210
osteoblast function and, 4
secondary hyperparathyroidism and, 208
synthetic derivatives, development of, 212–213
Glycosaminoglycans, 22
Gonadal dysfunction. *See also* Hypogonadism
bone loss, adult, 111–112
glucocorticoid effect, 209, 216–217
osteoporosis, men, 161
Granulocyte/macrophage–colony-stimulating factor (GM-CSF), 26, 27, 30
Grave's disease, 94, 116
Growth factor, fibroblast, 22, 32
Growth hormone (GH)
acquisitional osteopenia and, 92–93
estrogen replacement therapy and, 301
glucocorticoids and, 217
Growth hormone therapy
osteopenia, 93
osteoporosis, men, 188
Guinea pigs as animal models, osteoporosis research, 366

H

Haversian canals, defined, 1
Haversian remodeling, 338, 339
Health habits. *See* Alcohol use; Exercise; Tobacco use
Height measurement, crush fractures and, 51
Hematopoiesis, osteoclasts and, 25f
Hematopoietic progenitors, 22, 24
Hip bone loss, adult, 107, 109–110, 120
Hip fractures
costs, 127
ethnic differences and, 127–129, 128t
incidence, 128t, 129, 150–152, 151f
prevention, 349
tobacco use and, 115
Hip prosthesis placement, DXA and, 59
Homocystinuria, 179
Hormone replacement therapy (HRT)
bone loss, adult, 119

Index

392 ◄